Hospital Care and the British Standing Army, 1660–1714

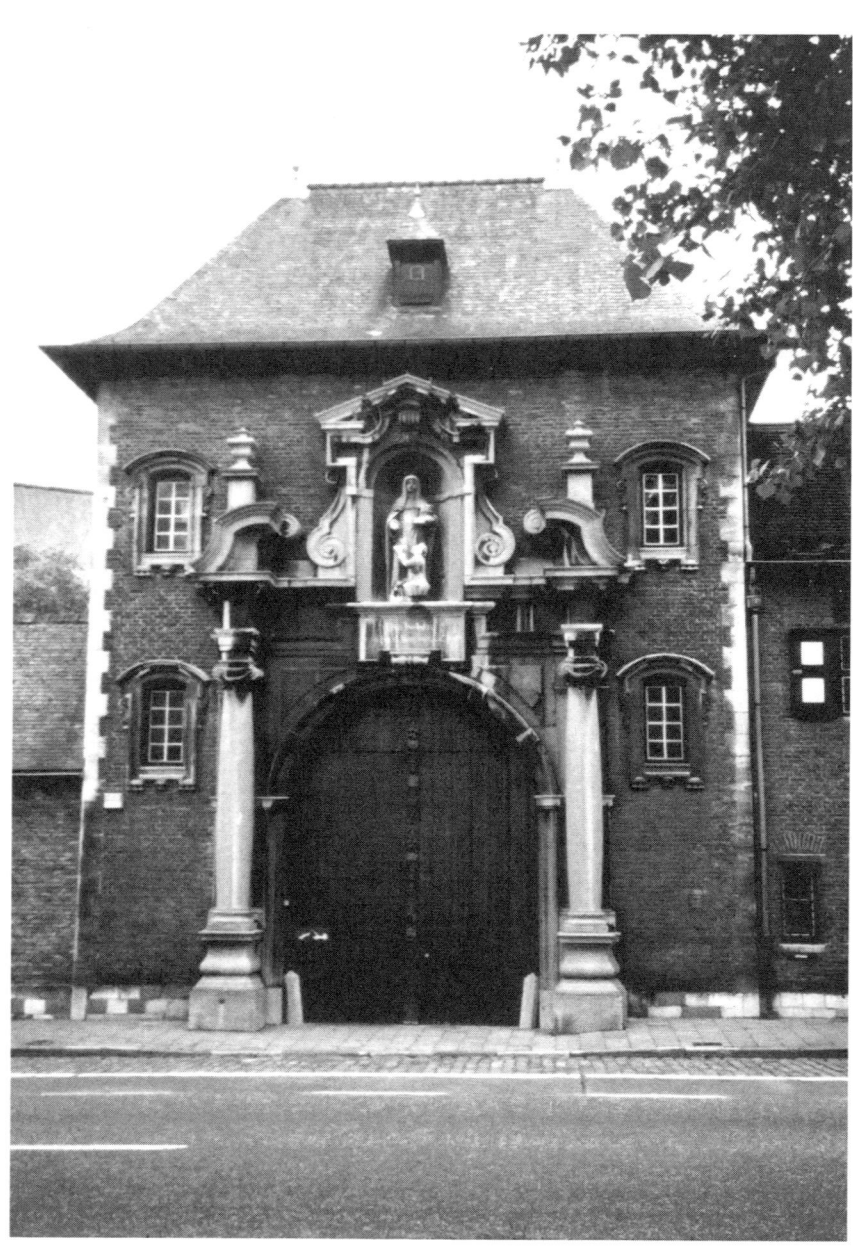

The Bijloke Hospital, Ghent
Main Entrance

Hospital Care and the British Standing Army, 1660–1714

ERIC GRUBER VON ARNI

ASHGATE

© Eric Gruber von Arni, 2006

All rights reserved. No part of this publication may be reproduced, stored in a retrieval system, or transmitted in any form or by any means, electronic, mechanical, photocopying, recording or otherwise without the prior permission of the publisher.

Eric Gruber von Arni has asserted his moral right under the Copyright, Designs and Patents Act, 1988, to be identified as the author of this work.

Published by
Ashgate Publishing Limited
Gower House
Croft Road
Aldershot
Hants GU11 3HR
England

Ashgate Publishing Company
Suite 420
101 Cherry Street
Burlington
Vermont, 05401–4405
USA

Ashgate website: http://www.ashgate.com

British Library Cataloguing in Publication Data
Gruber von Arni, Eric
   Hospital Care and the British Standing Army, 1660–1714. – (The History of Medicine in Context)
   1. Great Britain, Army – Medical care – History – 17th century. 2. Great Britain, Army – Medical care – History – 18th century. 3. Medicine, Military – Great Britain – History – 17th century. 4. Medicine, Military – Great Britain – History – 18th century. I. Title
355.3'45'0941'09032

US Library of Congress Cataloging in Publication Data
Gruber von Arni, Eric
   Hospital Care and the British Standing Army, 1660–1714 / by Eric Gruber von Arni
   p. cm. – (The History of Medicine in Context)
   Includes bibliographical references and index.
   1. Medicine, Military – Great Britain – History – 17th century. 2. Medicine, Military – Great Britain – History – 18th century. I. Title. II. Series.
RC971.G78 2004
616.9'8023'0941–dc22   2005010977

ISBN 0 7546 5463 X
Printed and bound in Great Britain by MPG Books Ltd, Bodmin, Cornwall

Contents

List of Illustrations	vii
List of Tables	ix
List of Abbreviations	xiii
Notes on Dates and Spelling	xiv
Acknowledgements	xv
Preface	xvii

	Introduction	1
1	The Garrison Hospital at Tangier, 1662–1683	9
2	Hospitals and Welfare for the Standing Army in Britain, 1660–1688	33
3	Hospital Provision in Ireland, 1689–1692	53
4	Medical Support during the Nine Years' War in Flanders	77
5	Soldier Patients in the London Hospitals	99
6	Hospital Provision during Marlborough's Campaigns	111
7	The Army's Hospitals in Spain and Portugal	157
8	Evaluation	181

Appendices

A	The Humble Report of Henry Shere to the Rt Hon. Lords of the Treasury, Touching the Hospital at Tangier, 1 March 1683	189
B	The Present Annual Charge of the Royal Hospital of King Charles II	193
C	Abstract of the By-Laws, Rules and Orders for Staff of the Royal Hospital of King Charles II near Dublin	195
D	Admissions to St Bartholomew's Hospital by Regiment, 1689–1697	199

E Inventory of Drugs, Medicines and Utensils for the Surgeon's Chests
   of Regiments of Horse and Foot, 1689   203
F The Hospital Establishment and Staff in Flanders, 2 April 1693   207
G Examples of Battle Injuries Received by Applicants for Admission
   to the Royal Hospital Chelsea, 1715–1732   209

Bibliography   211

Index   219

List of Illustrations

All illustrations are from the author's private collection unless otherwise specified

Frontispiece

The Bijloke Hospital, Ghent

Maps

1   Locations of hospitals and principal battles in Flanders and Brabant, 1690–1714   xix
2   Deployment route of the hospital for the 1704 campaign   xx
3   Locations of hospitals and main battles in Spain and Portugal, 1702–1711   xxi

Illustrations

Between pages 110 and 111

1   Plan of the garrison hospital in Tangier, 1662–1683
    Army Medical Services Museum

2   Plan of Sir Hugh Cholmley's proposed lazarette for the port and town of Tangier, April 1675
    Army Medical Services Museum

3   Sir Hugh Cholmley's design for the proposed mole, showing the intended site for the lazarette to the south of the mole and harbour (the cruciform structure on the extreme left of the drawing)
    The National Archives: PRO ref. MPH 1/1/ (18)

4   Sir Hugh Cholmley's proposal for a garrison hospital for Tangier, 1677
    The National Archives: PRO ref. MPH 1/1 (29)

5   Artist's impression of Sir Hugh Cholmley's proposed garrison hospital for Tangier, 1677
    Army Medical Services Museum

6   Artist's impression of the Hospital built for the encampments on Hounslow Heath, 1685–1688
    Army Medical Services Museum

7   A bijlander (or walenmajohl)
8   The River Maas looking east from the Citadel of Namur
9   An engraving of 1696 showing the Abbey of La Ramée
    Bodleian Library: University of Oxford, Douce L subt.24(1)
10 The Bijloke Hospital: Main gate looking north
11 The Bijloke Hospital: Main gate looking south
12 The Bijloke Hospital: Entrance to the Main Ward
13 The Bijloke Hospital: Roof beams of the Main Ward
14 St John's Hospital, Bruges, showing proximity to canal access
15 St John's Hospital, Bruges: Inner courtyard with main ward building on the right
16 The Hospital of Our Lady, Courtrai
17 The house of the Cell Brothers, Mecklin

List of Tables

0.1	Garrison establishments, 1661	5
1.1	Tangier garrison strength, 30 January–23 October 1663	17
1.2	Regulations for the hospital at Tangier	18
1.3	Tangier medical establishment, post 1668	22
1.4	Account of passengers aboard the *Diamond* bound for England as per the muster taken in Tangier Roads, 30 November 1683	26
1.5	List of victuals in store at Tangier compared with estimates sent from London, 30 November 1683	27
2.1	Disbursements to Colonel George Legge's Regiment, 17 July 1678	36
2.2	Payments to out-pensioners waiting for vacancies in the Royal Hospitals	40
2.3	In-pensioner daily allowance in the Royal Hospitals of Kilmainham and Chelsea	40
2.4	Officers and men wounded at Sedgemoor	42
3.1	Establishment of a hospital to attend the army in Ireland, 1 July 1689	62
3.2	Allied officers and soldiers killed at the Battle of Aughrim, 12 July 1691	71
4.1	Allied losses at Steenkirk, 3 August 1692	80
4.2	Average bed occupancy and numbers of deaths at Liège hospital 11 July–19 October 1695	89
4.3	Average bed occupancy and numbers of deaths at the Bijlocke Hospital, Ghent, 10 May–20 September 1695	90
4.4	Average bed occupancy and numbers of deaths at the hospital in Brussels, 24 June–20 October 1695	90
4.5	Hospital usage for the year 1695	91
4.6	Army statements of fitness, 4 September–4 October 1695	91

5.1	St Thomas's Hospital additional rules for service patients	100
5.2	Admissions and discharges of soldiers to St Bartholomew's Hospital, 1689–1697	104
5.3	St Bartholomew's Hospital: soldier admissions and discharges, 1689–1697	105
6.1	Sick and wounded in the British hospital at 's Hertogenbosch, 27 June–20 July 1702	114
6.2	Casualty list for the storming of the Schellenburg	127
6.3	Food items purchased for the Hospital at Kassel, 24 May–22 October 1704	129
6.4	The Blenheim Bounty allocation to sick and injured by rank as pensions	131
6.5	Annual pension allowance authorized October 1708 for the widows of officers killed on duty	133
6.6	Food items purchased for the hospital at Nordlingen, 26 June 1704–28 March 1705	134
6.7	Marching hospital food purchases, 17 May–11 July 1705	138
6.8	Mr John Craig's bill for drugs and materials used by him in treating the wounded on the field of Ramillies, 12 May 1706	140
6.9	List of stores sent to the hospitals in Flanders on 2 April 1708	144
6.10	List of stores sent to the hospitals in Flanders on 2 April 1709	147
6.11	Establishment for the officers of the standing hospital for Her Majesty's Forces in the year 1710	148
7.1	Staff list for the hospital in Catalonia, December 1705	161
7.2	Account of the effective men, including corporals, in each regiment of foot in Portugal, January 1707	163
7.3	English officers killed or taken prisoner at the battle of Almanza, 25 April 1707	164
7.4	Final payment to medical staff on disbandment of the hospital in Spain, for services provided between 25 December 1709 and 23 December 1710	177
8.1	Nursing staff numbers at the Bijloke Hospital, 1706–1712	184
8.2	Analysis of injuries suffered by applicants for admission to Chelsea Royal Hospital, 1706–1712	185

8.3 Age and length of service analysis of 503 soldiers applying for
     admission to the Royal Hospital, Chelsea, 1715–1732   186

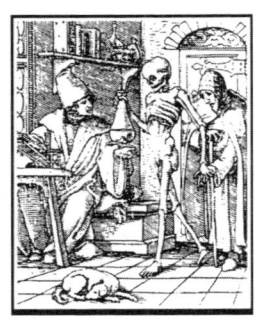

The History of Medicine in Context

Series Editors: Andrew Cunnigham and Ole Peter Grell

Department of History and Philosophy of Science
University of Cambridge

Department of History
The Open University

Titles in this series include:

The Making of the Dentiste, c. 1650–1760
Roger King

*'The Battle for Health': A Political History of the
Socialist Medical Association, 1930–51*
John Stewart

*Justice to the Maimed Soldier: Nursing, Medical Care and Welfare for Sick
and Wounded Soldiers and their Families during the English Civil Wars
and Interregnum, 1642–1660*
Eric Gruber von Arni

*The Irritable Heart of Soldiers and the Origins of Anglo-American Cardiology:
The US Civil War (1861) to World War I (1918)*
Charles F. Wooley

Florence Nightingale and the Health of the Raj
Jharna Gourlay

List of Abbreviations

Add. Mss   Additional Manuscripts
AMS Museum   Army Medical Services Museum
BL   British Library
Bod. L   Bodleian Library
Cal. S.P. Dom.   *Calendar of State Papers, Domestic*
Cal. Treas. Books *Calendar of Treasury Books*
HMC   Historical Manuscripts Commission
JRAMC   *Journal of the Royal Army Medical Corps*
JSAHR   *Journal of the Society for Army Historical Research*
LMA   London Metropolitan Archives
PRO   Public Record Office (now the National Archives)
RAMC   Royal Army Medical Corps
SCRO   Shropshire County Record Office
Staffs. RO   Staffordshire County Record Office
TNA   The National Archives

Note on Dates and Spelling

Throughout this work, the year is assumed to begin on 1 January and transcribed dates have been amended accordingly. Days of the month have not been altered and remain as originally expressed according to the Julian Calendar.

Idiosyncratic seventeenth-century spelling frequently resulted in the same word being written in different ways in the same passage. In this work the spelling of words transcribed from original documents has been standardized according to modern practice except where the original spelling assists in conveying the original sense or idiom of the text.

Acknowledgements

My grateful thanks and appreciation are extended to the following individuals who gave their time, knowledge and patience in assisting me to complete this work.

I have been very fortunate in the support given to me by three close personal friends. Mr Andy Phillipson has been a constant source of support, constructive criticism, advice and, frequently, transportation throughout the preparation of this work. My debt to him is incalculable, but above all else, I treasure his friendship. Two other very special pals, Alan Turton, Curator of Basing House, Hampshire, who has an amazing personal knowledge and understanding of all aspects of the seventeenth century, and Christopher Scott, lately Chief Education Officer at the Royal Armouries, were always ready to provide advice, guidance and suggestions when particularly knotty problems were encountered.

Much of this work could not have been undertaken without the support of the Army Medical Services Museum, Aldershot. The curator, Peter Starling, and his staff have provided continual practical support in the production of books, images and other material, not to mention innumerable cups of coffee.

Mrs Marion Rea, archivist at St Bartholomew's Hospital, was, as ever, extremely supportive in drawing the hospital's records of soldier admissions during the Nine Years' War to my attention and in facilitating my transcription of them. I hope that Chapter 5 of this current work assists in emphasizing the importance of these documents. Equally, Mrs Hilary Morris, friend, fellow museum trustee and a medical historian with a fathomless depth of knowledge in her subject area, has been more than generous in sparing time to read various drafts of chapters and offer her constructive advice and criticism. I am more than conscious of the pressures that this has placed upon her over-burdened schedule. My thanks are also due to Dr Mark Harrison, Director of the Wellcome Unit for the History of Medicine at Oxford University, for agreeing to read and comment upon my final manuscript.

The assistance of staff at the following Record Offices and Archive Centres is also gratefully acknowledged: The British Library, Department of Manuscripts; Bodleian Library, Oxford; Guildhall Library, London; The National Archives at Kew (in particular Hugh Alexander of the Image Library); London Metropolitan Archives; Portsmouth Record Office; Shropshire County Record Office; Staffordshire County Record Office; Liège Record Office, The Bijloke Hospital Museum, Ghent; St John's Hospital, Bruges and the Maritime Museum, Amsterdam.

Mr Wilfred Packer, a highly skilled draughtsman and artist, drew many of the images reproduced in this book, often from a bare minimum of information. The success of his efforts and achievements is visible in the end product. My thanks are also due to Richard Ellis, long-time friend and professional photographer, who generously assisted with photographic work.

Dr James Thomas of Portsmouth University provided a ready flow of advice, support, guidance and forbearance. His vast fund of knowledge on all matters historical and his wicked sense of humour have been a constant source of inspiration and delight.

Last, but by no means least, I have to record my love and thanks to my wife Elizabeth, research assistant, mentor, adviser and critic. Having agreed to read interminable versions of individual chapters with the minimum of complaint, she has frequently accompanied me on a variety of research trips within the United Kingdom, the Netherlands and Belgium, and endured long hours of isolation with unending tolerance and patience for which I am forever in her debt.

Preface

Throughout my thirty years' service as a nursing officer in the army it became glaringly obvious that no serious study had been made of British military nursing before the work of Florence Nightingale. When I retired from my appointment as Director of Studies for Queen Alexandra's Royal Army Nursing Corps in early 1996, I set myself the task of remedying this state of affairs. Along with most nurses of my generation I had been taught that military nursing did not exist before the mid-nineteenth-century Nightingale reforms. Finding this a difficult concept to accept, I decided to look deeper into the subject. With little understanding of the amount of material available for study, but continuing in the belief that whatever provision had been available must have been slight, I thought it realistic to embark on the task of producing a concise study of military nursing history. My initial intention was to cover the entire period from the formation of Parliament's New Model Army, through the formation of the British Standing Army, to the mid-nineteenth-century reforms in one volume. How ill informed I was.

Once work had begun it soon became obvious that the wealth of material that had survived relating to all aspects of the provision of care for sick and wounded soldiers was so vast that it was essential to trim my aspirations accordingly. As a result my first publication, *Justice to the Maimed Soldier* (2001), which was developed from my doctoral thesis, was restricted to coverage of the period from the outbreak of the civil wars in 1642 to the Restoration of the Monarchy in 1660. The book now presented relates to the years following the formation of the British Standing Army in 1660 to the end of the War of the Spanish Succession in 1714, and will, I hope, contribute significantly towards enabling me to achieve my original goal.

I have attempted to discuss Royalist and Parliamentary policy towards the provision of military casualty care and hospital provision during the formative years of the British Standing Army. In so doing it is impossible not to marvel at the work of seventeenth-century physicians, surgeons, nurses, apothecaries and other workers who struggled to care for their fellow men in far from ideal circumstances. Rather than the opprobrium that has frequently been heaped upon their shoulders, these people demand nothing but admiration from for their acheivements.

The nurses who were employed in the army's hospitals were wholly practical people with little or no time to document their work and, therefore, the majority are condemned to remain anonymous. The task of documentation was left to the hospital directors, physicians and surgeons to whom these women, and sometimes men, were subordinate and upon whom they were dependent for their livelihood. As a result, although my original intention was to describe the nature of nursing care during the period under discussion, such work cannot be viewed in isolation and, therefore, in order to provide an indication of the work undertaken by them, I decided to broaden the field of my research into an empirical study of military hospitals in general, including the wider aspects of official policy, administration, medical and pharmaceutical provision. The result will, I hope, not only demonstrate progressive developments but also identify various constant themes that remain valid to this day.

That so little has previously been written on this subject is reflected in the fact that most of the material presented in this work has been culled from original documents and is presented here for the first time. Any mistakes or misrepresentations are, therefore, entirely the author's responsibility.

Eric Gruber von Arni
Swindon, Wiltshire

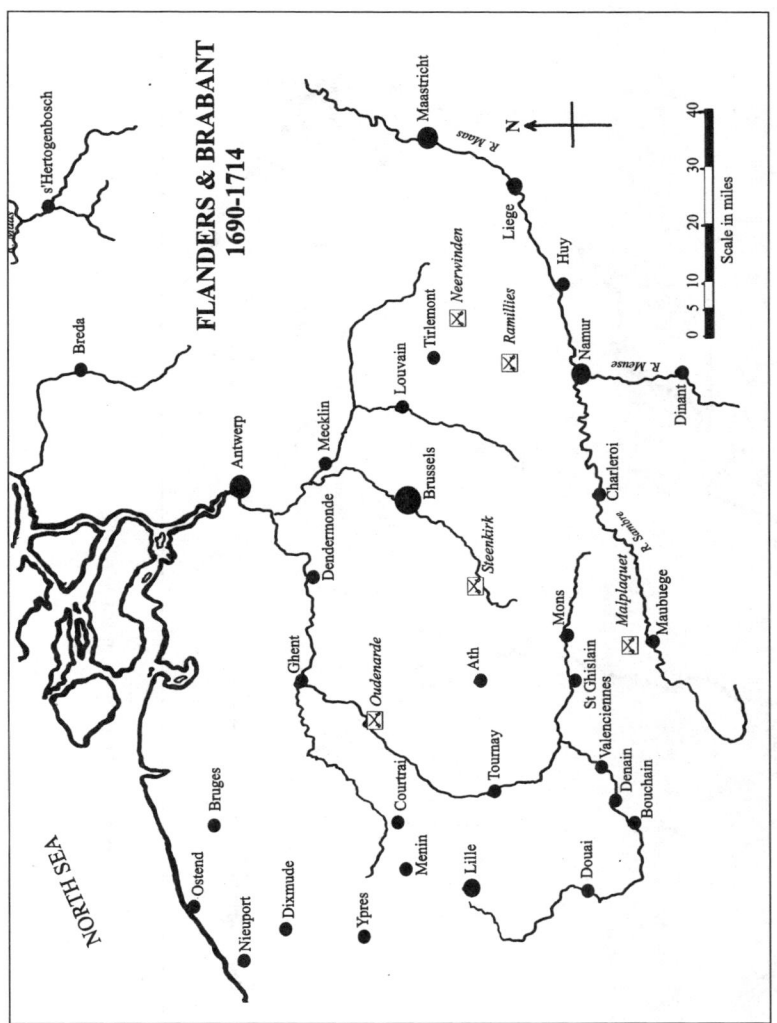

Map 1 Locations of hospitals and principal battles in Flanders and Brabant, 1690–1714

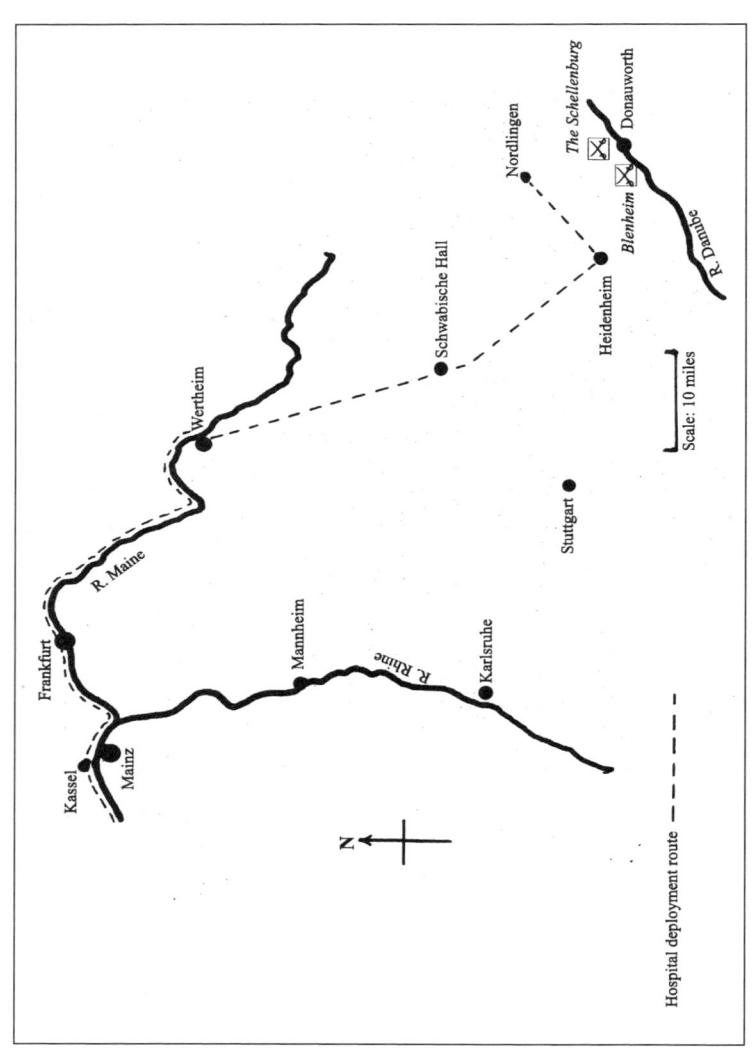

Map 2 Deployment route of the hospital for the 1704 campaign

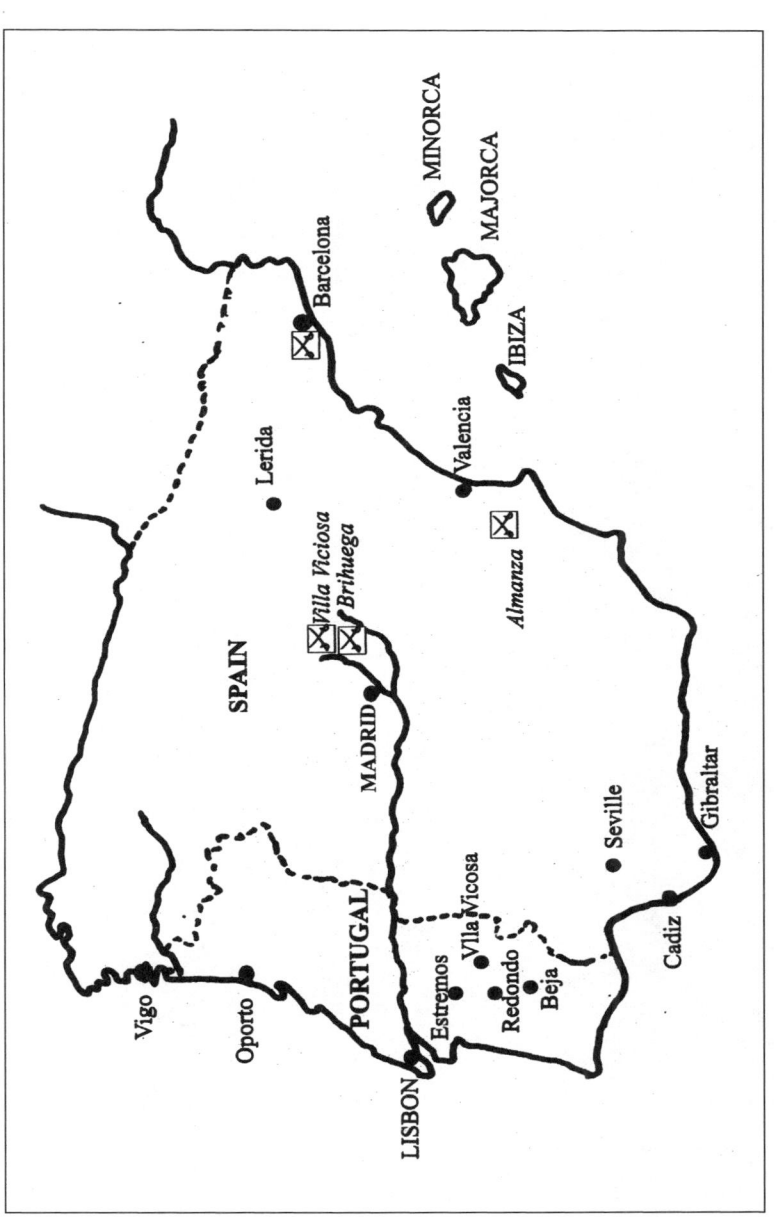

Map 3 Locations of hospitals and main battles in Spain and Portugal, 1702–1711

Introduction

> To the average professional officer, the military doctor is an unwillingly tolerated non-combatant who takes sick call, gives cathartic pills, makes transportation troubles, complicates tactical plans, and causes the water to smell bad.
>
> H. Zinsser (1878–1940)
> US bacteriologist

This work is an attempt to explore the nature and quality of medical, nursing and welfare facilities provided in hospitals for soldiers during the formative years of the British Standing Army between 1660 and 1712. To date, only two significant works have been dedicated to telling the story of the history of the British army's medical services: Gore's *Our Services under the Crown* (1879) and Cantlie's *History of the Army Medical Department* (1974).[1] The first was written during a voyage to India by a knowledgeable regimental surgeon who had identified the need for a history of the army's medical service. The latter was a more recent and bold attempt by an amateur military historian and former Director General Army Medical Services to describe the same subject. Both of these works attempted to give their subject a broad-brush treatment, but neither succeeded in producing an in-depth study of army hospitals and their work during the important and much-neglected period of the gestation and early development of the British Standing Army.

Despite the fact that it was written over a hundred years ago, the broad and minutely detailed study, *A History of the British Standing Army* (1894) by Colonel C. Walton, continues to provide the best study to date of the hospital organization that accompanied King William III's armies to Ireland and Flanders. No similar work has so far been attempted for the armies of Charles II, James II or Queen Anne, and the subject is barely touched in the erudite volumes of Professor J. Childs that address the broader aspects of the British army of the period.[2] A series of articles written by Colonel H.A.L. Howells that appeared in *The Journal of the Royal Army Medical Corps* between 1902 and 1911 provides a sound general synopsis of the history of military medicine and surgery from the earliest times to the Napoleonic Wars but, regrettably, the author failed to quote his sources.[3] Another article, this time written by former military surgeon and amateur historian George Gask, entitled 'A Contribution to the History of the Care of the Sick and Wounded During Marlborough's March to the Danube in 1704, and at the Battle of Blenheim', was published in the same journal in 1922. This was written without the benefit of access to Marlborough's personal papers that are now lodged in the British Library and, as a result, whilst Gask provides reasonable coverage of the hospital arrangements made prior to, and immediately after the battle of Blenheim, he neglects the later aspects of this campaign. The article is, therefore, limited to an incomplete narrative of the full story. Later, in 1939, Lieutenant Colonel G.A. Kempthorne published a useful, but also unsourced, article in the *Journal of the RAMC* entitled 'Some Notes on the Medical Service of the Restoration Army' that contains some useful biographical details of contemporary regimental medical officers. An attempt to provide a comparative study of world-wide developments in military medicine from antiquity to the end of the First World War was produced by F.H. Garrison in his *Notes on the History of Military Medicine* (1922), while a more recent but similar general coverage, including the seventeenth and early eighteenth centuries, is available in Gabriel and Metz's *A History of Military Medicine* (1992).[4] Of necessity, in such wide-ranging works, coverage of developments in British military medicine during the post-Restoration period, especially of hospitals, is reduced to no more than two or three pages in each case and is, therefore, extremely limited and of little worth in this respect. On the other hand, the contemporary French army medical service has been extensively documented in such works as Belhomme's *L'Armée Française en 1690* (1895), André's *Michel le Tellier et l'Organisation de l'Armée Monarchique* (1906), Chabané's 'Chirurgiens et blessés à travers l'histoire' in R. Baillargeat (ed.), *Les Invalides, Trois Siècles d'Histoire* (1975), Contamine's *Histoire Militaire de la France* (1992) and, most recently, by John A. Lynn in his magisterial *Giant of the Grand Siècle* (1997).[5]

It would appear, therefore, that an up-to-date review of the story of the army medical services, particularly acute casualty-receiving hospitals, during the early formative years of the British Standing Army is overdue. This present work aims to fill this void whilst, additionally, enquiring into the broader aspects of welfare facilities provided for soldiers and their families. In fulfilling this goal, no attempt has been made to describe contemporary developments in naval medicine, a subject that has already been given broad coverage in the four-volume *Medicine and the Navy, 1200–1900* by Keevil, Lloyd and Coulter.[6]

The current author's previous work, *Justice to the Maimed Soldier*, examined the same factors in the period spanning the years of the English Civil Wars and Interregnum. During that period of intense upheaval, both main factions in the struggle established hospitals for the sick and wounded of their armies but, assisted by superior administration, legislation and clerical support, Parliament's collective achievements far exceeded anything constructed by the opposition. The comprehensive and efficient system of centralized hospital care and welfare provision for those who had suffered in its service contrasted markedly with the relatively meagre facilities available to the Royalist forces, who maintained a traditional reliance upon the presumed benevolent concern of individual unit commanders in matters affecting their soldiers' health and welfare. Even though Parliament's ability to draw upon the City of London's extensive financial resources was a major factor in determining the quality of its achievements, the motivation of its members, driven by an altruistic desire to improve the lot of the 'commonweal', contrasted markedly with the Royalists' minimalist approach.

Sadly, when expeditions were sent abroad, Parliament demonstrated a singular inability to apply the same standards of casualty care that it had instigated at home.

A rudimentary contemporary understanding of waging international warfare, coupled with unfortunate delegation, resulted in hurried, ill-conceived and poorly co-ordinated planning.[7] Cromwell's over-ambitious foreign policy may have been remarkably successful in achieving significant territorial gains and an enhanced international status, but his failure to learn from previous mistakes and a reliance upon haphazard repatriation without adequate field hospital facilities resulted in catastrophic casualty morbidity in all of his army's overseas campaigns.

Even Parliament's domestic achievements in the field of military hospital support did not last. The latter years of the Protectorate were characterized by an unstable national economy, shrinking financial power and increased public debt. Following Cromwell's death in 1658, poor leadership and internecine quarrels brought real and increasing suffering to the population as a whole while the nation's administration was only maintained by a process of crisis management.[8] During the first six months of 1659 funding for the maintenance of Parliament's two military hospitals in London, at the Savoy and Ely House, failed entirely and, although the ensuing months brought a variety of emergency payments, an aggressive policy of discharging patients to service in garrison invalid units was instigated. Parliament authorized its final payment to the military hospital fund in November 1659, after which its accounting system fell into chaos.[9] Throughout that November and the following month Parliament was at loggerheads with the army. Attempts were made to rule the country through a temporary Committee of Safety while in Scotland, an exasperated General Monck, who had received the news of Lambert's expulsion of Parliament on 17 October, prepared to march south with his regiment. He crossed the Tweed on 2 January 1660 and, four weeks later, his troops entered London.

In the months immediately prior to the Restoration in May 1660, public administration and the nation's treasury remained in utter turmoil. Any remaining Parliamentary commitment to the welfare of its troops was submerged in a sea of financial difficulties. On 1 March Parliament was presented with a statement of the condition of the in-patients and pensioners of the Savoy and Ely House Hospitals.[10] This emotionally charged document pointed out that the numbers of patients and pensioners had recently been greatly increased by virtue of a continuing military presence in Flanders and the West Indies and, whereas many of those soldiers wounded in the early stages of the civil wars had been able to sustain themselves from their own resources, these more recent casualties were poverty stricken and unable to fend for themselves. By the end of April the accounts of the Committee for Sick and Maimed Soldiers were 49 weeks in arrears and patients in the military hospitals were in great distress.

Charles II had been proclaimed King two days earlier. Nevertheless, following a petition by 2,500 in-patients and out-pensioners, together with more than 3,000 widows, Parliament approved a fast day to be held on 10 May in order to collect parish donations for the sick and wounded of the Savoy and Ely House hospitals. In addition, an order was given for the release of £1,400 from the Exchequer for the use of sick and wounded soldiers and £2,000 for widows. It was obvious, however, that their situation was untenable under the new government. Inevitably any organization that supported soldiers who had only recently fought against the monarchy could not be allowed to continue. The restored King Charles II landed at Dover on 25 May and on 18 June a list of captains, officers or other senior in-patients of Ely House who were fit to be transferred to alternative hospitals was published as the first step in closing down the Parliamentary military welfare system.[11]

Eventually, on 13 September 1660, Parliament authorized the issue of £4,000 from excise monies to pay off all the remaining soldier-patients, pensioners, widows and orphans. Each was to be paid 12 weeks' pension and discharged with a certificate recommending them to the Justices of the Peace of their individual home counties for ongoing support under the terms of existing, earlier Elizabethan Poor Law legislation.[12] A final statement regarding the closure of the military hospitals was made in Parliament on 17 December 1660 which announced that four days earlier some 3,271 pensioners and in-patients had been discharged and paid off while 900 provincial pensioners still awaited settlement. Ely House was closed completely while the Savoy reverted, for a short time, to a civilian management before being converted into a barracks for troops of the Royal Household.

At the same time as pension payments ceased and military hospitals were closed, Parliament's army was progressively disbanded and London's suburbs became inundated with disgruntled soldiers waiting to receive their papers and back pay. On 15 November 1660 some 38 innkeepers of New Windsor had written to Parliament complaining that 300 soldiers from Windsor Castle were quartered upon them, with from six to twelve to a house, to each of whom had been loaned 6d a day together with heating, candles, food and lodging.[13] With the collapse of Parliament's hospital and pension structure, the only remaining recourse for soldiers and families seeking aid was an appeal to the Quarter Sessions or local parish officers.[14] It was into this situation that over 4,000 Parliamentary war pensioners were thrown and, for most, this meant an appeal to the charity of parishes which, for some, had not been their home for many years, and to whom they were unwanted and burdensome strangers.

The demise of the New Model Army and the final closure of the Parliamentary military hospitals were inevitable sequelae to the Restoration of Charles II. At the stroke of a pen, all the care and welfare innovations and improvements introduced during 18 years of conflict were swept away. The new Government had repudiated almost all of the legislation introduced during the Protectorate, including its social policies, and social support was reduced to the minimal provisions of the old Elizabethan Poor Law system. Inevitably, those who had fought for the Royalists were given preference and for years after the Restoration, whenever application was made by a pauper for relief to the County Quarter Sessions it was invariably stated, almost as common form, that the wound had been sustained fighting for the King at Worcester.

The need for some form of standing defence force was soon felt however when, only six months after the Restoration, the Fifth-Monarchy revolt of January 1661 pre-empted the final redundancy of the last regiment due to be disbanded, that commanded personally by General Monck. This regiment was the last remnant of the former New Model Army to remain embodied and, having successfully put down the revolt, its commander used his influence with the newly restored monarch to convince Parliament that the Royal Bodyguard should be expanded. Alongside Monck's Regiment of Foot, disbanded and reformed into the Duke of Albermarle's Regiment of Foot Guards, later to be retitled the Coldstream Guards, other newly raised regiments of Horse and Foot were organized into a body of Household troops numbering some 5,000 men that became the basis of the British Standing Army.[15]

In addition to the Household troops, thirty-one coastal fortresses and certain inland castles were occupied by garrison troops. Most of the thirteen major facilities included a surgeon and a minor hospital on their establishments but the remaining eighteen minor defences were only manned on a part-time basis by local volunteers who looked within their own local communities for medical care.

Table 0.1 Garrison Establishments, 1661

Major Garrisons

	Establishment	Surgeon
Berwick upon Tweed and Holy Island	637	n/k
Chepstow Castle	110	n/k
Guernsey Island	113	Mr Warner (1678)
Hull	664	Mr Hardy (1673)
Jersey Island	223	Mr Salanove (1674)
Landguard Point Fort[16]	113	n/k
Pendennis Castle	330	n/k
Portsmouth	707	Mr Grundy (1677)
Plymouth	223	n/k
Scilly Isles	328	Mr Price (1666)
The Tower of London	324	Mr Seele
Tynemouth Castle	223	n/k
Windsor Castle	338	n/k
Total	4,326	

Minor Garrisons

	Establishment
Arcliffe Bulwark	7
Carlisle	45
Chester	66
Cowes Castle[17]	4
Dartmouth Castle	22
Dover Castle[18]	20
Deal Castle	21
Gravesend	35
Hurst Castle	23
Moates Bulwark, Kent	13
Portland Island	13
Sandgate Castle	19
Sandowne Castle	19
St Mawes Castle[19]	16

Scarborough Castle	14
Shrewsbury	45
Upner Castle	29
Walmer Castle	3
Total	414

Source: H.J. Cook, 'Practical Medicine and the British Armed Forces after the "Glorious Revolution"', *Medical History* (1990), 34: 5.

In addition to the above units, a permanent garrison of approximately one thousand men was also maintained across the channel in Dunkirk, a town that had been ceded to England following its capture by Commonwealth troops in 1658.

Despite the semi-permanent nature of the newly constituted standing force, twenty years were to pass before any long-term public welfare provision for soldiers incapacitated by their service was reintroduced with the founding of the Royal Hospitals at Kilmainham, near Dublin, in 1679 and at Chelsea in 1680. Designed to mirror Louis XIV's Les Invalides in Paris, these palatial structures were intended to reflect the glory and beneficence of the monarchy as much as provide relief for old soldiers. They supplied, in today's terminology, 'long-term sheltered accommodation' for soldiers incapable of further military service but were not intended to offer acute surgical care for war wounded.

This then was the constitution of the nation's defence force during the first few years of the Restored Monarchy. With the nation settling into a semi-stable peace at home, it was inevitable that the newly formed army's first real test was conducted overseas, where the country's earlier performance in providing hospital and welfare facilities had been woefully inadequate. The following chapters will attempt, first, to determine whether any lessons had been learned from former experiences and then proceed to explore the nature and quality of nursing, medical and welfare provision for soldiers developed over the succeeding fifty years.

Notes

[1] A. Gore, *Our Services Under the Crown* (London, 1879) and Sir N. Cantlie, *History of the Army Medical Department* (2 vols, Edinburgh: Churchill Livingstone, 1974).

[2] Col. C. Walton, *A History of the British Standing Army* (London: Harrison and Sons, 1894); J. Childs, *The Army of Charles II* (London: Routledge & Kegan Paul, 1976); *The Army, James II, and the Glorious Revolution* (Manchester University Press, 1980); *The British Army of William III, 1689–1702* (Manchester University Press, 1987); *The Nine Years' War and the British Army, 1688–1697* (Manchester University Press, 1991).

[3] H.A.L. Howells, 'The Care of the Sick and Wounded during Marlborough's Campaigns', *JRAMC* (1908), 11: 526–38; 'The Story of the Army Surgeon and the Care of the Sick and Wounded in the British Army, from 1660–1688', *JRAMC* (1910), 14: 81–90; 'The Story of the British Army Surgeon and the Care of the Sick and Wounded from 1689 to 1702', *JRAMC* (1911), 17: 643–58; G.A. Kempthorne

'Some Notes on the Medical Service of the Restoration Army', *JRAMC* (1939), 72: 340–46.
4   F.H. Garrison, *Notes on the History of Military Medicine* (Washington, 1922, republished Darmstadt: Georg Olms, 1970); R.A. Gabriel and K.S. Metz, *A History of Military Medicine* (2 vols, New York: Greenwood Press, 1992), vol. 1.
5   V. Belhomme, *L'Armée Française* (Paris, 1895); L. André's, *Michel le Tellier et l'Organisation de l'Armée Monarchique* (Paris, 1906); R. Baillargeat (ed.), *Les Invalides, Trois Siècles d'Histoire* (Paris, 1975); P. Contamine, *Histoire Militaire de la France* (Paris, 1992); J.A. Lynn, *Giant of the Grand Siècle* (Cambridge: Cambridge University Press, 1997).
6   E.E. Gruber von Arni, *Justice to the Maimed Soldier* (Aldershot: Ashgate Publishing, 2001); J.J. Keevil, C. Lloyd and J.L.S. Coulter, *Medicine and the Navy, 1200–1900* (4 vols, Edinburgh: E&S Livingstone, 1958-1963).
7   C. Hill, *God's Englishman* (London: Pelican, 1970), pp. 144–64.
8   M. Ashley, *Financial and Commercial Policy under the Cromwellian Protectorate* (London: Frank Cass, 1934, second edition, 1962), pp. 174–8.
9   *JHC*, vol. 8, p. 667.
10 Ibid., p. 856.
11 Ibid., vol. 8, p. 66.
12 'Acts of Parliament 39 & 40. Eliz Cap.V. and 43 and 44 Eliz. Cap II' quoted in G.W. Prothero, *Select Statutes and Other Constitutional Documents* (Oxford: University Press, 1913), pp. 100–103; *JHC*, vol. 8, p. 667.
13 *Cal. S.P. Dom., 1660–1661*, p. 357.
14 G. Davies, *The Early History of the Coldstream Guards* (Oxford: Clarendon Press, 1924), pp. 110–12.
15 Lord Cotteslow, 'The Earliest Establishment, 1661, of the British Standing Army', *JSAHR* (1930), IX: 147–161 and 214–242.
16 At Harwich.
17 The defence of Cowes Castle was the responsibility of fifty men, selected from amongst the inhabitants of Cowes, who, by virtue of their office, were exempt from all other duties, together with another hundred men drawn from elsewhere on the Isle of Wight when the need arose.
18 The Lord Warden of the Cinque Ports had his headquarters here. The Cinque Ports garrisons did not come under the central administration of the Board of Ordnance.
19 St Mawes Castle was manned by a Company of one hundred volunteers from the local community who, by custom, kept the structure in repair and mustered only when a state of emergency was declared.

Chapter 1

The Garrison Hospital at Tangier, 1662–1683

When King Charles II married Catherine of Braganza in 1661 his marriage contract included a dowry that brought the colonies of Tangier and Bombay into the possession of the Crown. Whilst the latter was granted to the East India Company for further development of its pre-existing trading base on the Indian sub-continent, Tangier was an entirely new enterprise. In establishing an isolated garrison to guard the newly acquired territory on the north-west coast of Africa, the recently formed standing army faced a severe test of its abilities as it embarked upon its first overseas commitment.

The plan was to garrison the colony with a combination of fresh troops recruited in England and others taken from the garrison of Dunkirk. It remained under total military control for some six years until, in June 1668, a civil government was introduced and Tangier was incorporated as a municipality that survived until the colony was abandoned in March 1684. Ultimate control lay in the hands of the Committee for Tangier in London, a government body established by the Privy Council to administer the colony's affairs. The Committee was chaired by the King's brother, the Duke of York, with Samuel Pepys, the diarist, acting as Secretary until 1665 when, following reorganization, Pepys became Receiver General and Treasurer to the renamed Tangier Board. At first the colony was regarded as a potential toehold from which to develop an English empire in Africa based on trade. However, continual neglect, indifference, lack of investment and a failure to encourage the desired trade soon brought an end to these dreams.[1] How different things might have been if the enterprise had, as with Bombay, been placed in the hands of a mercantile body whose livelihood depended on astute commercial abilities.

Suspicious of the threat posed by the new colony to its trading empire, Spain tried its hardest to prevent England from gaining possession of Tangier but, on 16 January 1662, the first troops, some 300 marines of the Duke of York's Maritime Regiment and 200 seamen, landed from ships of the Royal Navy's Mediterranean flotilla under the command of Lord Sandwich to take possession of the colony from the Portuguese Governor, the Conde de Valdorez. At the time of the handover, Tangier consisted of about 500 houses, a parish church, a convent of Austin Friars and nine other chapels with between four and five thousand inhabitants, of whom two-thirds were women and children.[2] Within days all the street names had been anglicized and, after only two weeks, the Portuguese inhabitants, having taken great exception to the informal manners of the English soldiery, accepted the Earl of Sandwich's offer to convey them back to Portugal in his ships, leaving little more than empty buildings behind them.[3] Writing in 1672 Sir Hugh Cholmley, commenting on this episode, remarked that their dramatic decision to leave resulted from their:

> abhorrence of the free conversation which in Northern Countries is used between men and women ... was intolerable in a people that make jealousy their honour and therefore could not submit to those publick liberties which souldiers would take with their wives and daughters though this perhaps was more in innocency than might be at many other times.[4]

When the Earl of Peterborough arrived on 29 January 1662, accompanied by his newly raised permanent garrison of 100 horse and 1,000 foot, and assumed the grandiose title of 'Governor and Captain General of His Majesty's Forces in Africa', the absence of even the most basic facilities produced severe problems as the force had brought very few of the common necessities of life with them. Cholmley criticized the troops for contributing to the situation by their poor behaviour when he commented that:

> Many houses were destroyed to make fire for the pot and yet the souldiers had so little care or conveniences for the dressing of their victuals that, from want of watering [soaking] their salt meats or ordering their provisions as they ought to have done, appeared the bad effects of an ill diet in the great mortality which presently followed, the noise of which sufferings the poor souldiers endured.[5]

In reality it is difficult to know what else they could have done when little or no thought had been given to basic household equipment, logistics and supply. Within two weeks of the arrival the military council were complaining that 2,000 beds were urgently required along with 600 iron pots for the soldiers to 'boil their meat in', otherwise 'want of these necessities will bring sickness and diseases upon the souldier and, in a short time, the garrison will be destroyed'.[6] It was unsafe to venture outside the walls of the town, there were only limited supplies of fresh meat within and the little that was available was bad and sold at highly exorbitant prices. Water was piped into the colony from the hinterland and, as a result, supplies were severely limited and always subject to the threat of interference by local tribesmen. Conversely, wine was cheap, plentiful and, taken in large quantities, provided a readily available remedy for the sense of melancholy and home-sickness that permeated the inhabitants.

Inevitably, when news of these and other deficiencies filtered back to troops in England, Tangier gained a reputation as little better than a bad prison from which 'they could only hope to be freed by a grave, the common friend that put a speedy end to their misfortunes'.[7] The colony remained in English hands for some twenty-one years, continuously plagued by disease and continual harassment from local tribesmen while suffering the effects of corrupt and inept government both locally and from London. It is outside of the scope of this work to delve deeply into the political, strategic and tactical aspects of the colony's story except when these elements impinge upon the medical scenario. Anyone seeking to read further into the wider story of Tangier as an English colony can do no better than consult Enid Routh's *Tangier, England's Lost Atlantic Outpost, 1661–1684*. Although published in 1912, and not yet reprinted, no other work provides such comprehensive coverage of the subject.[8]

On 8 April 1665, Lord Bellasis arrived as Governor, sweeping into the colony like a new broom. One of his first actions was to order the construction of a barracks for the troops and the repair of houses damaged by the previous winter's heavy rains. He decreed that henceforth officers and soldiers were to receive their pay promptly, reduced the time spent on watch by each man and built roofs over the outlying forts thereby offering those on guard duty some protection from the elements. Orders were also issued that commissioned officers were to inspect their soldiers in quarters each evening to ensure that their needs were catered for and to check that they kept their quarters clean. He also established a Court of Justice that he regularly attended.[9] However, the new regime lasted only one year. Bellasis was a Roman Catholic and, finding himself unable to take the oath of conformity, he resigned his appointment and departed the colony in April 1666, leaving control in the hands of the Deputy Governor, Colonel Henry Norwood.

Tangier suffered from all the petty bickering and snobbery common to most colonial situations and small communities. This was particularly marked after 1668 when the colony's internal administration was changed from military government into a municipality with a Civic Corporation and a separate Grand Jury. Without prior experience or knowledge of how to manage a community, the Corporation, inevitably, struggled to fulfil its responsibilities. The maintenance of public health had been difficult even during the period of military government. In 1666 widespread and indiscriminate butchering of animals for meat, with the associated hazards to health, forced Lord Bellasis to prohibit the slaughter of animals anywhere except at the public abattoir. This establishment was subsequently funded by levying a charge of 6d for each beef carcass and 3d for every calf, hog, goat or sheep dispatched. Anyone ignoring his orders would be imprisoned and forfeit the carcasses of their beasts to the Provost Marshal.[10]

When the new Corporation was formed it automatically assumed responsibility for the market, public buildings, sewerage, water, pest-houses and for cleaning the streets. Initially the approach taken seemed sound and appropriate. A city scavenger was appointed and it was agreed that:

> those that would clense their owne doors or backsides [yards] might doe it, and that those that would have their durt, soyle or rubbidge carried out and taken away by the scavenger might agree with him by the month or quarter.[11]

Regrettably the system soon broke down. The large number of householders who had chosen to use the scavenger's services refused to agree to his monthly or quarterly charges and the rubbish and waste material built up until it completely fouled the streets, forming a noisome hazard to health. As time passed the Corporation's incompetence became obvious to all as their failures grew apace.

By 1678, after ten years in power, almost every Council session saw motions raised censuring their incompetence or inaction. They were still being criticized for failing to effectively clean the streets when, on 3 May 1678, the Corporation was held to blame for allowing 'hoggs to go about the streets, an inducement to infection and evil distempers'.[12] The earlier slaughterhouse regulations were ignored while other health hazards, such as mouldering heaps of rubbish, unpaved streets and open sewers remained unremedied. A long-standing feud arose between the Grand Jury and the Corporation. The Grand Jury continued to criticize the Corporation while the Corporation persisted in ignoring the directives of the Grand Jury. Not surprisingly, as the principal members of the Corporation were *ex officio* Justices of the Peace, they felt 'secure in the dignity of their office, content to survey the beastly scene and view with philosophic calm the streets they ought to clean'.[13]

What of the hospital? From the outset, a facility for the reception of sick and wounded soldiers was included in the colony's establishment but, sadly, only a limited amount of associated documentation survives. Initially, fifty regimental medical chests were provided by the navy, but from the earliest days, the hospital's reputation was so bad that men would suffer anything rather than admit to being ill for fear of being sent there.[14] Shortage or misappropriation of funds combined with lack of genuine concern or commitment to health care provision resulted in a varying quality of service to say the least.[15]

The building in question was a converted civilian house where the small windows, of typical Mediterranean design, helped to maintain lower internal temperatures but provided poor lighting and ventilation. In February 1665 Sir Hugh Cholmley, the engineer in charge of the colony's biggest project, the construction of a harbour mole, said that the hospital was so bad that 'the men fly from it as from the grave', regarding it as a place to go to be buried, not for the benefit of their health.[16] As late as March 1683, Henry Shere, who replaced Cholmley as garrison engineer, continued to describe the building as 'much too streight, so it is very incommodiously situated being built against an old Battery where the damp and cold in the winter season greatly annoy the sick people'.[17]

In 1667, when Deputy Governor Norwood suggested that some of the naval prize money should be used to construct a purpose-built hospital, his proposal was rejected. Less than a year later, when sickness broke out amongst the troops, he could not resist commenting, in a letter sent to Lord Arlington, Chairman of the Tangier Board in London, that:

> Had your Lordship thought fit to have gone thereon with the proposition I made to erect an hospital it would have turned to good account unto His Majesty I am sure, besides the charity ... of easing the sick.[18]

Two years were to pass before Norwood next commented on the work of the hospital. During a serious epidemic in the hot weather of 1669, he remarked, somewhat surprisingly, that 'great care was taken to nurse and cherish the sick with wholesome good accommodation' but, in reality, no permanent improvement had been achieved and even later, during Lord Inchiquin's term of office as Governor (1678–1680), the hospital was still being described as 'exceeding streight, without any garden or place of aire belonging to it, and also very damp'.[19] It stood on marshy ground and illnesses caused by neglect of sanitary precautions were aggravated by a lack of any decent facilities.

As hopes remained high for Tangier to be developed as a major trading port, logic dictated that measures should be taken in hand to protect the colony from ship-borne infection. In response to continual outbreaks of plague over the centuries, the European countries that bordered the Mediterranean had developed a long-standing and justifiable fear of ship-borne contagion and, as a result of rigidly imposed local precautions, British merchant vessels experienced considerable hindrance in their attempts to enter the ports of Spain, France and Italy where any ship suspected of trading with Turkish or Moorish outlets was automatically required to undergo forty days of quarantine before landing its goods. Many city states had developed sophisticated facilities in lazarettes or purpose-built isolation hospitals specifically designed to contain the disease and accommodate its victims.[20] In comparison, meanwhile, England's protective measures were basic in the extreme, consisting simply of identifying quarantine moorings in sheltered bays and creeks where infected vessels were required to moor until declared free from infection.[21]

As early as March 1665, probably spurred on by an embargo on trade imposed by the Governors of Cadiz, Malaga and Tarifa as a result of the Great Plague raging in England, a group of six local merchants wrote to the Commissioners for Tangier in London suggesting the provision of a purpose-built lazarette hospital for Tangier in the Mediterranean style.[22] The men who submitted the proposal were obviously familiar with quarantine arrangements elsewhere in the Mediterranean and they singled out those at Leghorn (Livorno) and Venice as examples worthy of emulating. Some reference is made to the presence of a 'lazarretta' (sic) in 1665 while, that same year, the newly appointed Governor, Lord Bellasis, was forced to issue a proclamation threatening banishment to anyone boarding vessels entering the harbour of Tangier before the vessels had been cleared and a licence to board issued.[23] Three years later, in 1668, part of the duties assumed by the incoming Court of Governors included 'the supervision of the local pest-houses'. It therefore seems likely that some elementary form of quarantine establishment was established fairly early in the colony's existence but, in practice, little heed seems to have been paid to the various associated regulations. Ten years later, Deputy Governor Norwood was forced to re-introduce legislation banning the unauthorized boarding of arrivals in the harbour before they had undergone a health inspection on pain of a penalty fine of fifty shillings or a month's imprisonment together with forfeiture of the vessel concerned.

Although, initially, Cholmley supported moves to build a lazarette, he was undoubtedly influenced by his own agenda for the wider development of the harbour area as a whole. On 7 April 1675, when he submitted his ideas for developing the port to the Tangier Board in London, he included a plan for an entire complex that would surround the mole and harbour, including buildings and warehouses large enough to service at least 20 small vessels, quarters sufficient to house 400 men, stables for 60 horses, a large smithy, a shop and a new garrison hospital for the sick.[24] Strangely, in view of his earlier support, Cholmley commented that 'until the trade of this place increases and the mole is nearer finished, there is no great necessity of a Lazarette' but, nevertheless, enclosed extensive drawings for just such a facility that entailed building on a site described as 'lying near the water side, on the sande that lays betwixt the first lime kiln and the present begun bastion near Cambridge redoubt'.[25]

His submission, costed at £1,000, even included a staff list for the proposed lazarette that included a Governor or Master who should be a man 'well versed in the condition or quality of the commodities usually put into such places' with a salary of £100 per annum, a Deputy Governor, or Registrar, who would act as the facility's accountant and, in the absence of any medical personnel, a Master Porter who would also serve when the hospital element was occupied as 'the keeper of those which may be appointed there to make their quarantine' assisted by four additional under-porters. More assistants could be employed as the need arose when, as hoped, the trade passing through the port increased.

More importantly, the plans for the purpose-built garrison hospital that were included in Cholmley's far-seeing plans for developing the port facilities also survive in the public records, These are remarkable documents insofar as they contain the first design for a military hospital for the Standing Army outside of England some two years before the foundation of the Royal Hospital at Kilmainham and four before that of Chelsea. His square, colonnaded building, surrounded by a central courtyard, was totally at variance with the linear concept of ward design familiar in medieval hospital architecture.

Indeed, the form of his proposed building contains many similarities to the general ground plan of *valetudinaria*, the military hospitals that, a thousand years previously, had been a common feature in the fortresses and northern border defences of the Roman Empire.[26] Equally, it might be noted that his drawings show a layout that relates closely to the open, airy patterns of Mediterranean and Ottoman designs and bear a considerable resemblance in both form and layout to those of the Italian master Palladio, as published in his work *The Four Books on Architecture.*[27]

The proposed building clearly demonstrates the widespread influence exerted by Mediterranean practices upon contemporary hospital design so clearly visible in the much grander concept of *Les Invalides* in Paris that was in the process of construction at the same time. The fact that, due to financial stringency and the subsequent closure of the colony, Cholmley's hospital was never built does not detract from the importance of his plans in the history of military hospital design.

Unfortunately, Cholmley was rather too outspoken for his own and the colony's good. His ideas for improving the overall worth of the colony were both expensive and couched in phrases unlikely to receive widespread acceptance at a time of almost universal corruption in public service. For example, when forming his '*Conclusions observing what may be of use for the future growth and welfare of Tangier'* he advocated a raft of proposals for improving both day-to-day life in the colony as well as its potential for the future. Amongst these he suggested that the civil government of the colony should adopt the attitude that there was at least some hope for the future that Tangier would, eventually, be something better than a 'little camp trading in drink' and, with equal vigour, he also published his personal suggestions regarding the attributes of any future prospective governor:

> Much depends upon the choice and qualification of the Governor that is sent, who ought to be a man of honour and know generosity, much as may render him above either open exaction or underhand contrivance to enrich himself by ways and means that will always be set afoot by men either desiring to share in the booty, or to ingratiate themselves with the Governor, what sorts of profit will be one way or other to the public prejudice of the place.[28]

Regrettably, but not surprisingly, Cholmley's plans, including those for the lazarette and hospital, were discarded, having been deemed too expensive and, in 1676, he was replaced as Surveyor General by a rival engineer, Henry Shere. In his turn, Shere also spent considerable time and effort in identifying the means whereby the colony's hospital facilities could be improved. As late as March 1683, he recommended that the 'Town House', a building 'very commodiously situate, with a large garden', that had been gifted to the corporation by Lord Bellasis for use as a municipal meeting house, be converted for permanent use as a hospital. The property had been used once before in that role during a prolonged siege of the colony in 1680 when it had been equipped as a hospital annex containing 60 beds.[29] His plan was to enlarge the premises by building an extension of sufficient dimensions to accommodate 140 patients in single beds that would then, together with the existing capacity, provide accommodation for 200 sick men, a figure deemed adequate for the colony's future needs. As an additional incentive, Shere added that the old hospital could then be vacated and become available for use as rent-free soldiers' quarters or stables to obviate the need for the hired accommodation in current use.

Unfortunately, these plans came only six months before the colony's final closure and, despite Shere's persuasive proposition and detailed costings, there is no evidence to indicate that these plans met with any greater success than those of Cholmley.[30] Even so, failure to upgrade the colony's hospital provision was only one factor in its decline. The general health of the colony was never good and for new arrivals life was particularly difficult. Civilian patients were always accepted into the military hospital for treatment when there was room for them yet, in view of its reputation, those who could cope in their own houses probably took little advantage of this privilege. In May 1667, the Lieutenant Governor, Colonel Norwood, told the Commissioners in London that 'the generality of the garrison are, God be thanked, in good health. Only the new recruits do fall ill fast'.[31] Nine years later newcomers were complaining about the strange blisters and pimples, similar to those of smallpox, that were generally attributed to the biting mosquitoes, described as being just like the gnats in some parts of England but a little more pert, and 'clinches' which resembled ticks but, when they were killed, they left an intolerable stink.[32]

In addition to sickness, trauma was a constant factor in the colony's daily life. The soldiers' lives were also endangered by the frequent attacks made by local tribesmen upon the garrison. In one engagement alone, that of 3 May 1663, the Governor's Regiment lost 207 casualties and Sir Robert Harley's Regiment 388; the following year, on 4 May 1664, the new Governor, Lord Teviot, was killed during an ambush by the Moors along with several officers and 500 men at a distance of only two miles from Tangier.[33] Notwithstanding wounds sustained during fighting, accidental injuries were a daily hazard. The construction of the aforementioned mole, a large jetty to enclose the harbour, was the most significant civic project undertaken during the colony's existence and a considerable number of labourers, assisted by garrison troops, were employed in its construction. A distinct mole community, including families, sprang up in residence as the work progressed. On 27 October 1683 a landslip on the site killed two or three men outright and several others sustained injuries, necessitating their admission to the hospital.[34]

Despite almost constant skirmishing interspersed by more significant brief but bloody encounters with local tribesmen, most military casualties were attributable to sickness and yet, amongst the 200 manual labourers on the mole, no more than eight people had been lost during the same period and of those, only half were due to disease. The only explanation that Cholmley could offer for the disparity between the health of the two elements of the community was that less care was taken of the soldiers than of the labourers. As contracted civilians, the labourers were paid regularly every month, and could pay for treatment when they were sick, whereas the soldiers went sometimes six, seven or even nine months without pay. Given the humdrum and boring routine of their lives, when the soldiers did receive their dues, their sudden wealth was rapidly spent on alcohol and intemperance. As a result they fell ill and, having spent all their money on drink, they had no money to help themselves. They were unlikely to be paid again for another six months and very few local merchants were compassionate enough to wait that long for payment. Many a soldier died for want of a shilling. Heavy, monotonous work became the soldiers' life style. In 1681, out of a total of some 1,200 to 1,400 men, 400 were needed to form the nightly guard. This meant that the soldiers were allowed no more than two or three consecutive nights in bed, a situation that was even condoned by the regulations that were against letting them 'fall into idle ways'.[35]

A letter, written on 28 February 1664 by the Governor's Secretary to the Commissioners in London, also described the general health of manual labourers working on the construction of the harbour mole as being generally much better than that of the garrison's soldiers and, on the basis that prevention was better than cure, recommended that, for the future, 'some public care was given to the health of the soldier, which would save His Majesty more in the recruits which must otherwise be sent every year'.[36] In truth, the psychological effects on a soldier of posting him to the colony for an unspecified period were severe. The Tangier

Regiment spent over twenty years in the colony and Cholmley was perfectly correct in suggesting that the ultimate remedy for the soldiers' health was a regular rotation of regiments through the colony which would 'keep the troops in good heart and cheerful in their duty' and minimize the time men spent exposed to the primitive local conditions.[37] Indeed, the Governor had good reason to make every effort to nurture the health and well-being of his troops as the previous twelve months had seen a rapid deterioration in the numbers of the original garrison. This is clearly demonstrated in the relevant muster lists where the returns for the period between 30 January and 23 October 1663 alone show an overall drop of more than 22 per cent in the garrison's strength in just nine months as shown in Table 1.1

Table 1.1 Tangier garrison strength, 30 January – 23 October 1663

Regiment	30 Jan	7 Apr	8 May	26 Jun	31 Jul	11 Sep	23 Oct
Governor's	1,000	986	960	859	815	778	793
Sir R. Harley's	947	913	667	623	617	602	559
Farrell's	381	373	380	392	372	379	371
Fitzgerald's	392	403	404	406	414	408	391
Total:	2,720	2,675	2,411	2,280	2,218	2,167	2,114

Source: J. Davis, *History of the Second Queen's (Royal West Surrey) Regiment* (6 vols, 1887–1961), vol. 1, p. 41.

Although he did not hold any individual officers responsible or directly to blame for the situation, Cholmley did complain about the frequent misappropriation of soldiers' money inasmuch as when soldiers died their officers would frequently retain any outstanding pay for their own pocket. As a remedy for this scandalous situation, he advocated that the dead men's arrears of pay should be set aside for the care of the sick, thereby assisting the hospital to raise standards and improve its reputation.[38]

Between 4 November 1662 and 20 March 1664, Thomas Povey, the Receiver and Treasurer for Tangier, issued only £203 16s 9½d 'to relieve and supply the sick in the hospital' and, as the colony grew, the financial support for the hospital barely kept pace with developments.[39] Even after the 1668 change in the colony's government from military to civil control, only £547 10s, just over £10 per week, was set as the hospital's annual budget although this sum was augmented by the pay of sick soldiers that was credited as a maintenance charge to the hospital during the period of each patient's admission. Indeed, despite its other serious shortcomings, shortage of funds was the principal cause of the hospital's poor reputation, especially when there were often as many as 400 men in the building, mostly soldiers and women suffering from venereal disease, at any one time.[40] As Pepys recorded, the largest group of patients being treated, barring those with dysentery, were 'rogues and jades that have the pox'.[41]

The Lords Commissioners in London seem to have suspected that all was not as it should be and, in 1675, appointed a hospital committee of four Overseers. The Mayor of the Colony assumed the role of Chairman of the Committee, assisted by the eldest alderman and two Field Officers of the garrison. Their responsibilities included the dispatch of regular reports to the Tangier Committee in London detailing their progress as well as implementing newly introduced hospital regulations. These are shown in Table 1.2.

Table 1.2 Regulations for the hospital at Tangier

1. The Overseers are to meet on the first Monday of each month to decide on the proportion and sort of diet the sick in hospital are to be allowed – not to exceed 9d per man per day.
2. The Overseers are to appoint such under-officers and attendants as are deemed necessary.
3. Sick soldiers are to be kept in their quarters until Monday morning, the day victuals are issued from stores. Sometimes the ill state of men has meant they have reported in the middle of the week but this has been avoided wherever possible.
4. Admission to the hospital is by ticket made under the physician's hand attested by the surgeon or, extraordinarily, by a note under the hand of any three of the Overseers.
5. Every Monday at noon the Commissary of the Musters takes the name of all sick soldiers sent to hospital and sees them personally. He is to submit a roll of their names to the Commissioners for Tangier. Ministers are to provide a weekly roll of those that they bury.
6. The Captain of the watch is to survey the hospital daily.
7. The Physician is to make daily visits and satisfy himself as to provision and usage of the sick and prescribe remedies.
8. Poor people of the town [the civilian labourers and their families] are in like manner to be admitted in such numbers as from time to time the Overseers find the established allowance will cover.
9. £200 per annum is allowed by the Commissioners for Tangier for putting to work the poor children of Tangier.

Source: *Cal. Treas. Books*, vol. 8, II, p. 1427.

The task of the Overseers was not an enviable one. The hospital, like everything else in Tangier, was constantly short of money and the patients suffered accordingly. Between December 1674 and December 1677 only £1,091 17s 4d was paid in.[42] In May 1683 the four Overseers, William Smith (the Mayor), Alderman Boynton, Charles Trelawny and William Staines, reported that their accounts for the half year's expenses between 1 February and 1 May showed an excess of expenditure over income of £264 9s 7¾d. They were forced to arrange an interest-bearing loan of £500, made up of £250 from Mr Lodington and Mr Onebie, merchants of London, and £250 from Mr Stone, a merchant of Cadiz, in order to pay immediate expenses, the Governor being 'verie bare of moneyes'.[43]

Their principal items of expenditure were food in the form of bread, wine, brandy and meat although, with the countryside around the colony barred to the residents by the aggressive local tribesmen, the supply of fresh meat was irregular and salt meat was the norm. Bread was baked locally and, in the first six months of 1683 alone, the baker was paid £214 7s 1½d. Obviously additional provisions for the hospital patients' dietary needs depended to a great extent on what was available locally. White biscuit, mace, oatmeal, tamarinds, French barley, cinnamon, currants, white and brown sugar and rice were all listed as purchases in the hospital accounts and a special allowance of 6d per patient was approved for the purchase of oranges and lemons.[44] More exotic foods were certainly available locally but at a price that put them well beyond a budget catering for patients regarded as recipients of charity. When Bellasis had occupied the Governorship he had made efforts to personally supervise the hospital's funds and frequently sent food from his own kitchen for the patients and, throughout its existence, however poor, the hospital diet was invariably superior to that of the common soldier for whom, given the colony's particular supply difficulties, dependent almost entirely upon sea-borne replenishment, the threat of malnutrition was ever present. Although contemporary understanding of the links between nutrition and health were rudimentary, an anonymous author writing in 1680 expressed the belief that although the sick in hospital received fresh victuals, a supply of fresh food for the whole garrison would bring long-lasting benefits in preserving its general health, adding that a continual diet of salt meat over two or three years led to various ailments such as 'obstruction, scurvy, diarrhoea and so forth'. He also warned that those who were cured by the healthier diet available in the hospital would, inevitably, relapse when their standard diet was resumed following their return to duty.[45]

Further insight into the establishment's diet is to be gained from a list of items compiled by Richard Burdett, Purveyor of the Royal Naval galley *Margaret* based in the harbour, that detailed the foodstuffs he sent to the hospital for men of his vessel that had been admitted between 13 July and 31 August 1675.[46] The crew that manned the Royal galley was composed of 'slaves, turks [primarily captured barbary pirates] and bonovolos' (volunteers), who, in common with the contemporary universal practice throughout the Mediterranean, had been allowed to establish a small trading area in the port area supervised by a sutler who also acted as translator for the local English community. That the hospital should open its doors to such people does not appear unusual in the twenty-first century; however, to contemporary eyes, the situation was exceptional. Burdett complained that he did not receive the same funding as that which was invariably provided by the Kings of France and Spain for their galleys to purchase both health-care for sick and wounded members of their crews and the recruitment of volunteers. As Burdett's galley did not carry a stock of medicines, and he had no means of purchasing medical care elsewhere, he was totally reliant upon the Tangier hospital for such provision although he assisted where he could by supplying it with articles such as large quantities of rags 'for the doctor to dress the maimed' and more than twelve barrels of oil of roses, a lotion used for cleaning and dressing wounds.[47]

Over the six-week period covered by his report, Burdett supplied 641 soft bread loaves, 423 bottles of wine, 273 portions of mutton, 183 pounds of rice, 2½ barrels of olive oil, 82 lbs raisins, four hens, almonds and 348 eggs for an average of 11 in-patients per day. It is noteworthy that particular care seems to have been taken to provide Muslim patients with food items such as rice, chickens, eggs and nuts that were compatible with the diet regulations imposed by their religion.

As well as numbering the patients admitted to hospital from his galley, Burdett's report also provides his classification of their status by categorizing them as marines, soldiers, slaves or 'woglies', a term (? derogative) that appears to refer to local volunteers or native labourers. In the six weeks covered, no marines and only one soldier were admitted but an average of seven slaves and seven labourers were to be found as in-patients at any given time during the same period. However, in one instance, the admission of several sick men from the galley may have been sufficient to overload the hospital's accommodation. A memorandum from Burdet survives that notes it 'might be necessary to send out twenty or thirty ammunition beds to be put into the hospital for the better accommodation of the sick people belonging to the said galley'. Of course, this might equally reflect a criticism of the poor quality of the existing hospital beds.[48]

Meanwhile, back in England, when the 4th Regiment of Foot were given orders to join the Tangier garrison, they were provided with an image of life in the colony that was far removed from truthful when they were told that their lot would consist of

> fresh and wholesome quarters with small gardens, coals for dressing their provisions they have out of the stores, at the King's charge; every Monday morning each man receives one piece of beef, one piece of pork, 7 lbs bread, a quarter of pease, a pint of oatmeal, besides butter and cheese for weekly allowance.

The reality that greeted them on arrival must have provided them with a rude awakening. The garrison was supposed to maintain a reserve store of six months' provisions in order that delays caused by stormy weather would not result in shortages. Yet, in October 1682, the victuallers were obliged to throw nearly 24,000 lb of Irish meat into the sea 'so extremely corrupted that it was not only unserviceable' but had also 'by reason of its noisome smell, become an unsufferable nuisance to the place'.[49]

Part of the problem in maintaining an adequate hospital service was the mismanagement, not to say misappropriation, of funds. The accounts of Samuel Pepys, the colony's Receiver General and Treasurer, show that between May 1666 and June 1669 Deputy Governor Norwood was paid more than £68,000 for the work of the hospital. As hospital standards were so grievously criticized it is not surprising that accusations were levelled against Norwood imputing that he had taken some of the hospital revenues for his own use. Pepys dismissed the accusations as baseless but, far from home and with time on their hands, the conduct of military officers was far from ideal, as Pepys himself recorded when discussing the behaviour of Colonel Percy Kirke, the Colony's last Governor:

> the governor is said to have got his wife's sister with child and that she is now gone over to Spain to be brought to bed. And that while he is with his whores at his little bathing house – which he has furnished with a jade on purpose for that use there - his wife, whom he keeps in by awe, sends for her gallants and plays the jade herself at home.[50]

At the heart of the matter lay the stark facts that the hospital was too small and that the level of finances allocated, which had remained at the original level set in 1662, was insufficient. Both elements failed to keep pace with an ever-increasing usage whilst judicious 'cooking' of the accounts was made possible by the colony's high mortality rate. The pay of deceased patients continued to be drawn by their officers for some time following their demise without much fear of discovery, as inventive accounting was standard procedure in public office.

In his journal, John Luke, the colony's Recorder, related that the Treasurer for the hospital, Mr St John, admitted to him in the course of conversation that he compiled the hospital accounts by adding a number of false extra patients to the total as he saw fit in the current circumstance. On enquiring about another account where a shortfall had been made up by the account holder personally, St John had muttered indistinctly, so, with gentlemanly discretion, Luke refrained from pursuing the subject, merely commenting that the Treasurer 'beganne to grow weary of my questions, so I excused him from further trouble, and tooke him into the cellar'.[51]

A steward conducted the day-to-day administration of the hospital whilst nursing duties were probably undertaken by soldiers' wives or widows. Exact numbers are not recorded. The contemporary weekly rate of pay for a hospital nurse in London was 2s 6d but, as that sum was the rate authorized for Tangier's surgeon's mate, it is highly unlikely that a nurse in the colony would have been paid as much. As the establishment allowed for a total sum of £42 per month for the payment of nurses, a nurse's wage would probably have been in the region of 1s a day and, therefore, up to 27 nurses may have been employed. As we are told that there were sometimes up to 400 in-patients, a nurse to patient ratio of one nurse to fifteen patients would have been regarded as normal and would have matched the authorized level present in the Parliamentary hospitals during the civil wars and Interregnum. As will be seen later in this narrative, the military hospitals that were to be deployed in Europe some twenty years later also used this figure as a guide to the allocation of nurses and, indeed, such a ratio would not be deemed inappropriate to modern eyes in such conditions.[52]

Medical officers were included in the lists of 'Field and Staff Officers' provided for in the overall establishment, two physicians and an apothecary being numbered among the Governor's staff. At first each of the four regiments present had its own surgeon and surgeon's mate but, when the colony's administration was civilianized in 1668, the regimental medical staff were abolished and the establishment was reduced to just one physician, Dr Thomas Lawrence, one surgeon, a surgeon's mate and an apothecary with an allowance of £1 10s per day allocated for the hospital. Thenceforth the medical establishment and pay structure was as shown in Table 1.3

Table 1.3 Tangier medical establishment, post 1668

Appointment	Daily Pay	Monthly Pay
1 Physician	10s 0d	£14 0s 0d
1 Surgeon	4s 0d	£5 12s 0d
1 Surgeon's Mate	2s 6d	£3 10s 0d
Nurses (total)	£1 10s 0d	£42 0s 0d

Source: TNA, CO 279/10, fol. 198.

As specified in the regulations, the garrison Captain of the Watch paid daily visits as part of his routine, as did the physician, who was required to satisfy himself that the patients were appropriately cared for and to prescribe treatments as needed. It was later deemed necessary to publish an additional directive that forbade the physician to enter into commercial business as a supplier of provisions since this would conflict with one of the principal functions of his duties as an arbiter and regulator for the correct provision of the patients' diet.[53] Occasionally an extra physician or two came over in attendance on a governor or ambassador, but the only effective and reliable assistance that could be called upon in times of need was that of ships' doctors serving in the Mediterranean squadron, some of whom came gallantly to the assistance of the wounded during the fighting of 1680. Payments recorded at that time included the sum of £18 15s 0d that was paid to seven surgeons loaned from naval frigates who assisted in caring for sick and wounded men. In one engagement alone, that of 27 October 1680, some 112 officers and men were killed outright, while 32 officers, 2 non-commissioned officers and 332 private soldiers were wounded and needed treatment.[54]

Held in lower social esteem than the physician, the surgeon and his mate had particularly onerous duties; their financial situation was frequently parlous and aggravated by the fact that they frequently experienced great difficulty in securing payment for their work. As early as 1664 surgeon Robert Farendale had brought an action against one Bartholomew Holgate, a former soldier, for medicines supplied for the treatment of gonorrhoea in both Holgate and his wife. Holgate rejected the claim, alleging that his wife had never received treatment from Farendale and rejected any assertion that he had himself had the infection. Holgate entered a counter-claim that Farendale had been the garrison surgeon at the time in question when Holgate had fallen down some stairs and sent for a doctor. Farendale had attended him and given him six pills but, when he realized that Holgate was a soldier, the doctor refused to visit him again even though 4d per month was currently being deducted from Holgate's service pay for medical treatment.[55] In that same year, James Wylie, the regimental surgeon of the Tangier Regiment, brought an action against one Simon Benjamin, claiming that he had refused to pay the twelve dollars fee agreed in advance for treatment of a 'dangerous wound upon his head, with a fracture of the cranium'.[56]

In June 1680 the situation became so bad that Colonel Fairborne, Deputy Governor under Inchiquin from 1675 to 1680, wrote to the Secretary of State in London, Sir Leoline Jenkins, complaining about the severe shortage of surgical staff. The two surgeons present in the colony had to double as surgeons for all the military units as well as providing a service to the entire civilian population. Not surprisingly they complained at their workload and sought either an increase in pay or permission to return to England. The colony could not possibly continue without them and, after commenting that both practitioners were competent at their work and, importantly, knew how the colony operated, Fairborne pointed out that their salaries were so low that noone else would take on the job. He recommended that their salaries be increased from 5s to 8s a day for the surgeon and from 2s 6d to 5s a day for his mate.[57] It is not clear whether these seemingly highly generous figures were agreed, but it seems that the men continued to work on in the colony until its final closure some three years later.

By 1683, after some twenty years of uphill struggle, time was running out. It had become obvious that, without massive financial support, the colony was an economic failure and the decision was taken to accept the situation, evacuate English nationals and leave the town to be re-occupied by the indigenous population. An engineer was dispatched to undertake an 'in-depth' assessment of the cost of repairing the city's defences but with covert instructions to ensure that his final conclusions would prove that the project was not financially viable. His role was, in truth, a thinly veiled face-saving exercise aimed at demonstrating that the retention of the colony was uneconomic, thereby providing the government with an ample excuse to abandon its interests in North Africa. The unenviable task was delegated to Lord Dartmouth, who was secretly briefed to assume the role of Governor. On his departure from England, he carried with him Charles II's sealed instructions regarding the true nature of his mission, which were to be made public only after his arrival in the colony. They included specific orders for him to ensure that the sick and wounded soldiers and officers of the garrison were safely evacuated aboard hospital ships especially provided and fitted out for that purpose with adequate provisions and attendants suitable to their needs. If any were too sick to make the journey, they were to be carried to Spain where the English consul would provide for them until their recovery.

In due course, the many invalids who required evacuation became one of Dartmouth's chief concerns. Initially, he was told that only one vessel, the *Welcome*, would be made available to him. In his estimation one would be insufficient for the task and, before leaving England, he wrote to the Secretary of State requesting that a second hospital ship be made available to him. He also thought that it might be necessary to dispatch the sick in more than one group, some accompanied by their families and effects, and for that reason alone, one ship would not suffice.[58]

Receiving no formal agreement to his request for a second hospital ship, Dartmouth took matters into his own hands when he arrived in Tangier and requisitioned the *Unity*, a merchant vessel originally hired for use by the ordnance department. He ordered its conversion by local workmen into a hospital ship and justified his actions by claiming that the second vessel was absolutely necessary as the numbers of sick were increasing daily. On 8 September 28 days' provisions for 200 men were taken on board and, on 16 October 1683, the *Unity* departed Tangier harbour with 114 infirm soldiers (one died), 34 civilian males and 104 females and children on board, most of them belonging to the senior battalion of Kirke's Regiment. At around the same time, another vessel, the *Virtue*, departed carrying those who had been in receipt of poor relief derived from the colony's charitable allowance of £200 per annum. These included several children, the orphans of soldiers killed in service in Tangier.[59]

According to contemporary terminology, the 'infirm' soldiers on the *Unity* were probably 'invalids' employed on the strength of the garrison to perform light duties in much the same way as invalid battalions were utilized to undertake sedentary garrison duties in England in lieu of pension provision. This hypothesis is strengthened by the knowledge that, unlike the *Welcome*, which departed much later, no special mention was made of nurses on the *Unity* but, instead, John Eccles, a gunner, who had performed the duties of usher and writing master to the school in Tangier, was put in charge of both the 'infirm' and the soldiers' families.

Dartmouth took the time to write to Secretary of State Jenkins on behalf of the evacuees requesting that upon their arrival in England they be placed under the protection of a competent person specially selected for the purpose. Embarrassed by the entire business, the government was determined to minimize any political fallout resulting from the loss of the colony and Jenkins reassured Dartmouth that the King had given special orders for their reception.[60]

Meanwhile, anticipating the need for ongoing support for the sick and wounded after they had returned from Tangier, Dartmouth wrote again to Jenkins on 19 October posing a variety of potential solutions.[61] He suggested that widows and children of seamen or any who 'had relation to the sea' should be cared for by Trinity House, to whom he had written separately. For others he recommended that Governors of Christchurch, St Thomas' and St Katherine's Hospitals might be approached for their support and ended by commenting that, as a last resort, the soldiers could always find relief through the Poor Law system in the established manner.

Four weeks later, on 12 November, the day before the *Unity* docked at Gravesend, Dartmouth was informed that Mr Pierce, a surgeon, had been ordered to go to Gravesend to wait for the *Unity* and to take care of all her passengers, a gesture intended to demonstrate to all concerned that the evacuees' welfare had been given a high priority.[62] In London, the King was advised to summon the Lord Mayor and instruct him to ensure that everything possible was being done for the evacuees. In the event, the 'infirm' evacuees did not arrive in the City but, instead, were admitted to the naval hospital at Deal where Surgeon Pierce was subsequently instructed to visit them to check on their welfare.[63] In a follow-up letter written on 19 November, Jenkins reassured Dartmouth that the planned reception had gone well:

> tomorrow will be a sen'night [week] since Captain Tucker came with his hospital ship [*Unity*] to Gravesend and Mr Pearse hath so well executed his orders that there is not one person of the whole hospital come up to complain hither to me, nor no more mention of them than if they were still at Tangier ... The King gave orders that the customs officers were not to interfere with the Tangerines ... Mr Mayor kissed the king's hand and was assured that the credit due to him in respect of monies given by him to the hospital in Tangiers would be duly repaid.[64]

Jenkins's letter did not, however, tell the full story. Not all of the *Unity*'s passengers had been satisfied with their reception. Some twenty-four men belonging to the Earl of Dumbarton's Regiment complained that no provision had been made for them. They were starving and without either money or clothing as a result of a classic example of petty bureaucracy. Mr Flowers, the agent appointed to administer aid to the returned troops, had been told to expect men from Kirke's Regiment and, in the absence of instructions for him to deal with anyone else, he ignored anyone from another regiment. In the event an officer, John Graham, was sent down to Gravesend with money to take care of them and, after John Gore, a 'slopfeller' of Billingsgate, had kitted them out with new clothes valued at 20s per man, the matter seems to have been finally settled. The invalid soldiers were eventually settled in the Royal Hospital at Chelsea and nothing more was heard of the matter.[65]

Decisions had to be taken regarding the ultimate disposal of remaining troops still in Tangier. Dartmouth was informed that Kirke's Regiment was destined to garrison Pendennis Castle in Cornwall and, on 19 October 1683, he confirmed that the officers' and soldiers' wives, their children and goods belonging to that unit had departed for England. He also requested Lord Arundell to take care that, on arrival, the party would be allocated quarters appropriate to their husbands' rank and station and that the soldiers' wives would be issued with money, at the rate of 3d a head per day, for their subsistence. Arundell was assured that this expense would be refunded once the battalion as a whole had arrived back in England.[66]

Eleven days later a second party of wives, families and servants, this time those related to the garrison's senior officers, including Kirke's wife and family, numbering some nineteen males and twenty females, departed on board the *Diamond*. The relevant passenger list, provided at Table 1:4, throws considerable light on the social structure of the colony's society as, included in the list, were twenty official Governor's servants, eleven for Kirke and nine for his wife, including five 'negro' children.

Table 1.4 Account of passengers aboard the *Diamond* bound for England as per the muster taken in Tangier Roads, 30 November 1683

Males	Females
Glond Burchie, Governor's steward	Madam Mary Kirk, Governor's wife
James Burch, Gentleman of Horse	Mary Kirk, Governor's daughter
Jno Boaman, Governor's servant	Diana Kirk, Governor's daughter
Daniel Mackly, ditto	Mary Oglesby, lieutenant's widow
Marmaduke Sadler, ditto	Ann Oglesby, lieutenant's daughter
Jno Muchely, ditto	Jane Goding, Lady Kirk's servant
Robert Browne, ditto	Frances Oures, ditto
Roger Jones, ditto	Elizabeth Boaman, ditto
William Forrester, ditto	Hannah Mackly, ditto
Henry Garden, ditto	Susan White, ditto
Henry Garden, junior, ditto	Frances Jones, ditto
Jno White, a negro boy, ditto	Frances Jones, a negro child, ditto
Tho White, a negro boy, ditto	Botshia Spottswood, schoolmaster's wife's servant
Farr Dunkan, a negro boy, ditto	Mary Mackly, a negro child, ditto
George Mercer, schoolmaster	Kallin Mercer, schoolmaster's wife
Alexander Spotswood, schoolmaster's servant	Sarah Culbroth, ditto
Jno Samms, burger	Sarah Samms, burger's wife
Tho Bayley, burger's servant	Sarah Samms, burger's child
	Elizabeth Samms, burger's child

Source: TNA, CO279/32.

Meanwhile, back in Tangier, conditions for the sick patients retained in the hospital after the departure of the *Unity* must have been grim indeed. As mentioned earlier, the colony's water sources lay outside the city and were controlled by the Moors who could, if they wished, stop them altogether. On 16 September 1683 the Secretary of State was informed that although the garrison had been relatively healthy until recently, the hospital was currently filled with near 400 soldiers as a result of impure water. The local springs were very dry as a result of a recent severe drought but, additionally, the townsfolk believed that the Moors had done something to the old aqueducts that brought the water into the town's reservoirs as there had never been any prior ill effects from drinking the water. The crews of the ships lying in the harbour remained healthy and, in order to maintain their health, locally hired ships were dispatched to fetch water for them from the Spanish coast.[67] Four weeks later a survey was made of the fortifications and its author commented on the distress occasioned by the continuing shortage of water, the poor quality of the little that was available, as well as the diseases that resulted from drinking it. The situation was so bad that had the Moors attacked, the garrison would not have survived.[68]

Food was in equally short supply. On 1 November several local traders petitioned for their dues, claiming that they were owed over £1,200 for bread, wine, meat and other goods supplied by them to the hospital. They were also very angry as a result of the treatment they had received at the hands of William Smith, an ex-Mayor of the city, who, despite having already claimed for his own expenses, told the traders that they should expect to suffer some loss in the circumstances and that their situation was not unreasonable. In effect, Smith dismissed their complaints with an order to be quiet and stop complaining.

On 30 November, a survey of the food remaining in the garrison stores was undertaken and, when the results were compared with a list sent from London setting out the Board's estimate of the remaining food stocks, discrepancies were discovered in several items as listed in Table 1.5.

Table 1.5 List of victuals in store at Tangier compared with estimates sent from London, 30 November 1683

Item	London Estimates	Item	Present in Tangier
Beef:	7 weeks	Beef:	3 weeks
Biscuit:	15 weeks	Biscuit:	11 weeks
Butter:	10 weeks	Butter:	4 weeks
Cheese:	13 weeks	Cheese:	12 weeks
Oatmeal:	10 weeks	Oatmeal:	10 weeks
Peas:	12 weeks	Peas:	12 weeks
Pork:	11 weeks	Pork:	11 weeks

Source: TNA, CO 279/32, fol. 364.

These findings meant that the colony was deficient by the equivalent of between one and two months' store of provisions and, although the victualler's agent accounted for the discrepancies by claiming that the calculations made in England failed to identify provisions lent to the navy and others supplied for the use of the sick at the hospital, waste had been a considerable factor due to the climate and storage failures.[69]

The second hospital ship, the *Welcome*, the vessel that had been officially converted specifically for use as a hospital prior to its departure from England, had been due to wait until the last soldier had been embarked and sail with the last group to leave the colony. However, in view of a threatened storm, she was forced to depart on 26 February 1684, two days earlier than planned.[70] The ship was carrying forty sick soldiers, two female nurses and Dr Thomas Lawrence, the garrison physician, who had spent twenty years of his life working in the colony. It is probable that the two nurses were former permanent members of the hospital staff.[71]

On 8 April 1684, after a voyage of 41 days, the *Welcome* arrived off the Isle of Wight opposite Sandown Castle whence, the following day, she sailed on to

London.[72] As with the *Unity* five months earlier, those who required continuing treatment were transferred to the hospital at Deal where Dr Pierce was, once again, placed in charge of their care. In the normal course of his work Pierce was reimbursed for the expenses that he incurred in treating sick and wounded seamen by charging his costs to a specific government fund and reassurances were now given that, providing he used the same procedures for the new arrivals, any associated costs would be refunded in the usual manner.[73] Unfortunately, no record has been found to show whether he did in fact receive his dues.

Throughout the years of the colony's existence, the sick and wounded of Tangier had, beyond doubt, often suffered from neglect and want although, from time to time, King Charles II had been moved to offer the occasional distribution of largesse in the form of a gift from his own limited purse, such as the £48 authorized on 10 February 1666 for Colonel Norwood to spend for the benefit of casualties sustained in the fighting of the previous year.[74] Later, the needs of families were remembered when the colony's Hospital Committee was charged with distributing a special fund of £200 per annum granted by the King for supporting and raising the orphaned children of soldiers and townsmen. As time went by this fund appears to have been more generally used for the relief of the poor, although the claims of soldiers' orphans were supposedly given first priority. Indeed, as late as 15 May 1683, the Hospital Committee wrote to assure the Lords Commissioners that 'care was not wanting in distributing His Majesty's gracious allowance to widows and orphans'.[75]

Although the former colonists had been promised restitution for any financial losses they had sustained, payments were inevitably delayed and squabbles over losses incurred continued for several years. It was, perhaps, poetic justice that Smith, the former Mayor, who had been quick enough to submit his own claim for losses while obstructing those of others, should be told that he would have to wait for reimbursement until everyone else had been paid. Among the payments that were issued during that summer was £20 to John Eccles, the gunner who had been placed in charge of the women and children transported from Tangier on the *Unity* hospital ship. Eccles had continued to hold that responsibility after his redeployment to Pendennis Castle, where he remained as a supervisor with the families. He was also authorized to receive their continuing allowance of 3d per person per day subsistence money.[76] Pendennis Castle was in a considerable state of disrepair and did not inspire the arrivals with any thoughts of a rosy future. Kirke, the Commanding Officer, did not take kindly to his regiment's new home and, on 3 April, wrote to Lord Dartmouth. He complained that his new accommodation was so bad that he had arranged to take his wife, and presumably her entourage, to London, where he was more likely to maintain a high profile at Court.[77] This was especially important to him in an age when royal patronage was necessary for any form of advancement in the service.

Such then was the sorry tale of England's involvement in its first African colony where the provision of medical care and military hospital facilities for the army reached its nadir. The ensuing chapters will show how succeeding generations met the same challenges with varying success.

Notes

1. E.M.G. Routh, *Tangier, England's Lost Atlantic Outpost, 1661–1684* (London: John Murray, 1912), *passim*; D. Ogg, *England in the Reign of Charles II* (2 vols, Oxford: University Press, 1934, republished 1956), vol. 2, pp. 658–9.
2. Sir H. Cholmley, *An Account of Tangier* (1787), p. 9.
3. Ibid., pp. 17–18.
4. BL Lansdown Mss, 192: Sir H. Cholmley, *A Discourse of Tangier* (1672), fols 27–8.
5. Ibid., fol. 29.
6. TNA, CO 279/1, fol. 93.
7. Cholmley, *Discourse*, fols 29–31.
8. Routh, *passim*.
9. TNA, CO 279/4, fol. 106.
10. Bod. L MS. Rawl. C423, fols 84 and 89.
11. TNA, CO 279/19, fol. 328.
12. Ibid., fol. 180 and CO 279/19, fol. 328.
13. Routh, pp. 299–300.
14. TNA, CO 279/1, fol. 102.
15. Ibid., fol. 93.
16. TNA, CO 278/4, fol. 43.
17. Staffs. RO, D.742/0/2/29.
18. TNA, CO 279/6, fol. 59 and CO 279/8, fol. 72.
19. BL Sloane Mss, 1952, fol. 19 *et seq.*
20. The first lazarettos had been built by the Northern Italian city-states between 1450 and 1470: T. Ranger and P. Slack (eds), *Epidemics and Ideas* (Cambridge: Cambridge University Press, 1992), p. 15.
21. Lazarettes were never adopted as a quarantine measure by Great Britain. As late as 1800 specified moorings were the method of choice when isolating infected vessels. For example, Portsmouth and Southampton identified Mother Bank, Plymouth used St Ives Pool, while London, the Thames and the Medway nominated Standgate Creek: *Naval Chronicle* (July 1800–January 1801), IV: 245.
22. HMC, *Heathcote Mss* (1899) pp. 206,10 and 213.
23. Ibid., p. 206; TNA, CO 278/12, fol. 163 et sec.; and CO 279/4, fol. 57; Bod. L MS. Rawl. C.423, fols 84 and 89.
24. TNA, CO 279/4, fols 57 and 65.
25. Ibid., fol.55.
26. G. Goodwin, *A History of Ottoman Architecture* (London: Thames and Hudson, 1971), *passim*; G. Majno, *The Healing Hand, Man and Wound in the Ancient World* (London: Harvard University Press, 1975), pp. 381–9.
27. A. Palladio, *I Quattro Libri dell'Architettura* (Venice, 1570).
28. Cholmley, *Account*, pp. 96–102.
29. Staffs. RO, D.742/0/2/29
30. The 'Town House' was normally used for municipal meeting, and, during the summer of 1683, was the venue for meetings of the Committee, consisting of Samuel Pepys, Dr William Trumbull (the Judge Advocate) and Frederick Bacher

31. (Recorder of Tangier), established to identify land ownership and value prior to the final abandonment of the colony: BL Rawlinson Mss, A.196, Minutes of the Land Survey Committee, 1683; E. Chappell (ed.), *The Tangier Papers of Samuel Pepys* (Navy Records Society, 1935), pp. 18, 31–2, 36–8, 42.
31. TNA, CO 279/8, fol. 72.
32. Bod. L Lister I. 18; G. Philips, *The Present State of Tangier* (1676), p. 16.
33. TNA, CO 279/3, fols 59–60; C. Dalton, *English Army Lists, 1661–1714* (6 vols, London: Francis Edwards, 1892–1904), I, p. 37.
34. Chappell, p. 50.
35. L.I. Cowper, *The King's Own, The Story of a Royal Regiment* (Oxford: Clarendon press, 1939), p. 15.
36. TNA, CO. 279/3, fol. 83.
37. Cholmley, *Account*, p. 102.
38. TNA, CO 279/4, fol. 41.
39. TNA, AO 3/117/1.
40. TNA, CO 279/32, fol. 138; J. Childs, *The Army of Charles II* (London: Routledge and Kegan Paul, 1976), p. 125.
41. Chappell, p. 90.
42. TNA, AO 1/310/1224.
43. TNA, CO 279/31, fol. 300, March 1684.
44. Col. J. Davis, *The History of 2nd Queen's (Royal West Surrey) Regiment* (6 vols, London: Bentley, 1887–1906), I, p. 180.
45. Cholmley, *Account*, p. 102.
46. TNA, ADM 106/308, fol. 240 and ADM 106/311, fol. 156; J.S. Corbett, *England in the Mediterranean, 1603–1713* (2 vols, London: Longmans, 1902), vol. 2, p. 77.
47. Ibid.
48. Ibid.
49. Cowper, p. 15.
50. Chappell, p. 90.
51. BL Sloane Mss, 1952, fol. 19 *et seq*.
52. One shilling per day was to be the authorized figure for a nurse's wage in Flanders some twenty years later during the Nine Years' War: TNA, WO 25/1318, fol. 376; Gruber von Arni, *passim*.
53. TNA, CO 279/17; HMC, *Report on the MSS of the Earl of Dartmouth* (2 vols, 1885), vol. 1, p. 104.
54. TNA, AO 1/437/161.
55. TNA, CO 279/5, fol. 160.
56. Ibid., fols 51–2.
57. TNA, CO 279/25, fol. 253.
58. Ibid., pp. 260–61; *Dartmouth MSS*, vol. 1, pp. 83–4.
59. TNA, CO 279/32, fol. 368.
60. *Dartmouth MSS*, I, p. 103; Routh, pp. 260–61; Davis, I, p. 240.
61. TNA, CO 279/32, fol. 263.
62. *Cal. Treas. Books, 1681–1685*, vol. 7, part II, p. 1090.
63. *Dartmouth MSS*, I, p. 99.
64. Ibid., pp. 83–4.

[65] Ibid., I, p. 101; TNA, CO 279/32, fol. 355.
[66] *Cal. S.P. Dom., May 1684–February 1685*, p. 87; TNA, CO 279/32, fol. 271.
[67] Ibid., fols 137–8.
[68] Ibid., fols 164–5.
[69] TNA, CO 279/32, fol. 364.
[70] Chappell, p. 290.
[71] Davis, p. 251.
[72] Chappell, p. 297.
[73] *Cal. Treas. Books, 1681–1685*, vol. 7, part 2, p. 1090.
[74] Ibid., Part 1, p. 649.
[75] TNA, CO 279/31, fol. 300.
[76] *Cal. Treas. Books, 1681–1685*, Part 2, p. 1262.
[77] Ibid., Part 1, p. 112.

Chapter 2

Hospitals and Welfare for the Standing Army in Britain, 1660–1688

In the aftermath of the Restoration, the closure of the former Parliamentarian military hospitals left a vacuum that could not be sustained for long. This chapter will examine the various attempts made to fill this void during the immediate post-Restoration years and also document the measures taken to define and improve the welfare and social condition of soldiers in an era of rapid change and development.

Unlike the Royal Navy, whose involvement in the two Dutch Wars had resulted in considerable combat experience, the newly formed Standing Army of Charles II undertook, as a body, very little fighting either at home or in Europe. British soldiers did, however, serve overseas in fairly large numbers throughout the 1660s and 1670s in mercenary regiments, formed in England and Scotland but serving in the pay and under the flags of foreign, particularly French, governments. Such service was condoned, and even encouraged, by the King and, as had formerly been the case during the Thirty Years' War earlier in the century, foreign service became the training ground that produced a core of experienced soldiers at little or no expense to the British government. It was by these means that the nation's future military leaders, who later came to prominence during the Nine Years' War and the campaigns of Marlborough, learned their trade. From August 1662 to February 1668, a British brigade operated in Portugal assisting the Portuguese to establish their independence from Spain. Between 1672 and 1676, another brigade, one that included the Royal English Regiment under the command of King Charles's illegitimate son the Duke of Monmouth, fought with the French army of Louis XIV in Flanders against the United Provinces.

Throughout the three Anglo-Dutch Wars fought variously between 1652 and 1674, troops were continually embarked aboard warships either to supplement the crews or to act as 'soldiers at sea' in the absence of a permanent, dedicated force of marine troops. As such these soldiers were treated as naval personnel and any casualties among them were treated according to the naval system. These wars had forced the government to take some interest in the care of sick and wounded seamen and placed responsibility for their care in the hands of a 'Committee for Sick and Wounded Seamen and for Prisoners of War'. Similarly named bodies were raised for the duration of each successive war and then disbanded at the cessation of hostilities. On 28 October 1664, following the outbreak of the Second Dutch War, one such committee was formed with four members, one of whom was the diarist John Evelyn. Evelyn's area of responsibility stretched from the North Foreland in Kent to Portsmouth, within which he was granted authority to appoint officers, physicians, surgeons and provosts martial.

One half of all the hospital beds in his domain were placed at his disposal but, as there were very few regional hospitals in existence, the value of this allocation was of minimal assistance and most of the casualties were dispersed to inns and private houses.[1] This necessitated the employment of far more surgeons and nurses than would have been the case had a centralized hospital facility been available, while Evelyn expressed his somewhat puritanical concern that indiscriminately boarding out the sick and wounded 'tempted the people to debaucherie'.[2] In a move to provide a short-term remedy, he was granted permission to temporarily reopen the Savoy Hospital as a military hospital but, regrettably, this arrangement lasted for only two years before the buildings were again returned to use as a barracks. Significantly, this was done at the express request of Evelyn himself who, in committee meetings, continually pressed, without success, for sufficient financial support to erect a purpose-built infirmary for the reception and treatment of sick and wounded seamen and 'soldiers at sea'.[3]

On reflection, it is not necessary to look far to identify the reasons dictating Parliamentary reluctance to contemplate the provision of long-term facilities for soldiers and sailors at that time. In the aftermath of the civil wars the country had developed an intense dislike of the concept of a standing military force of any kind and, as a result, the navy was neglected and Parliament exhibited extreme reluctance to tolerate anything more than a minimum expenditure on soldiers' needs, including their medical care. Even so, during Charles's reign the British army saw government-sponsored service in four overseas situations: Flanders, the Caribbean colonies, Bombay and Tangier. While the latter has been described in depth in the previous chapter, the medical support for English troops serving in Flanders, although not part of the regular Standing Army, provides additional evidence for contemporary attitudes to the provision of medical support in overseas situations. In order to provide interesting comparisons to be made with facilities provided for garrison forces in England, the situation in Portsmouth, where the King demonstrated both a keen personal interest and financial backing for the erection of a garrison hospital, will also be examined.

As is more than evident in today's society, medical care is expensive. The situation was no different in late seventeenth-century England. One of the first post-Restoration attempts to hold down the cost of providing medicines to soldiers of the English Standing Army was a Parliamentary instruction, published on 21 January 1673, backdated to the previous 20 September. While regimental surgeons of the First and Coldstream Regiments of Foot Guards were permitted to maintain a small stock of external applications, mostly ointments and lotions, valued at no more than 40 shillings, this new regulation also restricted expenditure on the more expensive internal medicines that were supplied by Richard Whittle, the Apothecary General, to £40 per year for internal medicines for soldiers of the Guards.[4] Meanwhile, in other regiments, surgeons were also entitled to the same 40 shillings a year for external applications but their spending power on internal drugs was now to be restricted to a miserly 20 shillings per annum. It was, however, conceded that troops on the march or on exercise away from their normal regimental medical provision could seek the services of a local physician or apothecary at public expense whereas the Guards spent their days almost continually in London barracks.[5]

This penny-pinching attitude contrasted strongly with that of the French, who were well organized. On the personal orders of Louis XIV, every garrison town was provided with a military hospital staffed by a Physician, Surgeon, Apothecary, an 'Aide-Major and a 'Controller' with nurses in numbers decided upon the basis of two nurses for every ten sick or wounded soldiers.[6] The traditional enmity between England and France had been submerged during the first fifteen years of the restored monarchy but, by 1677, the old antipathy had resurfaced. After more than twenty years of intermittent strife and three wars, the English Parliament and the States General of the United Provinces finally resolved their differences when, on 31 December that year, they jointly signed a treaty agreeing to work towards maintaining a long-term peace in Western Europe. The treaty was ratified on 20 February 1678 and was followed the next March by a more general alliance aimed at forcing France to return control of the fortified towns of Charleroi, Courtrai, Ath, Oudenarde, Conde, Tournai and Valenciennes, lost at the outset of the war, to the Dutch, a goal that was to be obtained by joint military action if necessary.

The French King, Louis XIV, was predictably reluctant to accept such demands and, with Parliament voting a million pounds for a war with France, the campaign that ensued differed from the earlier military involvements of Charles's reign inasmuch as the English expeditionary force, consisting of 11,000 foot and 1,000 horse, operated under British command and administration and remained an integral part of the country's Standing Army. The expedition's commander, the Duke of Monmouth, wrote to Thomas Forcade, the expedition's Surgeon General, authorizing him to demand reports from the surgeons attached to the regiments ordered to join the expedition informing him what medicines they had arranged to carry with them. He was also instructed to verify, to his own satisfaction, that the medicines so ordered were appropriate and that the surgeons carried out their duties in relation to the sick and wounded to his satisfaction.[7] Meanwhile, Elnathon Summers, Deputy Paymaster to the Forces, was authorized to allow the surgeons of the Guards regiments an extra ten pounds for additional medicines for issue to the battalions ordered to join the force.[8] Regrettably, however, medical support for the expedition was given minimal priority prior to departure and, whilst individual regiments were accompanied by their own regimental surgeons, no arrangements were made for a proper field or base hospital to accompany the expedition, nor was any agreement reached with the host nation for their medical facilities to be made available to British troops.[9]

The majority of the infantry crossed the channel in July and, in the process, large numbers of soldiers fell sick with dysentery even before they landed in Flanders. On 17 July one of the three regiments housed in barracks in Nieuport, that of Colonel George Legge, was reimbursed for expenses incurred in caring for the unit's sick as shown in Table 2.1.

Table 2.1 Disbursements to Colonel George Legge's Regiment, 17 July 1678

Paid to carry sick soldiers' necessaries ashore: 6s 6d
For cleaning the house of office: 7s
Linen for 40 pairs sheets for the sick soldiers: £14 7s 0d
Making the said sheets at 3d per pair: 10s
Making 40 beds, bolsters and rugs and bed cradles: £1 10s
Making and mending 1,200 bedsteads for the 3 battalions at 1s each: £60

Source: TNA, SP 44/52, fol. 173.

Legge's Regiment was eventually so decimated by sickness that his unit was sent into quarters at Mecklin. Conditions for the majority of the troops were poor, with most having to lie 'upon straw and never put off their clothes which occasions a great many of them to fall sick, every day more and more'.[10]

On 1 August the English force began its two-week journey inland en route to join the allied army camped south of Brussels. They travelled in locally hired flat-bottomed boats along the extensive inland waterways of Flanders but, during their journey, their sufferings increased. Soldiers exhibited the signs and symptoms of a variety of communicable diseases, such as typhoid, dysentery and respiratory diseases, and these were aggravated by exposure to the elements and unwholesome food.[11] Those unable to continue their march were left behind at an unofficial base hospital in Bruges where King Charles's personal surgeon Sergeant-Surgeon John Knight, Surgeon General to the Army, assumed responsibility for the sick and established basic facilities in whatever houses and lodgings the local people could offer, such as convents, private houses or tents.[12] This was almost the sole arrangement made to cater for the military casualties and it was totally inadequate. As the eight battalions passed through Brussels, over one hundred men in each regiment were reported sick.[13] The force finally reached the allied lines on 13 August, too late to join the war. The soldiers' deaths and sufferings had all been for nothing.

On 15 August, the day that the Duke of Monmouth began his journey back to England, Sir Richard Bulstrode, the English government's representative in Brussels, informed the Secretary of State, Sir Leoline Jenkins, that the eight battalions of the British force contained between eight and nine hundred sick in the most miserable condition that he had ever seen. However, with considerable effort, he had found a building in Brussels where they could be provided for and had arranged for doctors and surgeons to visit them daily – but that was all he had been able to achieve.[14] Eleven days later James Vernon, Secretary at War for Foreign Expeditions and Monmouth's private secretary, wrote to Lord Howard of Escrick, who commanded the First Regiment of Foot Guards and was the senior commander on the ground, informing him of the Duke's belated concern that 'there is not that order kept amongst the sick that ought to be, chiefly through the neglect of the officers appointed to attend upon that duty'. Howard was requested to conduct a thorough investigation into the situation.[15] At the same time Vernon also responded to Bulstrode's comments, reassuring him that the Duke was well aware of his concerns regarding the care of the sick and told him of the Duke's instructions to Lord Howard. The Duke had also written to Sir Charles Lyttleton, who commanded the garrisons at Ostend, Bruges and Nieuport, with instructions for him to send any recovered patients from Bruges to Brussels in the care of an officer so that they could safely rejoin their units.[16] Three days later, on his way home, the Duke of Monmouth passed through Antwerp and made a special detour to visit Colonel Sidney who lay sick and it was recorded that at that time there were some 2,500 persons sick 'of a new fever' in that town.[17]

By September Bruges had ceased to be the only hospital and over 1,000 sick were reported in Brussels and many more in the camp.[18] The English troops remained in Flanders for a further six months, until February 1679, when they were shipped home. An order for the return of the troops to England via Ostend included a requisition for as many wagons as necessary to be provided to convey such sick as were able to travel to Ostend in case they could not be carried by water.[19] They arrived in London to find themselves immediately disbanded and two months later the House of Commons declared all military forces in England illegal.

The King, however, decided to ignore Parliament's ruling. Earlier that year, in January, he had ordered Colonel John Legge, the Governor of Portsmouth, to repair that town's fortifications. At the same time the garrison, until then composed of only two companies of foot, was reinforced by ten additional companies, bringing the strength up to about one thousand men. Contracts were arranged valued at £6,000 for the reconstruction work and several huts were built to accommodate this increase in military personnel. The following August the King travelled by sea from Sheerness to Portsmouth to inspect progress but, on his arrival, the town and garrison were suffering from an outbreak of fever and Legge, encouraged perhaps by the fact that only the previous month Charles had approved the construction of the Royal Hospital at Kilmainham, Dublin, for disabled and retired soldiers of his Irish army, managed to convince the King of the need for a hospital to support his newly enlarged garrison.

On 7 February 1680 the Treasury called for an account of the expenditure on the Portsmouth sick and, in the following July, authorized the commencement of work on the new hospital but failed to cover the associated costs. Once building work had started, the King took a significant personal interest in the Portsmouth hospital and personally provided the necessary funds, amounting to some £1,500, by allocating the profits accrued from the sale of New Forest timber. Construction started in October 1680 on land chosen for the project which lay near the Land Port Gate on the landward side of the town, defences known locally as the 'Vicar's Close'. Sir Thomas Fitch and his brother John undertook the work on behalf of the Ordnance Board. Building work lasted for nearly three years although the hospital was probably completed by 6 September 1683, when Charles again visited Portsmouth and, during his tour, inspected the building.[20] The final edifice was designed to accommodate a total of forty soldier-patients and measured 192 ft by 24 ft externally with chimneys at either end and 'a great doorcase' with a 'fair ornament' of the royal coat of arms in bold relief mounted centrally above it.[21]

Sadly, no information has been found regarding the nursing personnel who cared for the patients admitted to the establishment, but there is sufficient evidence from which to visualize the nature of the structure. The building was of combined brick and oak-framed construction with the rooms divided into four distinct wards. Each of these measured 40 ft long by 30 ft wide with four massive pillars spaced evenly down the centre of the rooms to support the roof. The wards were fitted with enclosed beds, ten to each ward, measuring 4 ft wide, 6 ft 3 inches long and 8 ft high, with the mattress lying 18 inches off the floor. A cornice to which a curtain rail was attached surrounded the top, which was 'covered with whole deal board close jointed for the full breadth of the bedstead'. The beds were divided one from another by wooden partitions lined with split deal boards and permanently secured to the surrounding brick walls that were also lined with split deal timber. Under the beds the floor was to be paved with 'hard-burnt' brick laid in mortar while the central area between the two rows of beds was to be made of boards laid over oak joists. Fourteen glazed windows were fitted into the walls supplemented by an equal number of *lutheran lights* (sic) in the roof. A separate building accommodated the surgeon and sutler and the whole presented a similar image to that of Wren's design for the contemporary Royal Hospital at Chelsea.[22]

The Portsmouth garrison hospital was the only hospital built by the Ordnance Department between 1660 and 1750 and yet, despite the initial Royal interest shown in its construction, its lifespan as a hospital was remarkably short. By 1694 the hospital had been turned into a barracks and it was eventually demolished some time in the late 1720s.

Despite Charles II's initial interest in the hospital project in Portsmouth, the routine welfare of soldiers was given a very low status in the nation's financial priorities during the early years of the Standing Army. The comprehensive pension system constructed by Parliament during the civil wars and Interregnum had fallen into disarray by the time of the Restoration and was not revived afterwards.[23] The only source of official financial help was provided by a reversion to the antiquated system of poor relief, instigated during the reign of Elizabeth I, which required a distressed ex-soldier to appeal to the County Quarter Sessions for pension relief. Even when such financial benefit was approved the amount was limited by statute to an imposed maximum award of £20 per annum. There was, however, another less formal method of supporting old and disabled soldiers that existed alongside the statutory mechanisms. Throughout the reign of Charles II, a second option for rewarding a long-serving, faithful soldier who became unfit for further service, either through age or disability, entailed retaining his name on the muster roll of his company while excusing him from anything but the most sedentary duties. Inevitably, the inclusion of elderly and unfit soldiers on company strengths produced an inflated statement of the army's true worth as a fighting force. Large numbers of men recorded as available for duty were, in fact, incapable of active service.

Fortunately, towards the end of Charles's reign, certain financial steps were initiated aimed at improving the overall situation as regards soldiers' welfare. On 1

March 1684, in the aftermath of the King's foundation of the Royal Hospitals at Kilmainham and Chelsea, a deduction of one day's pay per annum from the remuneration of soldiers, guards and garrisons had been introduced as a contribution towards the cost of completing these establishments.[24]

Charles II died on 6 February 1685 and was succeeded by his younger brother who ascended the throne as James II. Following his accession, James supplemented the haphazard system of pensions by introducing a raft of standard payments payable to officers and soldiers who were disabled as a result of their service. Officers wounded in action were eligible to receive a one-off payment of a year's salary for the loss of an eye or limb or the loss of the use of a limb. For lesser wounds the amount payable was to be in proportion, depending on the nature of the wound and the merit of the officer. As a Catholic, James had spent many years under a cloud of suspicion and grew to regard the army as a means of safeguarding his position on the throne. In addition to the improvements in pensions for officers, James also introduced various moves aimed at enhancing his troops' loyalty to the crown by instigating several improvements in their terms of service and welfare facilities.[25]

At the same time, as a result of earlier practices, unfit men had been retained in service producing a situation in which large numbers of troops were incapable of fulfilling their role. The King decided to replace such personnel with newly recruited, active young men capable of carrying out any duty required of them whilst those deemed too old or unfit for further service were to be discharged. Many of these redundant veterans were entitled to placement in the Royal Hospitals at Kilmainham and Chelsea. Unfortunately, Kilmainham was in debt and could not take them and, even before it was completed, Chelsea proved to be too small to receive all who sought admission. From the moment that the latter establishment reached its capacity of 472 pensioners in 1687, it was found necessary to compile a waiting list of ex-soldiers awaiting admission. Fears were expressed that if applicants were summarily discharged they would be forced to go begging in the streets, the very situation that the hospital had been set up to avoid. However, the King remained adamant and insisted that the discharges were effected as soon as possible. In his view, admissions to Kilmainham or Chelsea for those who could not gain immediate entry could be arranged later, as and when vacancies occurred.[26]

As a result, and in order to protect the veterans from starvation, out-pensioner pensions were introduced whereby those waiting for admission to one of the two Royal Hospitals received a pension designed to cover their immediate expenses. The new regulation amounts are listed in Table 2.2. In addition, any soldier completing twenty years' service would automatically become entitled to a pension at the same rates as shown above. Compensation for non-incapacitating wounds was paid following a joint decision by the soldier's commanding officer and surgeons. If the soldier died from his wounds a sum not exceeding 10 shillings was available to cover his funeral expenses. This regulation also applied to those in receipt of an official pension awarded for wounds sustained on active service. The amount payable for burying a dead pensioner was set at 10 shillings.[27]

Table 2.2 Payments to out-pensioners waiting for vacancies in the Royal Hospitals

Cavalry	
Corporal of Light Horse	1s 6d per day
Trooper of Life Guards	1s 6d per day
Trooper of Light Horse	1s 0d per day
Dragoons	
Corporal of Dragoons	9d per day
Dragoons	6d per day
Foot	
Serjeant	11d per day
Corporal	7d per day
Drummer	7d per day
Private soldiers	4d per day plus 1d for clothing
Artillery	
Master Gunners	1s 2d per day
Gunner	7d per day

Source: Rev. N. Burton, *History of the Royal Hospital, Kilmainham* (Dublin, 1843), p. 33.

Once a vacancy in either Chelsea or Kilmainham had been secured, the individual soldier became an in-pensioner entitled to an ongoing pension dependent on his rank and station and these are shown in Table 2.3.

Table 2.3 In-pensioner daily allowance in the Royal Hospitals of Kilmainham and Chelsea

Cavalry	
Trooper of Light Horse	2s 0d per week
Foot	
Sergeant	2s 0d per week
Corporal of Foot	10d per week
Drummer of Foot	10d per week
Private soldier	8d per week

Source: Rev. N. Burton, *History of the Royal Hospital, Kilmainham* (Dublin, 1843), pp. 33–4.

Widows were to receive a lump sum equivalent to 11 months' pay but, if there were no widow, then a dead soldier's mother could receive the equivalent of a widow's allowance providing she was over 50 years of age and was herself a widow. If a soldier died a widower leaving orphans, any unmarried children were entitled to receive one third of the amount allowed for widows. In practice, the monies due to children were paid to the relevant parish Churchwarden, who was responsible for supervising their care and upbringing until the age of 12 years at which time children were placed in an apprenticeship to learn a trade.[28]

Meanwhile, national events intruded into the soldier's world. Any hopes for a seamless transition from one king's reign to the next were rudely shattered when the Duke of Monmouth landed at Lyme Bay in Dorset on 11 June 1685, four months after his father's death, and laid claim to the throne. Misinformed, in expectation of widespread national support that failed to materialize and short of funds, the Duke's aspirations were dashed when his cause met with disastrous failure. It would be inappropriate in this work to go into detail about the experiences and deprivations suffered by the wounded of the rebel army; they have been rehearsed adequately elsewhere.[29] Conversely, in comparison with the numerous narratives that survive to illustrate the fate of those who sided with the Duke's party, the medical care provided for the King's troops during the campaign in the West Country is sparsely documented. As a large proportion of the force raised to counter the invasion consisted of county militia who relied upon local medical resources, this is perhaps understandable, but the militia was bolstered by the addition of a significant force of regular troops. These included five battalions of Guards, five companies each of Dunbarton's Regiment and Trelawny's plus Kirke's Regiment of Foot, who marched with their normal complement of regimental surgeons who, disappointingly, do not appear to have left any notes or papers describing their work or experiences.

On 27 June, during their first significant encounter with the rebels at Norton St Philip's, the Royalist advance guard suffered one hundred casualties, most of whom were sent to Bath where they were cared for by George Bellamy, regimental surgeon of Viscount Lumley's Regiment of Horse. Nine days later, during the decisive battle of Sedgemoor, fought on 6 July, in which Monmouth's men were completely routed and dispersed, Thomas Hobbes, regimental surgeon of the Life Guards and personal surgeon to Lord Feversham, the Royalist commander, acted as the senior medical officer present, supported by George Bellamy, James Wylley, regimental surgeon of Kirke's Foot, who lost his medicine chest valued at £30, and Henry Musto of the King's Own Regiment.[30] Rebel casualty figures will never be accurately known although a figure of between two and three hundred killed on the field has been suggested, with many more dying during the pursuit.[31] Royalist casualties were relatively light, with the most reliable estimate being contained in a letter written by Feversham some three days after the battle in which he was sufficiently confident to write that he believed fewer than 50 of his own forces had been killed and around 200 injured.[32] Of these men, some 110 were transported to Bridgwater, where a temporary hospital was opened for their reception. It was there that Dr Thomas Lawrence, the Physician General, James Pearce, the Surgeon General, and the regimental surgeons Thomas Hobbes, James Wylley and Henry Musto established themselves and remained caring for the wounded for the next three months.

When the campaign was over and matters had settled once again into a relatively stable routine, Lawrence submitted his bill for the work he had undertaken throughout the campaign as well as, unsuccessfully, petitioning the King to the effect that he was

> by your Majesty's command, 81 days in the West attending the wounded and sick upon extraordinary charges which have ever been allowed to Physicians during all encampments. He prays his Majesty in consideration of his extraordinary expenses he may receive that favourable allowance from your Majesty's bounty which has formerly been granted to his predecessor Henry Chambers.[33]

Apothecary General Richard Whittle also served with the army in the West Country accompanied by two apothecary's mates and subsequently submitted a bill for £479 13s 4d in respect of his services in 'furnishing divers soldiers who were wounded at Weston [Westonzoyland] with meat, drink and other necessaries' at the field hospital in Bridgwater.[34] In return, he received a part-payment of £100 from the Paymaster General's office but the balance remained unpaid three years later.

With Monmouth defeated and the campaign over, the wounded of the King's army appear to have been reasonably well cared for. Those who required ongoing hospital care were eventually evacuated from Bath and Bridgwater to London, where their treatment continued at St Bartholomew's and St Thomas' Hospitals and, following a recommendation by the Surgeon General, James Pearce, special payments of 'smart' money were granted to the wounded, both officers and men.

Table 2.4 Officers and men wounded at Sedgemoor

Regiment	Number injured	Admitted Chelsea
Life Guards	37	1
Royal Regt. Horse	15	0
2nd Bn, 1st Foot Guards	70	12
Coldstream Guards	26	3
Dunbarton's Regt.	81	12
Queen Dowager's Regt.	4	4
Totals	233	32

Source: D. MacKinnon, *Origin and Services of the Coldstream Guards* (2 vols, London: Bentley, 1833), vol. 1, p. 182.

As shown in Table 2.4 the records of the payments made indicate the numbers of casualties suffered by individual regiments and correspond closely to Feversham's original casualty estimate of around 200 men. Of the actual amounts received, the 'smart' payments made to the First Foot Guards were typical. A captain received £100, four lieutenants were paid sums varying from £30 to £80 each, an ensign £20 whilst the non-commissioned ranks, numbering one sergeant, three corporals, two drummers and 46 private soldiers, received a total of £208 5s. The twelve men of that regiment who were admitted to the Royal Hospital at Chelsea each received £16.[35]

The Monmouth Rebellion had served to reinforce James's belief that his army required not only expansion but also training in weapon handling and other military skills and, between 1685 and 1688, he held a series of annual training camps for his army on the expanse of Hounslow Heath. These were not the first military camps to be held on that site. When, some ten years earlier, in June 1678, the diarist John Evelyn visited the Heath he was present when Charles II, accompanied by his brother James, reviewed the troops destined for the Duke of Monmouth's ill-fated Flanders campaign of that summer. Evelyn recorded on this occasion that he observed:

> The new-raised army encamp'd, designed against France, in pretence at least; but gave umbrage to the Parliament: his Majestie and a world of Company in the field & the whole Army in Batallia, a very glorious sight ...[36]

The first camp of James II's reign, held during the summer of 1685, was an *ad hoc* training camp for the six regiments of Horse, two of Dragoons and ten of Foot that had been hastily raised in response to the recently quelled rebellion. James visited the camp on 23 July and inspected 6,000 troops. He reviewed them twice in August and, after the second parade, wrote to his son-in-law, the Prince of Orange, 'on Saturday last I saw some of my troops at Hounslow; they consisted of ten battalions of Foot, of which three were of the guards, and the other seven new-raised regiments; of Horse there were twenty squadrons, one of grenadiers on horseback, and one of dragoons; and really the new troops of both sorts were in very good order and the horse well mounted'.[37]

The camp site was a barren expanse of scrubland that, more than one hundred years later, was still being described as wasteland fitted only for 'Cherokees and savages'.[38] The tent lines and buildings sprawled across the Heath for a distance of some three miles to the south and east of the river Crane between Hounslow and Feltham, south of the Great West Road and the modern-day M4 motorway. The land was owned by James's Catholic supporter Lord Bellasis, the former Governor of Tangier who had resigned that appointment rather than sign the Test Act. He had accepted an annual rent of £42, paid in arrears, in return for the King's use of his property.

Highly satisfied with his first camp, James decided to make the event an annual occurrence and, as the camps were now to be semi-permanent affairs, it was decided to develop the campsite with extensive and appropriate semi-permanent facilities. On 23 June 1685 Captain John Shales, a canny businessman, was appointed Commissary General of Provisions with wide-ranging responsibilities.[39] In addition to providing for the food and sustenance of the troops, through the normal supply of rations, issuing warrants for sutlers to set up their stalls and by establishing various local markets (from which he took the profits), Shales's terms of reference also required him to accept responsibility for funding medical care for those who fell sick or were injured in the camp. During the spring of 1686, a three-storeyed hospital was erected at the southern end of the camp on the site occupied today by Whitton School in Percy Road, adjacent to a bridge over the river Crane still known as 'Hospital Bridge'. A bakehouse and a large barn for storing grain were also built nearby, while elsewhere several semi-permanent barns or stalls for sutlers were provided. It is not known who was responsible for initiating the provision of these facilities but, with the campsite located at some distance from the usual source of hospital support in central London, the concept was probably inspired by someone with previous experience in either Flanders or in Tangier such as Thomas Lawrence.

On 13 January 1686, Shales received an initial advance of £200 towards the cost of building the hospital which, when completed, was to cost £926 14s 5d not including furniture and equipment, which were to add a further £189 18s 9d to the bill.[40] In addition to bedding, sheets, towels and napkins, the wards were issued with three or four dozen shirts for clothing new admissions while their personal garments were laundered. The construction and commissioning costs of these buildings were deemed sufficiently important for Sir Christopher Wren, Surveyor General of the King's Works, to be requested to view the completed structures and to certify that the bills were reasonably priced.

On 3 February 1686 James Pearce, the Surgeon General, who was also a Governor of St Thomas' Hospital, submitted his recommendations regarding the manner in which the hospital should be run.[41] His remarks, now contained within the Historic Manuscript Commission's publication, *The Dartmouth MS.*, are invaluable as they are tantamount to a set of contemporary hospital regulations. The hospital building contained three floors, with the ground floor containing offices for the physician, surgeons and clerical staff as well as the kitchens for preparing the patients' food. The upper two floors housed the wards capable of accepting fifteen patients per floor, each floor being placed under the supervision of one of two matrons, Margaret Harris and Mary Hopkins, who were employed at an annual salary of £18, approximately 1s a day. The two matrons were each allocated and supervised a maidservant or cook to prepare the food for the patients of their respective wards. Six nurses or tenders were personally selected by the matrons and worked, three to a ward, assisting in caring for the sick, washing linen, making beds and, when necessary, observing seriously ill patients at night.

The Hounslow hospital accounts were maintained by a clerk, Michael Bankham, who painstakingly recorded details of admissions, discharges, deaths and burials. When a soldier was admitted to hospital he brought with him a certificate signed by both his regimental surgeon and another officer. This certificate identified the soldier's name, regiment and company, as well as the disease or injury from which he was suffering. Nobody could be formally admitted to the hospital without being seen by either the hospital physician or a surgeon, and it was the clerk's subsequent duty to liaise with the regiments to obtain payment of the relevant subsistence money from individual captains of companies. Certificates were similarly employed when a patient was discharged from hospital in an attempt to 'prevent him rambling about the countryside when he is well and his relapsing into worse disease'.[42]

Dr Thomas Lawrence was in constant attendance at the camp, where the hospital rules required the physician to visit the sick once a day or more often if required, giving directions for the medicines required to the apothecary and informing the matron of the requisite diet for each man. In the bill submitted for his work during 1686, Lawrence clamed to have 'diligently attended the sick soldiers in His Majesty's camp at Hounslow from 26th May to 31st August 1686' and also reminded the King that his earlier petition for expenses incurred during the West Country campaign of 1685 remained unpaid. In response to this second request, the King finally agreed to Lawrence being paid an extra 10s a day over and above his salary in recognition of his work during both the recent rebellion and the financial loss that resulted from his inability to pursue his private practice while in attendance at the camp.[43]

The Apothecary General, Richard Whittle, who was entrusted to 'furnish the Regiments and the Military Hospital at Hounslow with good and wholesome medicaments', routinely provided medicines for the hospital.[44] Whittle was allocated a dedicated room for the storage of his drugs where, for security reasons, his assistant was accommodated and required to be in constant attendance. Prescriptions were to be signed by the Physician or, in his absence, either the Surgeon General, the hospital surgeon, or one of the regimental surgeons and retained for accounting purposes 'as His Majesty cannot pay for more than is administered'.[45] John Reed, Maurice Berkeley and John Seaborn, surgeons, are all quoted as receiving payment for work performed at the camp hospital.[46]

The cost of providing medicines, care and treatment for the troops was, then as now, proving expensive and Whittle was forced to continually press for payment of his bills. On 10 August 1687 he submitted a request for £318 3s 4d. He claimed that this amount remained outstanding from the original bill for £479 13s 4d that he had submitted six months earlier relating to his attendance, medicines, food and drink supplied by him at Bridgwater to troops wounded during the battle of Sedgemoor in the summer of 1685. In the event his bill remained unpaid in March 1688, when an invoice for medicines supplied during 1687 brought the total amount due to £345 16s 3d.[47]

The hospital wards normally contained beds for 30 patients, who usually lay one to a bed but, according to the Surgeon General, 'they [the beds] being pretty large, as men grow into a state of recovery, they may lie two in a bed' in which case the hospital could accommodate over 60 patients and, in an emergency, could be expanded to house 100. When the hospital first opened, patients were admitted indiscriminately on any day of the week but, when all of the beds had been filled, it became necessary to restrict admissions to a nominated day. Monday was identified as the day of choice as this was when patients requiring prolonged hospital care were transferred to one of the hospitals in central London, either St Bartholomew's or St Thomas'. It was also the day on which the Committees of Government of the London hospitals met with the physicians and surgeons to visit their in-patients. Monday was therefore the day on which decisions were made to discharge patients who were deemed either cured or incurable and vacancies were thereby created to accommodate the new arrivals.

The Surgeon General in liaison with the Commissary General, John Shales, made arrangements for transferring patients from the camp hospital to central London. These two officials were also responsible for identifying villages where arrangements could be made to accommodate patients who could not be cared for in the camp hospital due to lack of available space, and, subsequently, for notifying the regiments where they should send their sick soldiers for ongoing care.

In 1686 it had originally been intended to open the camp on 20 May but wet weather delayed this until, on the 25th, it was determined that the Heath was dry enough to erect the tents. This time the camp was to involve almost the entire army, both old and newly raised regiments. The troops began arriving on the following Thursday, 30 May, when 12 battalions of infantry marched in. On 2 June John Evelyn commented that the storms, rain and foul weather were highly unusual for the time of year and had been so bad that the soldiers 'either from sickness and other inconveniences of weather, [had been] forced to retire to quarters; the storms being succeeded by excessive hot weather, many grew sick'.[48]

The King was a frequent visitor to the camp and took a keen interest in its progress. It is open to question, however, whether he was as fully informed of the state of his troops as he thought he was when, on Tuesday 11 June, he wrote to the Prince of Orange informing him that during his visit to the camp in the previous week he had found everything to his satisfaction, including a comment that the camp was blessed with a good water supply and sickness was minimal.[49] An increase of sickness amongst soldiers is always bad news, as well as expensive and, in view of the many contemporary comments regarding the poor health of the soldiers in camp, the reality of the situation was either kept from or he chose to ignore it.

Thirteen days later the King and Queen again dined in their tent at the camp after hearing a sermon preached by the King's Catholic priest. On the same evening, several 'lewd women resorted to the camp to debauch the soldiers'. Twenty of them were caught and ducked in the nearby river whilst strict orders were issued that, in future, prostitutes and bawds were prohibited from entering the camp. These were wise precautions, as there are clear indications in the admissions lists of St Bartholomew's Hospital that a considerable percentage of the soldiers admitted at that time were treated for venereal infections.[50]

The King dined once more in the camp on 30 June, this time accompanied by the Queen, the Queen Dowager and Princes Anne but, shortly afterwards, in the middle of July, the weather deteriorated once more, necessitating the digging of drainage trenches to take away excess surface water. Sewage disposal in towns was primitive at the time and equally bad or worse in tented camps. With such weather conditions many of the large number of trench latrines required for such a sizeable camp would have overflowed, with a significant potential for an increase in the incidence of enteric diseases. As a precaution, some of the regiments of Horse were moved to alternative quarters in nearby towns and villages.[51] Despite these setbacks the King believed that the health of the camp was unaffected and subsequently informed his son-in-law that there had been no soldier deaths in the past month and that there were very few patients in the camp hospital.[52]

After an extensive programme of instruction that saw the troops exercising their arms every Monday, Wednesday and Friday, the camp was eventually broken up on 10 August when 140,000 soldiers marched away to their disparate quarters. The King was so impressed by the success of his 1686 summer camp that he determined that the following year's program would be even more ambitious in size, complexity and show. In the event John Evelyn was to comment on how the various commanders vied with each other 'in the expense and magnificence of their tents' while the troops were exercised in sham fights and in siege operations.[53] Regrettably, no information has been found from which the workload of the hospital may be determined or, indeed, how well the staff and administration coped with the inevitable casualties caused by such physical activities.

The camp of 1688 was the last to be held by James at Hounslow. It is not known when the last patients left the hospital, but evidence is available in the admission lists of St Bartholomew's Hospital to demonstrate that soldiers from the regiments present at Hounslow camp remained as patients in the London hospitals in early 1690, some having been transferred there from the camp at Hounslow during the previous year.

The autumn of 1688 saw the arrival of William of Orange at Torbay, which heralded the 'Glorious Revolution' and the end of James's reign. The new King's wars in Ireland and Flanders involved the army in constant active campaigning and the site on Hounslow Heath became virtually redundant. Nevertheless, although there were no remaining in-patients, the services of the two matrons, Mary Hopkins and Margaret Harris, were retained to maintain the hospitals in working order on a 'care and maintenance' basis. Unfortunately, their remuneration does not appear to have kept pace with their work effort. On 9 May 1690 Mary Hopkins complained to the Paymaster General, the Earl of Ranelagh, and the Secretary at War, William Blathwayt, that, having served as matron at the hospital ever since it was built, she had not received any pay since the new King had ascended the throne.[54] She also requested that her position as matron be clarified, either by her continuation in employment or, if it was decided that the hospital was no longer required, that she should be permitted to take payment in kind in the form of goods taken from the contents remaining in the hospitals.[55]

Hopkins had to wait for more than two months, until 30 July, for a response, but was, eventually, paid her dues for the year ending 3 February 1689. Naturally, her colleague, Margaret Harris, who was in the same situation, also demanded payment of her dues 'for want whereof she is reduced to great distress and prays payment thereof or some part thereof' but she had to wait until 10 August to receive her £18 for 'salary and coals' covering the same period as her colleague.[56] Both matrons remained in employment at the hospital during the following year although their ongoing financial difficulties continued until, on 17 October, they were forced to resort to a joint petition for their continuing arrears in pay and expenses. Even then it was not until 15 February 1692 that they received payment of their joint arrears of £58 18s 0d, representing dues owed to them up to 25 September 1691.[57]

On 18 September 1691, Shales was instructed to collect all the sheets, beds and bedding remaining in the custody of the hospital matrons and deliver them to the Commissioners for Sick and Wounded Seamen.[58] Mary Hopkins's appointment was terminated on 25 September although, even then, she was still not fully paid for her work as, a year later, the Earl of Ranelagh received yet another petition from her in which she submitted another request for payment of all the outstanding arrears due to her for expenses during her time at the hospital.

Regardless of the absence of beds and equipment, Margaret Harris continued to act alone in caring for the building and the two wards albeit at a reduced annual salary of £10, which, inevitably, remained unpaid. At some point prior to September 1693 she was forced, once again, to petition for payment of her dues, claiming that, had she not been present, 'the hospital building would have been pulled to pieces and gone to ruin'. On this occasion a statement by John Shales in which he summarized the situation as follows supported her petition:

> Whereas the two Matrons were allowed to take care of the sick soldiers in the hospital upon Hounslow Heath during the encampment there, and since have continued to look after the beds, sheets and other conveniences and necessaries to the said hospital belonging, which beds and sheets have been delivered to the Commissioners for Sick and Wounded Seamen by order of the Right Honourable The Lords Commissioners of the Treasury in September 1691. After which time there has been one Matron only, viz. Margaret Harris, to look after both wards of the said hospital for their preservation from damage and ruin, that they may be fit for his Majesty's service upon any occasion, who may deserve ten pounds per annum for her care of the same.[59]

Harris was not exaggerating when she claimed that her presence had saved the building from being ransacked. Most of the other buildings on the site had been broken up illegally during the intervening years and, on 6 March 1691, Sergeant Phillip Ryley, the Surveyor General of Woods, acting as bailiff, was ordered to take what remained, some 15,000 timber boards, into his custody and recover any that had already been surreptitiously removed. Eventually, Ryley collected over £200 from residents of Hounslow Heath who had bought or taken timber from the Heath, presumably taken from demolished encampment buildings. Despite the fact that her petition was strongly supported by the Commissary General, Harris had to wait for two years, until 17 June 1695, for the Paymaster General to approve her demands for her salary of £10 a year but, even then, her petition was marked 'rejected' by other Treasury officials.[60] As regards the hospital, bakehouse and barn, Sir Christopher Wren was eventually asked to survey them to ascertain their worth and to suggest how they could best be disposed of. As a result of Wren's report it was decided to dispose of all the remaining goods and properties left on the campsite. This was done over an extended period and many former camp items were still being sold off in 1698. The only effective acute hospital care remaining available to sick soldiers was provided by small regimental hospitals and the continued traditional use of the poor hospitals of London, St Bartholomew's and St Thomas' whose contribution to the care and treatment of sick and wounded soldiers is examined later in this work. Meanwhile, events in Ireland were to change the face of military hospital provision for ever, as will be shown in the next chapter.

Notes

1. E.S. de Beer (ed.), *The Diary of John Evelyn* (London: Oxford University Press, 1959), pp. 466.
2. Ibid., pp. 485–6.
3. Ibid., p. 476: The Savoy Hospital had been used as a Parliamentary military hospital throughout the civil wars and Interregnum. Following the 1660 Restoration of the Monarchy it had been emptied of military patients and, for a short time, returned to its use as a poor hospital for local citizens: Gruber von Arni, *passim*.
4. TNA, WO 25/3139, fol. 2.
5. Ibid.
6. Général H. de Perini, *Batailles Françaises* (5 vols, Paris: E. Flamarion, 1904), V, p. 54.
7. TNA, SP 44/52, fol. 41.
8. Ibid., fol. 43. James Vernon (1646–1727) acted as Monmouth's private secretary from 1674 to 1678. Later he became principal Secretary of State under William III (1698–1702): J. Childs, 'Monmouth and the Army in Flanders', *JSAHR* (1974), LII: 4–5.
9. Childs, *The Army of Charles II*, pp. 72–3.
10. TNA, SP 77/52, fol. 8.
11. Childs, 'Monmouth and the Army in Flanders', pp. 3–12.
12. TNA, SP 44/52, fol. 49.
13. TNA, SP 77/52, fol. 52.
14. Ibid., fol. 26; Childs, *The Army of Charles II*, p. 191.
15. TNA, SP 44/52, fol. 43. Thomas, Baron Howard of Escrick (1625–1678) was Lieutenant Colonel of the 1st Foot Guards and Colonel of the battalion of that regiment that accompanied the expedition in 1678. Howard died from disease later that year, as did Lord O'Brien, one of the regimental commanders: Childs, 'Monmouth and the Army in Flanders', pp. 4–5.
16. Sir Charles Lyttleton (c. 1629–1716) Governor of Jamaica from 1662 to 1664 and Colonel of the Duke of York's Maritime Regiment of Foot, 1668–1689: Childs, 'Monmouth and the Army in Flanders', p. 11.
17. Extract from Vernon's Diary of Monmouth's Campaign: TNA, SP 44/52, fol. 74. Henry Sidney (1641–1704) commanded his own regiment of foot in 1678 and held the appointment of Governor of Nieuport. Created Earl of Romney in 1694: Childs, 'Monmouth and the Army in Flanders', p. 5.
18. TNA SP 77/52, fols 28 and 31. See also fol. 8.
19. TNA SP 44/52, fols 167–9.
20. This was glebe land for which the Vicar of Portsmouth was promised forty shillings a year rent. In 1694 he complained that, after considerable effort, he had managed to receive just seven years' worth of rent and that was seven years in arrears. More of his tythe land was taken for the refurbished town defence for which he received no compensation: H. and J. Slight, *Chronicles of Portsmouth* (London, 1828), pp. 58–9.

21 Some confusion exists in the published material concerning this establishment. Dean, writing in 1947, described the building as still standing and in use as a store, albeit shorn of its attractive architectural features. The building that he described measured 120 feet by 30 feet externally. Barker, in his 1985 doctoral thesis, appears to accept these measurements as representing the final dimensions of the hospital as built, commenting that the final construction was smaller than those quoted in the original contract with the Fitch brothers. In reality, the original building was probably demolished in the early years of the eighteenth century. A map dated as early as 1716 shows the ground plan of the hospital with another construction superimposed on top of the site. A later map drawn in 1725 describes the hospital as 'in ruins' or 'fallen down'. Yet another map of Colewort Barracks drawn by the garrison military engineers in the 1860s shows later barrack buildings covering the site of the hospital and constructed with their linear axis at ninety degrees to the original hospital layout. The building described by Dean cannot, therefore, have been the seventeenth-century hospital, a mistake continued by Barker. In reality, there is no substantiated reason to assume that the dimensions of the hospital building were not as quoted in the original instructions issued to the Fitch brothers in 1681; C.G.T. Dean, 'Charles II's Garrison Hospital, Portsmouth', *Papers and Proceedings of the Hampshire Field Club* (1947), 16, 280–83; N.P. Barker, 'The Architecture of the English Board of Ordnance, 1660–1750' (unpublished PhD thesis, Reading University, 1985), pp. 318–20; C. Stevenson, *Medicine and Magnificence, British Hospital and Asylum Architecture, 1660–1815* (Yale: University Press, 2000), pp. 56–7.

22 Barker, pp. 318–20; TNA, WO 55/465.

23 Gruber von Arni, Ch. 3, *passim*.

24 TNA, WO 24/884, p. 31.

25 Ibid., pp 18r–20v.

26 *Cal. S.P. Dom., Jan 1686–May 1687*, pp. 162, 212 and 421: The Earl of Clarendon, Lord Lieutenant of Ireland, to the Earl of Sunderland, d. 8 June 1686.

27 R. Kane, *A System of Camp Discipline* (London, 1757), pp. 39–40.

28 Ibid., p. 35.

29 For details of the treatment of prisoners during and after the Monmouth Rebellion see original documents at Somerset Record Office, T/PH/Wig 2, fols 4 and 6; DD/PH/211, fols 40 and 248 and in secondary sources at D. Chandler, *Sedgemoor, 1685* (Staplehurst: Spellmount, 1985, reprinted 1999); R. Dunning, *The Monmouth Rebellion* (Wimborne: Dovecote Press, 1985); R. Clifton, *The Last Popular Rebellion: The Western Rising of 1685* (London, 1984).

30 TNA, T 4/3, fol. 349; *Cal. Treas. Books, 1685–8*, vol. 8, part I, p. 659.

31 B. Little, *The Monmouth Episode* (London: Werner Laurie, 1956), p. 187.

32 HMC, *Stopford Sackville Mss*, vol. 1, p. 21; G. Robert, *The Life and Progress of James, Duke of Monmouth* (2 vols, 1844), vol. 2, p. 91.

33 Ibid., fol. 285.

34 Ibid., part III, p. 1518.

35 Ibid., p. 182.

36 de Beer, p. 650.

37 *Cal. S.P. Dom., 1685*, p. 1079.

38 Lord Ernle, *English Farming Past and Present* (London, 1932), p. 154 quoted in H.C. Darby, *Historical Geography of England before 1800* (Cambridge: Cambridge University Press, 1936), p. 473.
39 *Cal. Treas. Books*, vol. 8 (3), p. 1358; *Cal. S.P. Dom., 1685,* pp. 1014 and 1050; *Cal. S.P. Dom. (Jan 1686–May 1687)*, pp. 26 and 309.
40 TNA, T 4/3, fol. 408.
41 HMC, *Dartmouth Mss,* (3 vols, 1887–1896), vol. 3, p. 143: F.G. Parsons, *The History of St Thomas' Hospital* (2 vols, London, 1930), vol. 2, pp. 116–17.
42 HMC *Dartmouth Mss,* vol. 3, p. 143.
43 *Cal. Treas. Books, 1685–1688*, vol. 8, p. 1459.
44 *Cal. S.P. Dom., 1686–1687*, pp. 132–234; L.I. Cowper, *The King's Own, The Story of a Royal Regiment* (Oxford: Clarendon Press, 1939), pp. 46–7; *Cal. Treas. Books*, vol. 3 (3), pp. 1133 and 1518.
45 HMC, *Dartmouth Mss* (3 vols, 1887–1896), vol. 3, p. 143.
46 TNA, AO/1/484, fol. 47.
47 *Cal. Treas. Books, 1685–1688*, vol. 8 (3), p. 1518.
48 W. Bray (ed.), *Diary and Correspondence of John Evelyn* (London, n.d.), p. 453.
49 TNA, SP 8/4, fol. 2.
50 St Bartholomew's Hospital Archives, Hb/1/9–13 and Hb2/1–2, *passim*.
51 TNA, SP 8/4, fol. 3.
52 Ibid.
53 Bray, p. 461.
54 TNA, T 4/6, fol. 164.
55 *Cal. Treas. Books, 1685–1688*, vol. 9 (2) p. 622.
56 Ibid., vol. 9 (3), pp. 1111 and 1257.
57 TNA, T 4/3, fol. 408; *Cal. Trea. Books, 1685–1688*, vol. 9 (3), p. 1348 and 9 (4), p. 1493.
58 Ibid., 9 (3, p. 1310.
59 TNA, T 1/16, fol. 246.
60 TNA, T/1/33.

Chapter 3

Hospital Provision in Ireland, 1689–1692

The wars fought by William III in Ireland hold a unique position in the history of medical support for the British army inasmuch as they witnessed the tortuous and painful gestation of a medical organization capable of providing support to the army in field conditions. England had maintained military hospitals in Ireland, especially in Dublin, ever since the Earl of Essex's campaign of 1599. During the intervening years the fate of the Dublin hospital is unclear but intriguingly, in 1644, a list of houses protected by the army included buildings in Back Lane annotated as 'belonging to the hospital and freed by the state', indicating that the Dublin hospital may have remained open at least until early 1644.[1] This establishment had, however, been closed before Philip, Lord L'Isle's appointment as Lord Lieutenant in 1646. When L'Isle took up his office he found both military and civil affairs totally disorganized and one of his first actions was to order the re-establishment of a military hospital in Dublin, 'which had hitherto not [even] been so much as thought of'.[2] The site of the re-established hospital was unspecified but later documents indicate that a former Catholic church, 'the mass house', in Back Lane, near the Cornmarket, was chosen. This would infer that the earlier establishment, previously closed in 1644, was simply reopened rather than a new build project undertaken. Almost no substantial evidence has been found relating to military hospitals at this time. Lord L'Isle's appointment lapsed in 1647 and little change occurred in the provision of casualty facilities during either of the succeeding governments under Parliamentary Commissioners (1647–48) and the Earl of Ormonde (September 1648–March 1649).

On 11 April 1649, after hearing the deliberations of a committee established to determine Irish affairs, the Council of State concluded that facilities for wounded soldiers, widows and orphans of troops serving in Ireland were inadequate. They decided that one or more new hospitals were needed, either in Dublin or elsewhere, and set about identifying the most appropriate means to fund their initiative.[3] Four months later, on 16 August, Cromwell was authorized to establish a second military hospital in the Archbishop of Dublin's sequestered house to supplement the existing 'mass house' in Back Lane. A previous Parliamentary ordinance had indicated that the Archbishop's former properties were to be administered by a committee formed to hold the buildings in trust for the benefit of Trinity College, Dublin, but the influence of committee member Jonathon Goddard, Physician General to the Army, was probably instrumental in swaying the decision in favour of using at least part of the buildings as a second military hospital.[4] It therefore seems likely that the hospital then established was the same as that known to have functioned in James Street during the latter half of the seventeenth century and which survived for almost a hundred years until it was replaced by the Royal Military Infirmary in the late eighteenth century.[5]

Material relating to the role and function of the hospital during the years following the Restoration of King Charles II in 1660 is equally scarce but payments made by the Earl of Anglesey, Vice-Treasurer and General Receiver for Ireland during the year ending 20 March 1662 included a salary of £50 to Adam Darley, the hospital's overseer, and £120 to George Carr for 'distribution amongst such of the soldiers in His Majesty's Hospital of Dublin as were by the late Committee thought fit to be continued and to the nurses and washerwomen there employed'. The only other known hospital personalities at that time are William Currer, who served as Physician General to the army in Ireland, James Fountaine, who held the dual role of Surgeon General in Ireland and Surgeon to the Hospital at Dublin, Robert Miller, apothecary at the 'hospital for wounded soldiers and lepers in Ireland', and Anne Shirley, the hospital laundress, who received £2 in part payment of her wages for the ten months between 14 January and 21 October 1661.[6]

Little of note occurred to disturb the existing medical arrangements for the army in Ireland for almost twenty years, but elsewhere the French were planning an innovatory development. In 1671, work began on constructing Les Invalides, an impressive retirement home for wounded and retired soldiers in Paris. Spurred on by the personal interest shown in the project by King Louis XIV of France, in 1679 the English King, Charles II, was convinced of the need to found his own hospital for invalids at Kilmainham, near Dublin. Building work started the following year and, by 1684, it was ready to admit up to 300 invalid pensioners.[7]

The rules and standing orders that governed the duties of the hospital staff provide an insight into the ways in which these functionaries were expected to perform their duties. A transcription of the original, extensive hospital staff table is shown at Appendix B and the rules at Appendix C.[8] Anyone appointed to a position on the hospital staff was administered an oath:

> You shall to the best of your skill and understanding well and truly exercise the Office of ... of the Royal Hospital of King Charles the second for antient [sic] and maimed officers and soldiers of the Army in Ireland and diligently and faithfully discharge the trust reposed in you according to such orders and instructions as you shall from time to time receive from the Governor and Master of the said hospital or other your superior officers. So help you God.[9]

A master or overseer was placed in administrative charge of the hospital but the physician, as the senior clinician present, was responsible for the day-to-day supervision of the apothecary, the nurses and anyone else concerned in caring for sick in-pensioners. The physician was required to attend the hospital at least twice in every week on such days and times as were stipulated. At such times the surgeons, apothecary and nurses were ordered to be present to receive any instructions 'as you shall think convenient and necessary for the assistance and comfort of the sick'. He did not, however, hold any powers of discipline and, in the event of any misbehaviour or neglect by the staff, he was required to report the same to the Master for any appropriate action to be taken.

The apothecary also held supervisory powers over the nurses who attended the sick pensioners in the hospital infirmary and was required to ensure that they 'do diligently attend and faithfully discharge their duty'. He was also appointed 'inspector of the mad-house', a contemporary term used to describe a secure unit set aside 'for the reception of sick soldiers as shall have the misfortune to become lunatics'. The provision of such a facility was in advance of the times as, in civilian practice, most psychiatric patients were cared for either by local general medical practitioners, their home parish or even in jails, dungeons or houses of correction. In Catholic countries a few monasteries and religious houses had a tradition of caring for 'mad' people but, until the end of the eighteenth century, mad-houses were not regarded as medical but as charitable institutions where a physician would pay infrequent visits to merely purge or bleed the patients.[10]

At Kilmainham, the apothecary supplied a variety of prescribed remedies for administration to the patients suffering from psychiatric conditions and also supervised the work of the nurses allocated to that facility. In their turn, the nurses were assisted by the hospital porter in washing the patients and also when carrying their food from the kitchen. The apothecary was especially enjoined to prevent the patients from being disturbed by the undue attentions of curious passing strangers. This was undoubtedly in response to an unedifying contemporary phenomenon whereby it was common practice for individuals to seek to view the patients as a form of entertainment. He was also required to ensure that the porter accompanied any patient from the secure unit who was granted permission to walk in the grounds.

Unfortunately, none of nurses who worked at the Royal Hospital have, as yet, been identified by name, but the hospital rules provide some insight into their duties and responsibilities. A senior or 'head' nurse was appointed to supervise the day-to-day work of the nurses. In keeping with an attitude prevalent amongst contemporary office holders, established hospital nurses viewed their positions as valuable personal assets to be rented on occasion to others for a percentage of the wages earned. It was also normal practice to employ older, usually post-menopausal, women as nurses in an attempt to reduce the risk of sexual misconduct between nurses and patients. The head nurse was therefore specifically warned not to allow any nurse to employ others to undertake the work in their place, except when, through age or infirmity, prior permission had been obtained from the master. For similar reasons, she was also to ensure that the nurses did not entertain visitors in their rooms. Security was a high priority at the hospital and everyone was reminded of the need to ensure that strangers and others found in the building without authority were to be removed.

The head nurse had a role to play in the recruitment of nurses and acted as the master's adviser on suitable applicants for appointment when vacancies occurred. Given the existing local climate of civil conflict and religious prejudices it is probable that, in the selection of women for employment as nurses at the Royal

Hospital, the criteria used were affected by the same contemporary prejudices prevalent in London. For example, on 9 September 1689 at St Bartholomew's Hospital in London, 'Lettice Pyne, widow, being a person that hath lived well and an Irish Protestant', was elected to a post as one of the sisters of the Hospital to work on 'Dyett ward'.[11]

Additional elements of the head nurse's work included overseeing the general state of cleanliness and hygiene of the hospital as well as the supervision of the hospital linen in ensuring that it was correctly accounted for and maintained in good repair. She was also required to be on the lookout for 'idle or loose women that frequent or lie in the hospital' soliciting for business and to evict any that were found from the premises. This could be a very real problem, as was proven two years later when the staff of the regimental hospital of the Guards accommodated in the former Savoy Hospital were driven to submit a petition in which they requested that action be taken against layabouts and 'lewd persons' who had committed violence in their grounds.[12]

The ward nurses' duties included cleaning and maintaining their wards in good order. Each bed was to be made up every morning and the rooms supplied with a sufficient quantity of clean water. At the appointed time they were to take soiled linen to the 'chamberlain' for washing and collect items that had been laundered. They were not only to ensure that the pensioners in their care received all of the allowances to which they were entitled, but were also particularly reminded of their duty to care for those who fell sick, notifying the physician or surgeon accordingly, and arrange the patients' rapid transfer to the infirmary for urgent treatment.

If any pensioners were unable to attend meals in the great hall, the nurses were responsible for collecting their food from the cook on their behalf at midday. At the same time they would also collect the pensioners' food for that evening's supper and breakfast the following day. The diet provided for pensioners was prepared according to a rigid and monotonous menu. This consisted of a daily allowance of one pound of bread, one ounce of butter, one and a half pints of porter (ale), a pint of cocoa, three quarters of an ounce of sugar and one eighth of a pint of milk.[13] On Sundays and Tuesdays these items were supplemented by thirteen ounces of mutton, a pint of broth and an ounce of oatmeal. On Wednesdays and Fridays these additional items were changed to a quarter pound of butter and two pounds of potatoes whereas on Mondays, Thursdays and Saturdays the supplement was thirteen ounces of beef and a pint of broth. On Christmas Day, St Patrick's Day and the Monarch's birthday these allowances were doubled and an extra two quarts of ale were provided instead of the routine porter.[14]

In addition to their weekly pension of 1s 6d the in-pensioners were entitled to a weekly payment that varied according to their rank for the purchase of tobacco. Every other year the pensioners received a new full suit of clothes with an allowance for replacement of 'half clothing' every year. Meanwhile the hospital apothecary was allowed the annual sum of 2s 6d per man, with an overall maximum sum set at just under £1,800 for supplying drugs to the 430 pensioners. Similarly, the pensioners' laundry was paid for as long as the total cost did not exceed £322.

Various other staff appointments included Moses Davis, a chaplain, Doctors

Corning, Patrick Dunn and John LeCaan, physicians, John Purvis and William Hunt, master surgeons, William Morris and Thomas Chetwind, master apothecaries. The clerks, Nathaniel Boyle and Matthew Gunn, maintained the hospital account books while Frederick Matthewson fulfilled the same function for the hospital stores. Peter Thopp and William Moore held the appointment of purveyors, John Jeffrey and James Lynam worked as butlers, and William Ryley and Mary Watkins were listed as cooks. Other minor office-holders included William Hamilton, who was listed as a 'fueler', and Samuel Nacup, the clerk of the chapel.[15]

Once he had founded the hospital, the King's interest in the project soon waned, especially when his attention was diverted to the establishment of a similar establishment at Chelsea in London. By 17 July 1686, only two years after the opening and some seventeen months after Charles's death, the circumstances of Colonel John Jeffreys, the first Master of Kilmainham, had become so reduced that he was forced to submit a petition to the new King, James II, in which he complained that during the intervening two years he had lost many of his original benefits and requested their reintroduction. In return, James II agreed that Jeffreys could retain his position as Governor of Kilmainham under revised and improved terms of service, but only two years later much greater demands were imposed on Ireland's military hospitals.[16]

The sequence of events that followed William of Orange's landing in England and King James's subsequent flight to France changed the nature of the army's position in Ireland for ever. James received considerable moral and some material support from the French King Louis XIV. Richard Talbot, the Catholic Earl, afterwards Duke, of Tyrconnel, whom James had appointed his Lord Deputy in Ireland in 1687, quite rightly foresaw the potential importance of that country as a sympathetic military base for James to use for any attempt to regain his throne and set about organizing the formation of an Irish Jacobite army. In Dublin, with James's blessing, he took control of the Royal Hospital, turned out the in-pensioners and began the process of converting the building for use as an acute casualty receiving hospital. It was not to revert to its original purpose until the war's end in 1692.

In due course, with the assistance of Louis XIV, James landed at Kinsale on 12 March 1689 with 5,000 troops.[17] As a result of Tyrconnel's efforts, a force of 53,716 men lay at James's disposal and he decided to initiate his campaign by moving north to take control of Strabane and then move north to besiege Londonderry. There, the Governor, Robert Lundy, was an ardent Jacobite who, along with his fellow officers, deserted the town but not before he had ordered the easily befuddled Admiral Herbert, who had arrived with a naval force intended to reinforce the local Protestant garrison, to return to England together with his complement of troops.

The siege lasted for 105 days, from 19 April to 30 July 1689, and the deprivations experienced by the town's population and garrison during their ordeal were appalling. All of the town's children died and the population, which exceeded

6,200 at the outset, had been reduced by sickness and starvation to 4,508 by the time that the siege was finally broken.[18]

Meanwhile, the Jacobite camp had also been forced to consider what other means could be taken to maintain the health of the troops. Dr Archbold was appointed Physician General to the Irish army and Patrick Archbold (? a relative) their Surgeon General.[19] On 5 August representations were made to James for a collection of money to be taken up for the sick and wounded soldiers of his army. In a reply reminiscent of his father's approach to the same problem some 45 years earlier, and probably lacking a viable alternative, James fell back on the traditional solution of recommending that his nobility and gentry should exercise their patronage and contribute to a fund for the relief of the sick and wounded.[20] Archbishops and bishops, both Roman Catholic and Protestant, were ordered to appoint collectors to demand and receive the 'benevolence and charity of all good Christians for the use of the said sick and wounded soldiers in such proportion as they shall think fit' in their respective dioceses. The monies so accumulated were to be handed to Luke Hore of Dublin, a merchant authorized to receive the same.[21]

Back in England, the long delay in bringing relief to Londonderry had revealed the weaknesses and ineptitude inherent in the nation's military organization. Following the coronation of William and Mary, a considerable portion of the English army had been disbanded whilst the majority of the troops that were retained had been loaned to Holland. When, in March 1689, news of the worsening situation in Ireland arrived in London, orders were issued for the immediate raising of eighteen new regiments of foot and four of horse but, when it was discovered that there were insufficient arms remaining in the various armouries, immediate steps had also to be taken to procure replacements from Holland in a great hurry, at considerable trouble and expense.

On 25 April, when Admiral Herbert arrived back in England from Londonderry, the Secretary of State, the Earl of Nottingham, was assured that the town had fallen and ordered the admiral to stop any further attempt to relieve the town. However, shortly afterwards, when the King became aware that the town still held out, he ordered an advance party of four regiments under the command of Colonel Percy Kirke, formerly of ill repute in Tangier, to sail to the relief of the town. After some delay Kirke's force departed but, even though he entered Lough Foyle without difficulty, Kirke proceeded to waste more time in establishing a base and failed to take any aggressive action for several weeks. It was not until 30 July, when two of Commissary Shales's store ships finally broke through the boom stretched across the Lough, that Londonderry was finally relieved.[22] John Shales, the same man who had managed the camps on Hounslow Heath during the previous reign, had been sent to Chester and Whitehaven on 14 May as Commissary of Provisions with a brief to establish an embarkation and supply facility for both Kirke's force and for the coming campaign in Ireland.[23] Naturally, the provision of good medical care for any army is directly in proportion to the quality and efficiency of the supply and financial organizations that form the essential supporting pillars for any war or campaign. A significant proportion of blame for the medical and other disasters that accompanied William III's war in Ireland can be attributed to the failings of those elements.

Overall command of the army now gathering in England was given to Herman, first Duke of Schomberg and a former Marshal in the French army, who was over 80 years of age. As a result of Parliament's parsimony and dislike of permanent armies, there were pitifully few regular troops for him to command and, in order to raise the required new regiments, the summer months were spent in a frenzy of hectic recruiting and training. An efficient army cannot be produced overnight and, with the exception of a few experienced Huguenot and Dutch troops, when Schomberg finally sailed from Hoylake on 12 August, his chaotic army of 10,000 men consisted only of very poorly trained and badly equipped levies.

Tellingly, some three weeks after their departure, Thomas Tyrer, the Mayor of Liverpool, submitted a bill for reimbursement of the money that he had paid out of his own pocket towards the exorbitant costs incurred in caring for the numerous sick soldiers that had been left behind.[24] Equally, it also appears that a temporary hospital was established in Chester where the sick who could not travel were treated as, on 16 March 1691, some six months after Schomberg's departure, Thomas Seaborne, a 'lycentiate in physick and chyrurgery who had been appointed master of the hospital for sick and wounded soldiers' in that town, petitioned for reimbursement of the £239 10s 11½d that he claimed was due to him for his work in that capacity.[25]

Meanwhile, having landed at Bangor, Schomberg's army spent its first night in Ireland standing at readiness prior to moving off at dawn in the direction of Carrickfergus, which fell to them on 16 August. However, after taking Carrickfergus, Schomberg refused to give battle to James and, moving via Belfast, Lisburn, Hillsborough and Newry, he established an entrenched position at Dundalk to await reinforcements. The army arrived in Dundalk on 7 September, where Schomberg sited his camp to the north of the town on extremely wet ground.

The erection of the camp was completed in about a week and formed a large rectangle flanked on all sides by a ditch between eight to nine feet broad and six to seven feet deep, with redoubts at the corners. On 21 August, just before the autumnal rains set in, the General ordered his troops to build themselves huts but, whereas the foreigners in William's pay, those few experienced Huguenot and Dutch troops, worked with a will, the ignorant, raw recruits that composed the English regiments, whose officers were no more experienced than the men, would not take the trouble to run up shelters or dig trenches to drain their camping ground. The majority had never seen a gun fired in anger, the officers were mostly very young, there was widespread over-consumption of alcohol, in one regiment the weapons were useless, and several regiments were short of shirts. In fact, many were almost naked despite the soldiers having been charged twice over for clothing and, in the circumstances, it is not surprising that, even amongst those who did not catch the fever raging through the camp, many were suffering from trench foot. In their commander's own words, 'there were many who had limbs mortify in camp and some had their toes and some whole feet fall off as the surgeons were dressing them'.[26]

Blame for the fiasco fell on the shoulders of John Shales, who was particularly censured for the absence of adequate horses and transport for the movement of stores and equipment, but the Commissary of Provisions was not alone in his failings. Regimental colonels at that time were regarded as proprietors of their regiments which were, in turn, viewed as a property, as much for the enhancing of personal fortunes as for achieving a military objective. The colonel was responsible for feeding, clothing, paying and arming his troops and corners were frequently cut so that savings could be made against the standard allowances paid to the colonels by Parliament in return for these services. As Schomberg admitted in a letter to the King, 'if the regimental colonels were as good at fighting as they were at pillaging and withholding their soldiers' pay, the king would be better served'.[27] The colonels were taking so little care of their regiments that weapons were continually being broken, the captains were cheating the men out of their pay and, as a group, the officers were perpetually requesting leave to the point where, had all that was requested been granted, very few officers would have remained with the army. When leave was subsequently denied, they pretended they were sick in yet further attempts to absent themselves.

Although the camp at Dundalk was reasonably easy to defend and close to the sea with easy access for resupply by the navy, little consideration was given to sanitation or the health of the troops. A surgeon and two surgeon's mates accompanied every regiment. They could cope adequately with wounds and injuries but, in the absence of a physician to personally advise the commander on health matters, an outbreak of fever could strike with devastating effect. Inevitably, sickness was quick to appear. Schomberg later claimed, perhaps with good reason, that the infection had been brought to his force by the survivors of Londonderry but the deplorable state of disorganization, lack of training and incompetent general staff administration certainly exacerbated the situation.

Casualty figures were poorly recorded at the time and those that do survive are confusing to say the least. The following statistics are believed to be as full and accurate as can be expected in the circumstances. When Schomberg had arrived at Dundalk his command had numbered some 14,000 troops. Of these, sickness quickly claimed some 1,700 who died on the spot, a further 800 perished in transit to Belfast and yet another 3,800 died in that city's hospitals.[28] The late arrival of Shales's wagons had inevitably compounded the problem but, nevertheless, on 6 October Schomberg told the King that 'there are in this army about 1,000 sick [including] some wounded men left at Belfast: these begin to come back from thence and few of them die'. Over two weeks later, the Paymaster General, William Harbord, told the King that 'the sick here and at Carlingford have been sent to Carrickfergus and so to the hospital at Belfast where it is believed there will be at least 200'.[29] This suggests that both Schomberg and Harbord were either in complete ignorance of the truth or were attempting to paint as rosy a picture as possible by glossing over the realities of the situation. Equally, they may have been deliberately lying to the King.[30]

On 13 October an order was issued for all of the sick to be sent on board ships in Belfast harbour while officers were to be nominated to supervise the provision of huts for the soldiers who remained well. There was no immediate response until additional instructions were issued for all the army surgeons to meet with the Physician General, Dr Thomas Lawrence, the next day at 10 o'clock to consult what methods were to be implemented to prevent further spread of dysentery and fever which, by then, had become widespread.[31]

Many of the sick were dispersed amongst local townsfolk and Dr Henry Scardevill, the General's personal chaplain, was later refunded money that he had expended in providing some form of recompense to local ministers in both Dundalk and Carlingford who had supervised the local care provided to the sick and wounded. Dr Sylvester, one of the hospital physicians, was also reimbursed for his expenses at Dundalk that included £10 paid to Dorothy Boyd, presumably for care that she had provided in nursing sick soldiers.[32] At the beginning of November, probably as a result of Lawrence's conference with the surgeons, orders were once more issued for the sick to be collected together for evacuation from Dundalk in wagons to Carlingford and Newry for onward transportation by sea to hospital in Belfast. The appalling state of command and control exercised by regimental officers is indicated by the fact that it was even felt necessary to issue an order instructing the colonels, lieutenant colonels and majors of each regiment to be present personally to see that the sick men were properly taken care of and given money for their journey. In addition, it was ordered that a nominated officer from each regiment, accompanied by a detachment of fit soldiers, was to attend and care for the sick during their journey to the point of embarkation.[33]

The following day the sick were indeed carried to the wagons but despite their instructions the field officers failed miserably in their duties and, as a result, the subsequent journey through the snow-covered countryside turned into a nightmare. Many soldiers died in transit and every time the wagons jolted, their corpses were quickly thrown off into the wayside hedgerows. It was later reported that the roads from Dundalk to Newry and Carlingford were full of bodies. Schomberg suggested that some 1,600 to 1,700 had succumbed in the camp, another 1,970 en route to or in Carlingford, and a further 1,100 died later at sea. When the ships, full of sick and dying men, eventually arrived at anchor in Belfast Lough it was found that on board several ships all of the sick passengers had died.

The troubles of the sick did not end with their arrival in Belfast. As they lay on board ship at anchor there was no one to look after them until, on 4 November, orders were issued that required every regiment who had sent sick men on board the ships was to send a junior officer accompanied by ten men to provide elementary care. In addition, the Commissary General was instructed to respond favourably to any request for necessaries for the sick, and a stock of army tents, previously stacked along the dockside by returning regiments, was taken on board to assist in keeping the sick men warm.[34]

In his subsequent report, Schomberg attributed the entire catastrophe to 'nothing else but the bad weather, the moistness of the place, the unacquaintedness of the English to hardship and their lazy carelessness'. He rejected the concept of any failure on the part of the military authorities and laid the blame firmly at the feet of the inexperienced English soldiers, comparing their performance unfavourably with that of the experienced Dutch troops who had managed to provide themselves with adequate huts and shelter from the weather and of whom only 11 had died during the whole campaign.[35] Whilst there is some validity in these remarks, there can be no excuse for Schomberg's personal neglect in permitting the situation to continue for as long as it did without remedy.

The last remaining troops were withdrawn from Dundalk between 4 and 7 November 1689 and dispersed into winter quarters in Carlingford, Newry, Armagh and Antrim. Unfortunately, when they departed, in the absence of any means of moving them, a few sick were left behind but, reassuringly, they were not ill treated by their enemy. Shales later claimed that two days before the camp was evacuated Schomberg had ordered 70 wagons to carry the sick to Carlingford but these had not been dispatched in time due to a shortage of horses and drivers.[36] Of the survivors who actually managed to find a hospital bed in Belfast, some 3,762 died there between 1 November and the following May, according to tallies submitted by the men who buried them.

By his own estimate, Schomberg had lost half of the force with which he had started his campaign a mere three months earlier but his enemies had also suffered.[37] Throughout that dreadful autumn of 1689 the Irish army had also been riven with sickness and, according to a French officer taken prisoner near Dundalk, all of the large colleges in Dublin were full of sick soldiers and many more lay in Drogheda.

The causes for the failure of the disastrous campaign of 1689 were manifold and not merely limited to the shortcomings of the raw untrained soldiers or even of the supply system. Some limited preparations for receiving casualties had been taken prior to the commencement of operations as, on 1 July 1689, a staff establishment list for the English hospitals in Ireland was published with, for the first time, a surgeon general, Charles Thompson, appointed to the headquarter staff.

Table 3.1 Establishment of a hospital to attend the army in Ireland, 1 July 1689

Two Physicians, one to be Physician General, each at £200 per year
One Surgeon General, at £365 per year
Four Master Surgeons, at 10s each per day
Two Chaplains, one to be Chaplain-General, each at 6s 8d per day
Three Purveyors, at 6s each per day
Two Clerks for the accounts, at 5s each per day
Twelve Surgeons-Mates, at 3s each per day
Three Cooks, at 3s each per day
Two persons [Butlers] to look after the Bread and Beer, at 3s each per day
Twelve Nurses or Tenders, at 2s 6d each per day
One Apothecary-General, at 10s per day
Three Apothecary's Mates, at 3s per day each

Source: TNA, WO 24/884, pp. 108–9.

The establishment was based on an anticipated casualty load of 300 patients and, although a proviso was added that more attendants could be taken on in excess of the establishment should the need arise, arrangements were obviously woefully inadequate in execution. Even though an extra four surgeons, two apothecary's mates, a butler and a cook were taken on in December, the overwhelming numbers of sick soldiers who flooded back from Dundalk camp found the meagre facilities totally unprepared and grossly insufficient.[38]

In addition to the above, twenty horses were supposed to be provided for the hospital's use, attended by four carters and four stable boys but, as a result of Shales's inadequacies, these probably did not materialize. To pay for these facilities, every soldier admitted to hospital after 29 July had a specified amount deducted from his pay – 2d a day for the sick and 3d for the wounded – in return for food, medicines and other expenses. Unfortunately, the money collected for this purpose by the captains of companies was misappropriated and, starved of funds and adequate equipment, the hospital staff deployed without even the most basic equipment. The few items that were available had been supplied personally by individual surgeons. Just how ill prepared the army's casualty care system was may be deduced from the surviving accounts of Paul Buissiere, one of the surgeons attached to Schomberg's force, who eventually submitted a bill for the huge sum of £2,234 0s 9d in respect of a variety of instruments, equipment and household stores that he had personally provided prior to the start of the campaign. These included such basic items as 1,200 straw beds (palliasses), 20¾ cwt flocks for making quilts and bolsters, 600 pairs large blankets, 1,400 pairs of sheets, 800 shirts and night caps, 72 napkins, 6 table cloths, 6 cwt fine tow, 143½ pairs of old sheets to be converted into lint and bandages, several pieces of grey, blue and white linen for use as towels, as well as surgical instruments and kitchen equipment.[39] In a letter sent to the King on 3 March 1690, Schomberg remarked on the serious state of affairs in the hospital and commended Buissiere for his work at Carlingford. As a result, Buissiere replaced Charles Thompson as Surgeon General, the latter having been deemed to have failed to respond adequately to the emergency.

Although Shales and his commissariat were undoubtedly corrupt from top to bottom, they were not solely responsible for the many ills experienced by the troops. The Paymaster, William Harbord, was equally at fault, a fact that was well known to Schomberg who, on 14 November, had written to the King commenting that the Paymaster 'makes great profit out of the musters, the hospital, the artillery and the payment of troops' whilst other reports tell of his tendency to abscond whenever his immediate funds were insufficient to pay the troops.[40] His junior staff assumed the role of regimental agents, responsible for providing the money to pay the troops. In reality only very small amounts were actually issued and what little that was received by the regiments had an exorbitant rate of interest levied upon it as a 'service charge' or 'expenses'. The only unit that received regular issues of pay was Harbord's own non-existent independent troop of dragoons for which the Paymaster himself drew pay as if it had been manned to a full establishment. In fact the unit consisted only of himself, two clerks who were listed as officers, and a standard that he kept in his own bedroom.[41] When questioned regarding his failings, Harbord claimed that 'it was not fault of his if the army was destroyed' and attempted to pass the entire blame onto John Shales. Incredibly, Harbord later admitted that, had he known as much about hospitals at the beginning of the campaign as he did at the end, he might have saved two-thirds of those who died but, in reality, he retained the funds designated for the hospitals use for his own pocket.[42] Regrettably, whilst Shales was arrested and spent six months in prison, Harbord escaped without punishment and, incredibly, was later appointed Lord Treasurer for Ireland!

Starved of funds and equipment, it is not surprising that the medical organization failed although the problems for which it was severely censured were not entirely of its own making. Not everyone was totally concerned with greed, profit seeking and self-interest. In some instances local people made valiant attempts to alleviate the plight of the troops. One such was Thomas Pottinger, the Mayor of Belfast, who, as late as 4 July 1691, submitted a petition in which he claimed that most of the city's inhabitants had fled to Scotland when the Irish army under Tyrconnel had originally moved north. He claimed to have 'negotiated the preservation of the town at vast personal expense' and, when the Duke of Schomberg arrived, furnished horses and vehicles for the carriage of bread and provisions. Later, he had visited Schomberg at Dundalk where, without seeking payment, he had arranged for one of his storehouses in Belfast to be converted into an overflow hospital where many of the sick were placed when the army went into winter quarters. Having emptied his purse on such matters, he sought reimbursement from the Lords Justices for the services that he had rendered but, unfortunately, it is not known whether his request was answered.[43]

In the spring of 1690, frustrated by the disastrous situation in Ireland, King William decided to take personal command with Dr Thomas Lawrence and Paul Buissiere appointed to his personal staff as Physician General and Surgeon General respectively. In the wake of his decision, a warrant was issued on 1 March authorizing the introduction of a revised hospital establishment for the army. Under the terms of this document, base hospital facilities were to remain in Dublin while two new types of mobile hospital were to be formed equipped to enable them to move wherever the army deployed.[44] One, termed the fixed hospital, would establish itself in a town or village some distance behind the forward troops where it would act as a staging point on the rearward evacuation chain. The other, known as the marching hospital, would accompany the troops as near as possible to the scene of fighting and receive casualties directly from the battle or siege lines. Although standard practice in the Netherlands, this was the first occasion in the history of the British army that such a concept was planned in support of English fighting troops and is an indication of the personal influence exerted by William III on the structure and management of his forces. Nevertheless, mismanagement and incompetence conspired yet again to prevent these plans from being fully implemented that year. Poorly documented, hindered by financial shortages and repeated misapplication of funds, the full extent to which the intended hospital formations were implemented and used during the 1690 campaign remains obscure.

Despite the best intentions to improve medical provisions for the army, matters remained unsatisfactory. Atrocious weather, defective clothing, lack of pay and a shortage of food combined to sap the soldiers' health and morale. Whatever hospital facilities were brought into being had, by September, been inundated with casualties when Count Solms, the officer that William had left in charge of the army after the King returned to England, wrote 'we have to move a great many men into the hospitals and, on account of the sickness, [more] doctors are wanted'.[45] Responsibility for many of the continuing medical problems remained with the Paymaster General, Harbord, who, at the beginning of the year, had been advanced £770 for general expenses and another £750 for medicines.[46] Additionally, on 10 March, he had also been authorized to receive £1,000 'in part payment of the £1,952 9s 2d needed to provide beds and furniture for the various hospitals' with the balance of £952 9s 2d being paid four days later.[47] With such funds at his disposal matters should have improved but Harbord continued in his old habits of embezzlement and misappropriation and, despite the authorization to establish the new hospitals, it is impossible to confirm the form they actually took. Salaries remained unpaid and the marching hospital remained unserviceable until July and even then it could only function on a very limited basis. The confusion that surrounded the hospital appears to have been general as, in March the following year, treasury officials were instructed to investigate a petition submitted by at least two hospital officers, possibly surgeons' mates, who claimed that £69 due to them for their services with the marching hospital during 1690 remained unpaid.[48] Naturally, as a result of this invidious situation, the medical services continued to attract ongoing criticism for, once again, failing to achieve the intended service standards.

On 6 March, Doctor Thomas Lawrence was appointed 'Physician General to the Army in Ireland' and he, together with another three physicians, Doctors Ferguson and Silvester and one other, joined the hospital staff alongside Paul Buissiere, now Surgeon General, two additional master surgeons, one of whom was Charles Thompson, and eighteen mates. Richard Thomas, William Trant and John Segard were appointed hospital chaplains alongside the Chaplain General Dr Henry Scardevill. The Dutch chaplain, Theodor van der Browig, was appointed specifically to minister to his countrymen in William's army. A huguenot apothecary, Monsieur Angiban, was one of the two apothecaries to the hospitals in Ireland in company with five mates, one of whom was Richard Johnson.[49]

In addition to the hospital staff, some 45 additional surgeons' mates, one for each regiment, were added to the army's establishment prior to William's landing at Carrickfergus on 14 June. The successful campaign that ensued culminated in victory at the battle of the Boyne on 1 July.[50] Drogheda was captured on 2 July and Dublin was entered three days later. Naturally, when the army arrived in Dublin, the existing hospitals that had functioned as such for James's army were taken over by William's army and henceforth, for the remainder of the war in Ireland, the provision of base hospital facilities for the English army continued to be provided by the Royal Hospital at Kilmainham in its role as the army's main referral and base hospital, supported by the hospital in James Street.[51]

The governorship of the Royal Hospital at Kilmainham had lain vacant since the death of John Jeffreys in the spring of 1689, albeit the functions of the post were performed by an Acting Deputy Governor, John Falconberg, during the intervening period.[52] On 8 July 1690, three days after William's entry into Dublin, Colonel Samuel Venner was appointed to that position and, fortunately, his accounts for the period between July 1690 and 13 March 1691 survive. They contain the only surviving indication of the mobile hospitals' whereabouts during the 1680 campaign by virtue of entries that indicate the deployment of medical staff for specific duties.[53] In one instance the former Surgeon General, Charles Thompson, was reimbursed for his expenses in providing for three surgeons' mates, two apothecaries' mates and a wagoner who were sent to Cork while, in another, Dr Lawrence is shown as having been involved in the establishment of a hospital in Drogheda. In October, £3 12s 7d was spent on providing boats and carts to convey sick and wounded from Waterford.

Other entries in Venner's accounts provide a fascinating insight into the hospital's day-to-day running costs, particularly catering. Between 20 July and 30 October 1680, £1,108 8s was spent on food for the in-patients based on a basic *per capita* allowance of 4d a day. This sum was deemed sufficient to cater for both in-patients and also those who remained unfit for duty until they were able to return to their units. One particular entry recorded that £3 13s 6d was expended on providing bread for sick and wounded prisoners, indicating that enemy soldiers were also seen and treated. Other items of expenditure included soap, coal and candles, the purchase of 90 close stools (commodes), the washing of blankets and rugs and the purchase of shoes, stockings and coats for soldiers discharged from the hospital. Interestingly, two separate payments of £10 10s and £7 5s respectively were made to 'old soldiers' in October and December 1690 while another, of £2 18s 4d was paid in January 1691 for 'making old soldiers' coats'. These entries would appear to indicate that the pensioners who had earlier been ejected when Tyrconnel had taken over the hospital and converted it from a 'retirement home' into an acute receiving hospital continued to receive pension payments in some form from Kilmainham.

Throughout that year the routine provision of drugs and medical equipment had remained the responsibility of the College of Physicians which, with the Apothecary General, held a monopoly for their supply. An order for the supply of medicines, drugs and utensils for the year's campaign had been placed with the college the previous November and an associated bill, submitted by two of the college censors, indicates the broad spectrum of items provided to the hospital during the campaign. They included 600 lb fine tow, 183½ pairs of old sheets and some old linen for converting into lint and bandages, several pieces of grey, blue and white linen for use as towels, turned wooden, pewter, brass and other kitchen wares as well as furniture and some unspecified surgeons' instruments. Four different apothecaries were involved in supplying a variety of drugs, spreading knives, spatulas, cloth, paper, mortars and pestles, scales and weights and an alembic (an apothecary's still), all of which were packed securely into 50 chests.[54]

Meanwhile, following their defeat at the Boyne, the Jacobite army had retired southwards to establish a defence line along the River Shannon. On 7 and 8 July, King William held a grand review of his army at Finglas before dividing his force into two parts for a renewed attack on his enemy's forces. Two days later one of these columns departed under the command of General Douglas with the aim of capturing Athlone. Douglas arrived at his destination on 17 July but, a week later, finding himself facing almost the entire re-formed Jacobite army, he gave up the siege and marched away to rejoin William. Meanwhile, the King had successfully captured Wexford, Waterford and Duncannon fort and now, accompanied by Douglas, marched to besiege Limerick. The trenches around Limerick were opened on 17 August and an artillery bombardment commenced. It is noticeable that Dr Lawrence was personally present in these trenches throughout the siege.[55] On 27 August a 27-yard-wide breach was made in the walls and, at 3 p.m., an assault was attempted. The subsequent fighting lasted some three hours, during which William's troops sustained between 1,500 and 2,000 casualties before the decision was taken to abandon the attack. The garrison's loss was said to have been a comparatively low 400.

On 31 August the King decided to call a halt to the siege and returned to his primary goal of pursuing the war against France in the Low Countries. Overall command in Ireland passed to General Godart van Ginkel (later 1st Earl of Athlone). Before the 1690 campaign ended, Cork fell to the Earl (later Duke) of Marlborough on 28 September followed by the capture of Kinsale on 15 October. Dr Lawrence had returned to England as part of the royal entourage. This was arranged at the specific request of the King, who presumably wanted Lawrence's extensive experience in the role of senior medical adviser close at hand for the forthcoming campaign in Flanders. Patrick Dunn, one of the former staff physicians at Kilmainham, took over as Physician General to the Army in Ireland.

Back in London, the expense of providing even a minimal care system continued to attract predictable complaints that the expense occasioned by military hospital facilities could not be borne out of public funds. The King's Treasury eagerly sought some means of offsetting these outgoings and they did not take long to arrive at a solution. As ever, it was the common soldier who was to suffer. On 1 June 1690, it was decided to raise the money by increasing the amount taken from the pay of soldiers who used the hospital services. For a private soldier this meant the loss of 2d from his basic pay of 8d a day, with other ranks suffering a commensurate loss. When a soldier died in hospital he was buried at a cost not exceeding 2s 6d and his clothes were returned to his company commander for reissue to another soldier.[56]

On 6 November, at the close of the year's campaign, the army went into winter quarters as usual and the field hospitals were disbanded 'by reason that the establishment of 1 June last … [had] not answered the services which the King expected from them'.[57] During the ensuing winter the hospitals in Dublin, augmented by another that was set up in Waterford, attempted to cater for all of the medical needs of the army in Ireland but, on 31 December, some preliminary plans were made to replace the marching hospital with another 'for as much as it is necessary that due care be taken of all sick and wounded soldiers in [the] said

Army in Ireland furnished with medicaments and attended with the requisite officers and soldiers'.[58] To provide sufficient funds for these additional changes paymasters were instructed to make yet further deductions from soldiers' pay (commissioned officers excepted) of one farthing per day for the infantry and a halfpenny per day for the cavalry.[59]

Matters did not rest there, however. Henrik, Graaf van Solms, an aristocratic professional soldier and a great-uncle of the King who now shared command in Ireland with Ginkel, wrote a memorandum to William concerning the hospitals in Ireland in which he claimed that both officers and men had complained of the manner in which the hospitals were conducted.[60] He remarked particularly upon the invidious system by which the authorities raised money for the hospitals by deducting sums of money from the soldiers' pay when they were wounded. In reply, the authorities pointed to the inefficiency of the officers but, in view of the general dissatisfaction expressed by all sides, Solms recommended that a full enquiry into the previous year's failing be instituted.

George Story, chaplain to the Earl of Drogheda's Regiment, who had observed the shambles at close hand, put it more strongly and cast doubts on the qualifications and experience of many of the army's medical practitioners.

> The troops suffered much towards the end of the campaign, and consequently the number of them will be found considerably less than that number sent in originally, this may be accounted for by three reasons. Firstly, the mortality amongst them has been very great, secondly some have deserted, and thirdly the commissioners gave in a larger number than that which really existed ... Many officers and men have perished for want of doctors and proper care being taken of them in the hospitals; the men in charge of the hospitals pass for doctors, but they are not so. The hospitals must be governed differently ... [it requires] careful industry to recover and heal the sick and wounded which no doubt must be a great encouragement to the poor soldiers when they know that if any misfortune attend them they shall undoubtedly be taken care of.[61]

Goaded into action, the King responded by asking his Physician in Ordinary, Dr John Hutton, assisted by his personal surgeon, van Loon, to produce a thorough report and to make appropriate recommendations, with authority to implement them, for 'establishing hospitals for the sick and wounded, and magazines and stores of medicine, with all other conveniences necessary for the ensuing campaign'.[62] The resulting report, submitted on 1 April 1691, made several pertinent recommendations. The main hospital should continue to be sited in Dublin co-located with the main medical and equipment stores. Kilmainham and the building in James Street would answer these roles, whilst a marching hospital should be established, ready at all times to move with the main body of the army to the front line. In imitation of the previous year's failed plans, the fixed hospital should be set up in a convenient town at an appropriate distance in the army's rear along the lines of communication to receive sick and wounded patients evacuated from the marching hospital, the most forward medical unit. It was further requested that a physician be allocated to each hospital, that there should be a master surgeon present in each of the forward hospitals, and that the Surgeon General, accompanied by a master surgeon should be co-located with the headquarters of the army, or wherever the General placed himself, in order that they might receive his instructions directly. The report also recommended that an overall establishment of 18 surgeons' mates should be dispersed throughout the three hospitals according to the workload and that a master apothecary be allocated to each hospital accompanied by six apothecary's mates, the latter to be employed where their services were most required.

It was also recommended that there should be a purveyor to each hospital who would perform the duties of butler, that is to say assume responsibility for distributing provisions to the sick and wounded, except in the hospital of Kilmainham, where both a butler and an assistant were required. Each hospital would require a clerk, a cook with an assistant and, in the case of the fixed hospital, a butcher would also be required.

Although 20 nurses were already employed in the hospital at Kilmainham, it was recommended that there should be 40 nurses or 'tenders' distributed between the three hospitals with authority for this number to be increased should the situation require it. In addition, there should be 15 washers spread between the three hospitals in proportion to the number of sick patients present.[63]

In addition to the Physician General's report, Colonel Venner, the Governor at Kilmainham, was also asked to make certain recommendations for the future, particularly with regard to the manning and equipment of the marching hospital. In his answer Venner specified that there should be a total of 25 tents, each measuring 10½ ft high, 8½ ft wide and 20 ft long, constructed so that they could be joined to each other end to end, with tent poles sited at 10 ft intervals. Liners for the tents could be made out of material obtained from some old unserviceable tents that Venner claimed were readily available at Kilmainham. Individual tents would contain four beds, each about 4 ft wide and designed to accommodate two sick or wounded men. Using Venner's tent and bed dimensions, the hospital would, when assembled, be able to accommodate up to 200 patients, a figure that Venner deemed sufficient for the coming campaign despite the fact that some 2,000 casualties had been suffered in the three-hour assault on Limerick alone.

As a counter to Hutton's recommendation for 40 nurses, Venner suggested that 25 men-servants be allocated to replace an equal number of nurses on the grounds that he felt men could more readily help to put up the tents, or, when necessary, take them down and carry heavier loads such as wood, water and other necessaries for the sick and wounded. On the other hand, Venner felt that the marching hospital alone would require 10 washerwomen to cope with its needs.

Venner then turned his attention to the hospital transport and here, perhaps, it is possible to gain an insight into his knowledge of the subject and why his views were so readily sought. He recommended that there should be 12 horse-drawn carts provided to carry the tentage and that the carts should be capable of carrying the sick and wounded to the fixed hospital. Obviously the wagons would require drivers, some 25 in number, assisted by eight stable boys. The drivers or wagoners should be paid 18d per day and be armed with firelocks in order that they should serve as a guard for the hospital. Two conductors should be appointed to take command of the 25 wagoners and, unusually for the period and particularly noteworthy, Venner also recommended, for the first time, that the wagoners be clothed in a specific, recognizable uniform. In addition to the aforementioned transport, he also suggested that a further eight larger wagons, with four horses to each wagon, should be required to transport the medicines, bedding, and other stores that needed to be kept dry.[64] The esteem in which Venner's recommendations were held can be judged further by the speed with which they were implemented. On 21 April Viscount Sydney, the Secretary of State, wrote to the Lords Justices of Ireland with a copy to General de Ginckle informing them that the King had approved both Dr Hutton's report and Venner's proposals and directed them to put the recommendations into immediate effect. This was done three days later when an order for their establishment was published. Apart from an obvious improvement in the quality of service these changes could bring, their importance can also be demonstrated in financial terms. Hospital staff salaries now totalled just over £6,250 annually. This represented an increase of some £1,750 and a 28 per cent rise in costs for hospital pay. In addition there was a much more generous allocation of equipment.[65]

Many additional lessons were being learned. The Secretary at War, William Blathwayt, was requested to call upon the President of the College of Physicians and ask him to ensure that the medicines ordered for the army's use were dispatched with all haste. He was also instructed to ensure that the medicines destined for the hospital during the coming campaign season were purchased early and paid for in cash. In another highly significant instruction, clearly indicating a growing awareness of the importance of an efficient field medical service, orders were given for the officers of the hospital, especially the surgeons, to depart early so that they could travel in an unhurried manner and arrive fresh with time to acclimatize to their situation and overcome any lack of experience.[66] In addition, changes were made to the soldiers' everyday diet following recommendations that biscuits should be issued in place of the uncertain supply of bread. The recent short campaign in Scotland during 1689 had demonstrated that the timely provision of Cheshire cheese and biscuits had been nourishing, simpler and had kept the marching soldier in better health that would have been the case had they been forced to rely upon sporadic supplies of stale bread. Individual soldiers could carry sufficient biscuits for ten days supply, and the biscuits could be safely stored for six months or longer, which was not possible with bread.[67] Significantly, it was also cheaper and easier to acquire large stocks of biscuits on campaign.

The reorganization of the army in Ireland began in earnest during March 1691 and, by 7 June, van Ginckel was ready to begin his advance against Athlone, where a second siege was opened on 18 June. Part of the town was captured on 20 June but it was a further nine days before the entire town fell. After the town had been taken, the sutlers in Dublin were ordered to go to the marching hospital in Athlone, collect the sick and wounded and convey them to either Kilmainham or James Street. Ginkell noted that he had personally observed how greatly improved the care of the sick and wounded had become since the changes introduced over the previous winter and praised the work of the surgeons.

After repairing the town's defences, van Ginckel decided to press on to Limerick but, on 12 July, he came face to face with the Jacobite army at Aughrim. During the severe fighting that followed, the English and their allies lost some 450 killed and around 1,000 wounded, as shown in Table 3.2. Aughrim saw the destruction of the Irish army as an effective field force and the end of the Jacobite struggle to retain Ireland for their cause quickly followed.[68] Galway fell to van Ginckel on 20 July, followed by Limerick on 27 September after a prolonged siege.

Table 3.2 Allied officers and soldiers killed at the Battle of Aughrim, 12 July 1691

Soldiers			
Foot:	Killed 337	Wounded	781
Horse:	Killed 63	Wounded	125
Officers			
Foot:	Killed 24	Wounded	95
Horse:	Killed 35	Wounded	13
Totals	Killed 459	Wounded	1,014

Source: G. Story, *A Continuation of the True and Impartial History of the Wars of Ireland* (1693), pp. 139–40.

The final articles of surrender were signed on 3 October but it was not until the following 3 March 1692 that a proclamation was published announcing the end of the war in Ireland. The hospitals had already been disbanded. On 6 January an order was issued declaring that 'there be no further use of a marching hospital in this Kingdom [Ireland], and the same being expensive to the Government', the physicians and others associated with the unit were discharged. Straight away, the hospital treasurer was issued with £975 12s so that he could pay the outstanding dues of the hospital's principal officers, but the surgeons' mates had to wait a further week for the £45 needed to complete their wage bill.

At this point some explanation is perhaps needed regarding the contemporary use of the titles of Physician General and Surgeon General. Confusion can arise because, at that time, more than one individual could hold the title at the same time. For example, Paul Buissiere and a Dutchman, van Loon, are both listed as 'Surgeon General' in contemporary accounts although Buissiere was the senior surgeon of the army's two mobile hospitals and van Loon, King William's personal surgeon, remained with the headquarters and also worked at the Royal Hospital at Kilmainham. It would, perhaps, be more useful to regard the title as meaning Physician or Surgeon to a General, a terminology that indicates more exactly the nature of their position as the chief medical advisers to a commanding General.

However when, on 20 October 1691, a warrant was issued to Dr John Hutton who, during the previous year, had been responsible for investigating the Irish medical establishment, he was appointed 'Physician General of the Army' with the authority and power 'to examine and approve of all such persons as shall be recommended for physicians or surgeons to the land forces and to inspect and approve of all medicines, internal and external'. The following day his position was further clarified by another document that described him as 'sole Physician General of the armies, land forces and hospitals erected and to be erected for the use of the army' – a position much nearer the present day role and function of the Director General of the Army Medical Services.[69] It would therefore appear that Hutton became the army's most senior physician, technically placing him in a senior position to that of Lawrence, whose role was limited to the direction of medical services in Flanders although he retained the title 'Physician General'.

Although the war in Ireland had been won, the need for mobile field hospitals and their associated staff had been firmly established. The early disasters were clearly brought about by lack of foresight and planning coupled with incompetence and corruption in the supply and provisioning organization. These deficiencies were further exacerbated by widespread corruption among regimental officers who expected to make a profit out of their office holding. This was a direct result of a system in which a regimental commission represented both an investment and a potential source of increased wealth to the owners, many of whom ruthlessly undercut costs, robbed their own troops, defrauded the government and thought only of lining their pockets.

It is highly significant that, as has been shown, the Dutch troops who fought alongside the English adapted far better to the climate and their situation. This was a direct consequence of the lessons that they had learnt earlier during the many years of conflict in their home country. It is to the Dutch system of medical support, transported to Ireland by William III, that the British army owes the foundation of its hospital organization and medical services.

Once King William was free to pursue his main priority, that of countering the threat of French expansion into the Low Countries, England's army found itself increasingly involved in a continental war. Many of the medical personnel who had gained invaluable experience in Ireland were now transported to the Continent of Europe where their services were, once more, urgently required. The revolutionary changes that had taken place in the provision of the army's medical services in Ireland were not lost but carried forward into the Low Countries, suitably adapted to fit local conditions. How the service developed will form the basis of the ensuing chapters.

Notes

1. HMC *Duke of Ormonde's Mss* (2 vols, first series), vol. 1, p. 150; Gruber von Arni, pp. 92–8.
2. Henry Whalley to Lord Mayor and Aldermen of the City of London, 22 February

1647: HMC *Earl of Egmont's Mss*, p. 367; J. Haydn and H. Ockerby, *The Book of Dignities* (1890), p. 554.

3   Ibid., p. 80.

4   Ibid., pp. 281 and 581; J. D'Alton, *The Memoirs of the Archbishops of Dublin* (Dublin, 1838), p. 274; *Cal. S.P. Dom., 1649–50*, p. 80.

5   The Royal Military Infirmary was built in 1786 at Parkgate near Phoenix Park under the direction of Board of Works architect, William Gibson. It now houses the Department of Defence.

6   *Cal. S.P. Dom., 1649–50*, p. 407; HMC *Ormonde MSS* (8 vols, new series, 1904), vol. 3, p. 416.

7   C. Stevenson, *Medicine and Magnificence, British Hospital and Asylum Architecture, 1660–1815* (London: Yale University Press, 2000), pp. 46–61.

8   G. Burston, *Abstract of the By-Laws, Rules and Orders of the Royal Hospital of King Charles II near Dublin* (Dublin, 1752), pp. 21–3, 59–60 and 114.

9   Ibid.

10 R. Porter, *The Greatest Benefit to Mankind* (London: HarperCollins, 1997), p. 493.

11 N. Moore, *The History of St Bartholomew's Hospital* (2 vols, London, 1918), vol. 2, p. 765.

12 *Cal. S.P. Dom., 1693*, p. 153.

13 The nature and strength of 'porter' is not known as there is little technical information on brewing surviving from that time. A beer known as porter is said to have been produced some twenty-five years later, in 1722, although porter is not mentioned in the 1735 edition of the *London and County Brewer*, a standard work on the subject. It has been argued that the original porter had a gravity of around 1070 (7–8° ale by volume) and was therefore much stronger than the later Victorian product. I am grateful to Andrew Phillipson for this information.

14 Burston, pp. 1920–23. This dietary system continued until at least the 1740s.

15 TNA, AO 1/1503/199.

16 Burston, pp. 172–3.

17 D. Ogg, *England in the Reigns of James II and William III* (Oxford: Clarendon Press, 1955), pp. 247–8; HMC *Marquis of Ormonde Mss* (2 vols, old series, 1899), vol. 2, pp. 409.

18 J. Mackenzie, *A Narrative of the Siege of Londonderry* (1690); E. Macartney-Filgate, 'The War of William III in Ireland', *Transactions of the Military Society of Ireland* (Dublin, 1905), pp. 8–9.

19 A. Peterkin and W. Johnston, *Commissioned Officers in the Medical Services of the British Army, 1660–1960* (2 vols, London: Wellcome, 1968), vol. 1, p. 1; J. D'Alton, *King James's Irish Army List* (Limerick: The Celtic Bookshop, 1855, republished 1997), p. 38

20 Gruber von Arni, pp. 21–38.

21 HMC *Ormonde Mss* (2 vols, 1899), vol. 1, p. 409.

22 Ogg, p. 250.

23 Ibid., p. 252.

24 *Cal. S.P. Dom., 1689–90*, p. 236.

25 Ibid., p. 239.

26 Ibid.

27 *Cal. S.P. Dom., 1689–90*, p. 288.

28 Lt. Col. G. le M Gretton, *The Campaigns and History of the Royal Irish Regiment* (London: Blackwood, 1911), pp. 5–6.
29 *Cal. S.P. Dom., 1689–90,* p. 300.
30 Sir J. Dalrymple, *Memoirs of Great Britain and Ireland* (3 vols, London, 1773), Appendix to Book 1.
31 G. Story, *A True and Impartial History of the Most Material Occurrences in the Kingdom of Ireland during the Two Last Years* (London, 1693), p. 29.
32 TNA, AO 1/313/1246 and 1248, both n. fol.
33 G. Story, A Continuation of the True and Impartial History of the Wars of Ireland (London, 1693), pp. 35–9.
34 TNA, AO 1/313/1246, n.fol.
35 Ibid.
36 *Cal. S.P. Dom., 1689–90,* p. 276.
37 E. McCartney-Filgate, 'The War of William III in Ireland', *Transactions of the Military Society of Ireland* (Dublin, 1905), pp. 16–17.
38 TNA, AO 1/314/1248, n. fol.
39 TNA, AO 1/1503/200 and E 351/1786.
40 *Cal. S.P. Dom., 1689–90,* p. 288.
41 J. Fortescue, *A History of the British Army* (20 vols, London: Macmillan, 1899–1932), vol. 1, pp. 346.
42 Ibid., pp. 346–8.
43 *Cal. S.P. Dom., 1690–91*, p. 434.
44 BL Harl. Mss, 7441, fol. 25v; C. Walton, *History of the British Standing Army, 1660–1700* (London, 1894), p. 755.
45 *Cal. S.P. Dom., 1690,* p. 120.
46 *Cal. Treas. Books, 1689–92,* vol. 9, part 2, p. 372.
47 Ibid., p. 375.
48 Ibid., p. 1051.
49 Ibid.
50 TNA, WO 24/884, fol. 193.
51 Gore, p. 69.
52 TNA, AO 1/1503/199.
53 *Cal. S.P. Dom., 1689–90*, p. 95.
54 TNA, E 351/1787.
55 *Cal. S.P. Dom., 1689–90*, p. 95.
56 Ibid., fol. 193.
57 *Cal. Treas. Books*, part 3, p. 875.
58 Ibid.
59 Ibid., Cowper, p. 58.
60 J. Childs, *The British Army of William III, 1698–1702* (Manchester: Manchester University Press, 1987), p. 175.
61 Ibid.; Story, *Continuation*, p. 115.
62 *Cal S.P. Dom, 1690–1*, p. 341.
63 Ibid., pp. 110 and 356.
64 Ibid., pp. 356–7.
65 *Cal S.P. Dom, 1690–1*, pp. 119 and 341.
66 Ibid., p. 74.

[67] During the Cromwellian campaign in Flanders 1657–8, considerable difficulties had also been experienced in feeding the English troops due to their aversion to eating rye bread: see Gruber von Arni, pp. 131–9.
[68] Story, *Continuation*, pp. 139–40.
[69] *Cal. S.P. Dom., 1690–91*, p. 549.

Chapter 4

Medical Support during the Nine Years' War in Flanders

In September 1688, fearful of threats to his eastern borders, and using a disputed succession to the Electoral Archbishopric of Cologne as an excuse, Louis XIV of France had invaded the Rhineland in an attempt to establish a fire-break between himself and his enemies, particularly the myriad states that made up the Holy Roman Empire and his traditional foe the Dutch. By this action, Louis repudiated a truce that had been signed four years earlier at Ratisbon and, with William of Orange on its throne, England found itself inexorably drawn into the continental struggle.

For King William III, the Irish war had been an unavoidable interruption to the main thrust of his life-long opposition to the French King's expansionist policies in the Low Countries. The nine-year conflict known to history variously as 'The War of the League of Augsburg', 'The War of the Grand Alliance' or the 'Nine Years' War', was characterized by summer campaigns of interminable marching and counter-marching during which the combatants attempted to out-manoeuvre each other like chess players while avoiding destructive direct confrontations whenever possible. Formal sieges of fortress towns became commonplace, but set-piece battles were rare. Each year, between late September and the following April or May, both armies moved into winter quarters. As a general rule, little or no active fighting took place during this period. In the autumn, men were frequently released to assist in harvesting crops, as the winter progressed the weather deteriorated, roads became quagmires and travel, especially by wheeled vehicles, became almost impossible. The winter months were therefore spent consolidating, repairing, and replenishing stores and manpower. Whole battalions were sent from England to Flanders as reinforcements for depleted units serving on the Continent. Having delivered up their men, the officers, NCOs and drummers of these replacement units then returned to England to begin the process of recruiting their battalions back up to establishment.[1]

In early 1690, despite the fighting in Ireland, William felt secure enough to dispatch a small initial force of English troops, numbering some 10,000 men, to Flanders as a token of his ongoing commitment to the continental struggle. For the majority of the men, however, their sojourn in Flanders was short lived as the King later decided that the situation in Ireland demanded the withdrawal and redeployment of the entire cavalry component of this force together with five battalions of foot. This action reduced the English contingent to some six ill-trained battalions with an effective strength of only 3,600 men. As a consequence, Graf von Waldeck, commander of the Anglo-Dutch forces in Flanders, decided that his best course of action was to employ the English troops on garrison duties throughout the campaign, thus the majority of the English were manning fortified towns when the remainder of the allied forces met with a severe defeat at Fleurus on 1 July.

Apart from regimental surgeons, the troops sent to the Continent in 1690 were almost totally reliant upon local resources and the Spanish or Dutch forces for hospital care. The medical facilities of their continental allies were relatively well organized as the Spanish had maintained a large, well-established military hospital of 330 beds in Mecklin since 1585 and the Dutch had established several military hospitals scattered throughout the United Provinces. The Dutch *Grootlegerhospital* in Brussels served as a clearing station for the immediate reception of their own sick and wounded, subsequently transferring those cases that required ongoing care to permanent military hospitals in Bergen-op-Zoom, Breda, Dordrecht, Gorinchem, Gouda, Maastricht, Namur and Rotterdam and the largest of their facilities at 'sHertogenbosch.[2]

The movement of casualties rearwards from the battle lines to base hospitals was facilitated by the nature of the terrain. Flanders is a country interspersed with rivers running in roughly a south to north direction, each interconnected by a series of canals that make movement by water frequently easier and quicker than by land, especially in bad weather. This comprehensive waterway system facilitated the transportation of large numbers of casualties over significant distances in the relative comfort of boats hired specifically for the purpose. In view of King William's Dutch affiliations, it is not surprising that the English Parliament's initial approach to the provision of care facilities for English casualties in Flanders was to make the naïve assumption that their allies would naturally offer the use of their facilities for the benefit of the English troops. Probably at the King's request, von Waldeck wrote to the Dutch authorities in Brussels requesting them to accept the English sick into their military hospitals. Initially, the admission of English troops to these establishments was accepted, albeit reluctantly, but, when subsequent reimbursement of charges was not forthcoming, creditors in Brussels seized medical stores and equipment sent from England and attempted to bar English soldiers from these hospitals.[3]

In the spring of 1691, even though his Irish campaign was far from over, William was anxious to return once again to his primary objective of countering Louis XIV's ambitions in Flanders and began to transfer the bulk of his military resources to the continental struggle. After a triumphal entry into The Hague on 5 February, some three years after his earlier departure as Stadtholder, William immediately assumed the role of Commander in Chief of the forces of the Grand Alliance. The only significant operation during the year was the successful siege of Mons by the French and, although this was an action that saw the most intense bombardment of all Louis's wars, no English units were present. The remainder of the campaign season was spent in fruitless manoeuvring until the armies went into winter quarters in September.[4]

Some of the hard lessons learned in Ireland had been noted and it was realized that the deployment of such large numbers of troops into the field made it imperative to provide them with more substantial medical facilities, including dedicated English military hospitals. On 20 October 1691, a warrant was issued to Dr John Hutton, the King and Queen's chief physician, appointing him Physician General of the Army and authorizing him to 'examine and approve of all such persons as shall be recommended for physicians or surgeons to the land forces and to inspect and approve all medicines, internal and external'.[5] The following day his responsibilities were extended by another warrant that clarified his position as 'sole Physician General of the armies, land forces and hospitals erected and to be erected for the use of the army'.[6]

In the spring of 1692, the medical personnel who had previously been employed on service in Ireland were utilized to provide the staff for the newly established hospitals in Flanders, initially in Brussels, Breda and The Hague. These facilities were to be furnished by private contract with a civilian entrepreneur, the Dutch apothecary Francis Keggelaer. In return for an advance of 15,000 guilders (£1,500) and a per-capita payment of 9 styvers per day, equivalent to 4½d, for each soldier admitted and treated in these hospitals, the contractor undertook to supply and manage a hospital system. In addition, from 2 May 1692, every soldier had to suffer a deduction from his pay to offset the costs of maintaining the hospitals in the Low Countries. Each private soldier and non-commissioned officer of the foot and dragoons regiments lost 1d per week while 2d per week was taken from the pay of every trooper of horse. The 'gentlemen' of the Life Guards were exempt from paying this sum although their attached troop of horse grenadiers, who were not classed as 'gentlemen', were required to pay the same rate as troopers of horse.[7]

Keggelaer immediately assumed the title 'Intendant of Hospitals' but problems soon arose as The Hague and Breda facilities were sited too far from the combat area and were subsequently moved to Mecklin and Louvain.[8] A marching hospital similar to the unit previously used in Ireland was also deployed in Flanders for the 1692 campaign, to act as a casualty collection and sorting unit situated between the battle lines and the static hospitals, but whether this unit had a separate establishment or was manned by detachments from the base hospital is unclear.[9]

The 1692 campaign started with the French besieging the fortress city of Namur, which capitulated on 30 June. July brought continuous manoeuvering between the opposing armies but, after William divided his command, sending some of his English troops to act as garrison troops, only half of the English contingent was present during the one major field action of that summer, at Steenkirk on 3 August. After one of the bloodiest of contemporary engagements, fighting was eventually broken off, with the allied army retiring in good order despite having suffered losses totalling the 8,258 casualties as listed in Table 4.1. It should be noted that the accuracy of these figures may be questioned in view of the fact that they indicate that more soldiers were killed than wounded, but this could be a reflection of the hand-to-hand nature of the action. French losses, estimated at some 7,000 killed and wounded, were equally severe.

Table 4.1 Allied losses at Steenkirk, 3 August 1692

Rank	Killed	Wounded
Colonel	10	11
Field Officers	17	18
Captains and Lieutenants	139	281
NCOs	138	105
Private Soldiers	4,409	3,130
Totals	4,713	3,545

Source: BL Add. Mss 28926.

After the battle, many of the English wounded were treated in the marching hospital at Anguine before being evacuated to Brussels. Here the hospitals of the various allied contingents were soon so crowded with patients that many wounded were left lying in the streets awaiting attention. The story is told of the Princess de Vaudemont* taking charge of the situation and making several journeys with her coach to collect and carry them to the Great Hall of her palace where, with the help of her ladies, they were dressed and cared for until hospital beds could be found for them.[10] Meanwhile, the wounded who had been left on the field were honourably cared for by the French, who carried them to their base at Enghien. On 11 August 1692, a week after the battle, it was reported that a considerable number of English wounded left on the battlefield, including Lieutenant Colonel Colthrop of the 1st Guards, had been collected and treated by the French and now lay dispersed among several of the enemy's hospitals.[11] Shortly afterwards, the French decamped from Enghien leaving their wounded prisoners unguarded. Many of those fit enough to walk returned to the English camp while wagons were sent to collect those who were incapacitated.[12]

On 2 August 1692, the day before the battle of Steenkirk, on the King's instructions, medical salaries had been halved but, after complaints from Dr Lawrence, including charges of corruption against Keggelaer, this decision was reversed and the original pay scales restored. Subsequently, a hospital inspection commission was appointed, consisting of Regimental Colonels, O'Farrell, Godfrey and Fitzpatrick, together with Richard Hill, Deputy Paymaster General to the Army. They were ordered to visit the hospitals at Brussels, Mecklin and Louvain to examine the conduct of the hospital officers, the accommodation, bedding, patients' diet, hospital transport, including the horses, and to make an inventory of the appointments, equipment, furniture and prize goods that had been issued to the hospitals for their use.[13] They were also instructed to appoint a wagon master to supervise the provision of vehicles to all the hospitals. This order emphasized the importance of the innovatory measure of providing transport solely for the hospitals' use that was not merely loaned to them, as and when available, from the

---

* The wife of Duke Charles IV of Lorraine, Commander in Chief of the Army of the Spanish Netherlands, a confidant and trusted subordinate of William III.

army's general transport pool.[14] Regrettably, the commission's subsequent report has not been discovered.

On 21 August 1692 Dr Lawrence could no longer tolerate the abuses being perpetrated by Keggelaer and wrote to the Secretary at War, William Blathwayt, to inform him that the situation in the hospitals was verging on mutiny, particularly among the locally employed surgeons who had threatened to desert their posts if they were not paid, as they were experiencing the greatest difficulties in supporting themselves financially. The apothecaries were experiencing the same financial distress but, thus far, had 'cheerfully and with patient expectations of relief' continued to carry out their duties. Keggelaer had adopted an extravagant life-style and maintained a particularly high level of personal comfort and catering inasmuch as he frequently entertained regimental officers to dinner at the hospitals' expense.[15]

Regrettably, in his complaining letters to Blathwayt, Lawrence only provided minimal information regarding the state of the patients other than to say that dysentery was their main complaint, aggravated, in his opinion, by the troops' inexperience combined with consistently poor, wet weather. However, he also added the comment that 'several' had recovered sufficiently to return to their units and others continued to improve.[16]

The army's hospitals closed in September when the army went into winter quarters but on 10 September a report circulated that Keggelaer had refused to pay two women who had worked for the hospitals. This seems to have finally brought matters to a head and, in a subsequent report written on 4 November, Colonel O'Farrell, the chairman of the Hospital Committee, informed Keggelaer that he could not understand his 'ill ordered and dark' accounts and ordered the Intendant to submit a revised, full and comprehensive account of all of his receipts and expenditures for the entire campaign.[17] At the same time, O'Farrell wrote to Blathwayt informing him of the situation.[18] In fact Keggelaer's accounts were so badly maintained that one of Deputy Paymaster General Hill's clerks had to completely re-draft them. Not surprisingly, Keggelaer's services were subsequently terminated.

When the hospitals closed, the majority of in-patients were transferred back to England and the beds and equipment put into store at Mecklin and Ghent under the supervision of Mr Creuger, a local official who had offered to arrange for a honest storeman to mend and repair the equipment as necessary.[19] Those patients who could not be repatriated were moved into local civilian religious establishments, notably the Bijloke Hospital in Ghent, the Hospital of St John in Bruges, the Hospital of Notre Dame in Brussels and that of the Cell Brothers in Mecklin.[20] Between 3 September and 19 October, at St John's Hospital in Bruges alone, there were 479 sick soldiers admitted, each of whom spent an average of 18 days in hospital before either being discharged or repatriated to England. This resulted in a bill for 5,491 soldier/days spent in hospital calculated at the standard rate of 9 styvers (4½d) per soldier/day plus additional charges. With a bill for almost £230 covering two months' work at just one of the civilian hospitals involved, these figures indicate the true nature of this 'cost-saving' arrangement that was based upon a premise that only minimal casualties would be suffered during the winter.

In reality, the policy was erroneous as it ignored the increased risk of infection and sickness among the troops posed by the cold winter months when they spent longer periods closeted indoors, for warmth and companionship, in close proximity to one other. The local civilian populations were similarly exposed to a higher risk of contracting communicable diseases, thereby compounding the risk of cross-infection and the outbreak of epidemics. In his study *War and Rural Life in The Early Modern Low Countries*, Myron Gutmann has comprehensively apportioned the cause of excessive deaths among the population of the Low Countries during the seventeenth century to cluster outbreaks of epidemic diseases during the months of September, October and November.[21] Inevitably, civilian admissions to hospital would have peaked during the same months in which the English closed their army hospitals. The transfer of the more severely ill soldiers into local civilian hospitals would have increased their work-load, with many resultant ramifications for supplies and patient care.

A more in-depth study of the reasons behind the adoption of winter closure policy is obviously appropriate at this point. Throughout the 1690s the financial state of the European nations was in a continual state of flux. An economic boom enjoyed during the 1680s and early 1690s would be followed by a stock market crisis and, in England, the Great Recoinage of 1696–99. King William was a frugal man, conscious of the parlous state of both his own and the nation's treasury. He regarded hospitals as areas with significant potential for a great deal of waste and was keen to keep their expenditure to a minimum. As a result, his attitude towards the provision of casualty care was ambivalent.

The financial cost of providing hospital care to the sick and wounded was frequently censured by the King, who demanded that everyone involved in military health care should avoid waste in an attempt to reduce expenditure to the minimum but, in practice, the closure of the hospitals each autumn may well have been a measure of false economy. Although the food stocks, such as meat, butter and cheese, that remained in the hospitals upon closure were sold back to the suppliers, even the grease (? dripping) from the hospital kitchens being regarded as a resaleable commodity, and the clothes of dead soldiers returned to their units for a nominal fee of one guilder per suit, it is questionable whether such receipts ever outweighed the losses incurred by the considerable waste and damage sustained every time equipment and stores were laid up for the winter.[22] Poor supervision and neglect invited further losses that had to be replaced each spring when the hospitals were reopened. The lack of an adequate supply network from England also entailed a constant need for the local purchase of such items as beds, bed linen, towels, paper, ink, clothing and medical equipment. This suggests that the potential benefits, financial or otherwise, of keeping the hospitals open may well have outweighed the monetary savings accrued by their closure.

In the campaign season additional expense arose when members of staff from the base hospitals were detached or redeployed to man the temporary facilities frequently set up to provide medical cover for sieges. In such cases a building would be requisitioned for use as a hospital and local labour recruited to clean the rooms and repair the windows and roofs and dig latrines. Carpenters would be tasked with constructing a variety of fitments and, invariably, a bricklayer would be called upon to construct a base for a common hot-water boiler as well as the ubiquitous tisane boiler, an indispensable item of equipment used in the preparation of the herbal drinks that provided an important element in contemporary medicine and treatment.

Locally employed labour also provided a significant contribution to the medical and nursing staff in order to maintain sufficient numbers. It was established contemporary practice to allow one nurse to every sixteen patients. This figure had varied little since the time of the English Civil War and seems to have become an established norm when calculating requisite numbers.[23] Both men and women, sometimes husbands and wives, were employed as nurses or 'tenders', as is evident from the various wage bills contained in Hill's accounts. Their numbers grew from around 30 per hospital during 1692 to upwards of 60 the following year, two-thirds being hired from the local population and the remainder either brought over from England for the purpose or recruited from the groups of soldiers' wives who had accompanied their husbands. There was also an army of additional 'servants' who carried out a variety of functions such as maintaining the boilers, general work around the buildings and, in one case, two men to 'watch the clothes and washhouse to keep them from being stolen'.[24]

The winter of 1692/3 was exceedingly wet and, in an unusual out-of-season action, the French managed to surround and raid the towns of Furnes and Dixmude where, among other stores, a considerable amount of hospital equipment was lost. The hospital commission was re-established the following year as a permanent feature, with Major General Sir Henry Bellasis, Brigadiers George Ramsey and Charles Churchill and Deputy Paymaster General Richard Hill as members. One of its main tasks was to keep costs to a minimum and ensure that the limits laid down for the numbers of personnel employed in military hospitals were held at the lowest possible level. Additionally a revised medical establishment was also promulgated and is tabulated in Appendix E below.

The Intendant of Hospitals' post, vacant since the sacking of Keggelaer the previous year, was filled by Colonel Samuel Venner, while the people to fill the revised establishment were recruited in England and in Flanders.[25] Venner had previously served at the head of a regiment of foot in Ireland where, towards the close of that campaign, he had additionally been appointed Governor of Kilmainham Hospital. That he should choose to adopt the same title following his move to Flanders came as no surprise to those who had known him in Ireland, where he had gained a reputation for adopting a lofty, superior attitude towards his subordinates. In particular he was known for the regal manner that he adopted during his rounds of inspection when he would frequently tap his gold-mounted tortoise-shell snuffbox or consult his gold turnip-watch embossed with scenes of the Goddess Diana hunting.

As discussed above, in Chapter 3, Venner had contributed significant comments during the process of army hospital reorganization in Ireland during 1691. To obtain his new appointment he may well have benefited from powerful patronage or have been in a position to exert influence at court but, as Governor of Kilmainham, he may have simply been regarded as the most experienced person available. Whatever, the situation, once he was in post the avaricious side of his personality soon came to the fore and he quickly demonstrated a talent for emulating his predecessor's penchant for spending money that was not his own as he strove to improve his personal style and comfort. This did not pass unnoticed and by June, by way of response, the Commissioners were forced to introduce a variety of additions and deletions to the hospital establishments that clearly reflect their successive attempts to reduce or curtail Venner's profligacy. These included the employment of hospital butlers and washerwomen in an attempt to improve the service to patients by providing an in-house service to replace the former system that entailed the hospitals' and patients' laundry being sent out to local entrepreneurs who had bribed Venner for their contract. At the same time, the Commissioners eliminated a purveyor's appointment that Venner had created specifically to cater for his personal needs and service.

The 1693 campaign season had opened with a further increase in the English contingent to a total of 13,200 men. During the year, hospitals were established in Brussels, Bruges, Ghent, Dixmude, Mecklin and Liège, together with two evacuation units in the ports of Antwerp and Rotterdam for the accommodation of casualties awaiting repatriation to England.

William delayed until 8 July before attempting an attack upon the French defences that had been constructed between the Scheldt and Lys with a force numbering some 8,000 infantry, and 6,000 horse. After the Engliah troops suffered severe losses in the storming of redoubts around the villages of Espierre and Dotignies, their assault was successful. Unfortunately, the victory was followed by appalling scenes during which English troops joined with other allied soldiers in the frenzied sacking and pillaging of more than twelve villages. Meanwhile, on the same day, the French surrounded the town of Huy, which surrendered four days later. This action threatened Liège and, to protect that city, William attempted to draw his enemy into action near the villages of Neerwinden and Landen.

The battle of Neerwinden was fought on 19 July, during which two French assaults on the Allied line were repulsed although a third concerted assault succeeded and Neerwinden fell, forcing the English and Dutch to withdraw in considerable confusion across the river Gheet. The riverbanks were very steep and the horses could not get out. D'Auvergne claims that as many men were drowned in the river as were lost in the fighting, including several men and women that he describes as attendants upon the army, such as servants, soldiers' wives and sutlers.[26] Neerwinden was a severe defeat for the allies and it was several days before the army was able to re-muster. By the evening between 20,000 and 25,000, including 5,000 to 6,000 English, were casualties; French losses were said to be in the region of 8,000 to 9,000.[27]

Many of the allied wounded were captured but, as a result of an arrangement whereby either side submitted bills for the care and treatment of captured wounded to their opponents for reimbursement, they were reasonably well cared for. In all, the total charge levied by the French for the care and treatment provided to English troops after Neerwinden came to 33,059 livres, a sum roughly equivalent to £3,500 in contemporary seventeenth-century English money. On 15 September, a party of captured wounded Englishmen was sent in two boats to the French hospital at Namur, for which a charge of 355 livres 4 sous (about £35) was levied. Another bill submitted on 24 January 1694, some six months after Neerwinden, quoted a charge of 11,968 livres (about £1,200) for providing care, treatment and food for 68 men from the time of their capture, and throughout the time they remained in the French camp prior to their departure for the hospitals at Maastricht and Namur. These were significant amounts of money but the wounded do seem to have been provided with a reasonably high standard of care as the supplies included 1,200 lb meat 'for feeding, and for stock', 55 pots of brandy and the hired services of three Swiss *vivandières* who were employed to run a kitchen for the English wounded throughout the time they remained in the camp. The bills also listed the payment of ten nurses who cared for their needs as well as charges for sundry linen items and, finally, the cost of hiring a man named Durre whose job was to ensure that everything necessary was indeed being provided for the men.[28]

Meanwhile, those troops who had survived the battle unscathed were still at risk from infection and disease. Colonel Bellasis summed the situation up in stark detail in a letter written to Blathwayt from Bruges on 16 December:

> The three French [Huguenot Regiments in William's service] and Tiffin's, being cantoned betwixt Ostend and Newport [sic], and their quarters straight and ill, and the place very unwholesome, I'm afraid many of them will fall sick, and therefore would be glad to know the King's pleasure about them. None of the Spanish Hospitals will take them in for less than 9 styvers a day which is extraordinary expense that the officers are not able to bear and for the want of an extraordinary allowance or [the provision of our own] hospitals I'm satisfied will be the loss of many soldiers of his majesty's troops this winter which might do good service the next campaign.[29]

Equally, the effects of the battle were not simply limited to the armies that fought. The great number of bodies that were left scattered around the countryside after the battle fomented an outbreak of sickness among the local population, the effects of which were felt over the entire 40 kilometres between the battlefield and Liège.[30] Even after the French army had left the area in mid-August a disease called 'hot fever' decimated the population of the community of Montenacken, lying halfway between the river Meuse and Neerwinden.[31]

Apart from the French capture of Charleroi there was no further significant military action that autumn and the forces retired into winter quarters and the hospitals closed once again. As usual, the care and treatment of the sick and wounded did not cease with the onset of autumn. On 10 November Mathew Prior, Secretary to the English embassy in The Hague, wrote to William Blathwayt requesting instructions on how to deal with more than 500 sick and wounded English soldiers awaiting repatriation at the ports of The Brill and Helvoetsluys. They could only be transported at the rate of 50 or 60 in each packet boat and, to cover their accommodation and expenses while waiting, Prior had issued them with 200 guilders (£20) and requested that the Dutch government provide them with lodgings and heating.[32] In another letter written the following month Prior described how he had arranged for someone to distribute food to the wounded who remained in Helvoetsluys as Blathwayt had told him that his expenditure on the casualties would be refunded in due course.[33]

Meanwhile, a decision had been taken regarding the conduct of Samuel Venner who, having attracted widespread and severe criticism of both his methods and accounts, was obviously totally unsuited to his appointment and, in the footsteps of Keggelaer, he was formally relieved of his post. The following year he was charged with bribery and corruption involving regimental agents and, regardless of any patronage that he may have earlier enjoyed, he was relieved of the command of his regiment and cashiered.

The enormity of Venner's punishment, which entailed considerable financial loss, as well as severely damaged social standing and personal prestige, cannot be over-emphasized. Nevertheless, financial mismanagement was widespread and not simply restricted to hospital intendants and, as in Ireland, regimental officers were also involved in fiscal abuse. On 7 March 1694, Bellasis told Blathwayt that he was

> very glad to find that Colonel Venner has no more to do with the next summer's hospitals, of whom I have had many complaints since I came into winter quarters of his having over-charged the regiments in his hospital accounts. Officers of several regiments have made their complaints to me that part of the subsistence for their regiments has been [collected] in England by their Colonels which has put them to great straights here and is a prejudice to the service. [I request that the Earl of Ranelagh] be ordered not to issue subsistence in London without just cause.[34]

After two years of fraud, mis-management and incompetence, responsibility for the provision of medical facilities for 1694 was placed in the hands of Patrick Lamb, the King's Master Chef. Lamb was a long-standing and trusted member of the Royal Household and, as both Intendant of Hospitals and Contractor for the Hospitals, he was given wide-ranging powers. Nevertheless, although his background had given him experience in the management and direction of menial labourers, similar to those employed as helpers in the military hospitals, the government and the army were, understandably, both worried about his administrative competence. This is not surprising as his new appointment exposed him to considerable personal financial risk. The remainder of this chapter will attempt to assess his part in the development of an efficient army medical service.

The onset of the 1694 campaign season brought yet greater increases in the strength of the English contingent to a total of 54,925 men.[35] A revised annual establishment for the hospitals was published on 25 March 1694 in which the controllers for the army's three main hospitals were named as John Hudson, James d'Ayrolles and Richard Hampton. Dr Thomas Lawrence remained as Physician General while three additional physicians, Dr Prelone, Dr LeCaan and Dr Oliphant, were employed one at each of the hospitals at Bruges, Brussels and Ghent. There were also three chaplains, Dr Edward Paget, Dr Henry Shute and Dr George Grey, three master apothecaries, with Isaac Teal as Apothecary General assisted by William Morris and Peter Chambron. The Surgeon General was named as George Pringle, with Hannibal Hall, Frederik Zichorius and William Wallace as additional master surgeons. The vacancies for hospital clerks were filled by Samuel Keck, Benjamin Sweet, Herbert Price and Gowen Paige, while the 24 English surgeons' mates were joined by eight locally employed Flemish or Dutch colleagues. The number of authorized apothecaries' mates was increased to nine.[36]

Those who travelled from England made their way across the channel either individually or in groups over the next four to six weeks. For example, Dr John LeCaan, one of the physicians who had gained previous experience of military medicine as a member of the staff at Kilmainham, was recorded as travelling on 4 April accompanied by his servant Daniel Moe. Doctors Shute and Paget, two of the three hospital chaplains, delayed a further six weeks until 17 May.[37]

Almost immediately, the surgeons complained about the quantity of the contents of the surgeons' chests supplied through official sources, claiming that the drugs they contained were not worth 10 guilders (£1), let alone their supposed regulation value of £25. Eventually one of the Hospital Commissioners, General Bellasis, felt it necessary to intervene by writing personally to Blathwayt asking him to take the necessary steps to ensure that the quality of the contents, as well as the quantity, was correct.[38]

The port hospital at Rotterdam was reopened in support of the three base hospitals of St John at Bruges, Brussels and the main facility in the grounds of the Bijloke Hospital in Ghent, a religious foundation in the south-west of the city that was to function as the army's main base hospital for the remainder of the war. The accounts of Richard Hill, the Deputy Paymaster in Flanders, indicate that, by this time, the English army no longer relied upon the good offices of the overworked resident hospital staff in such places but employed its own work force, including nurses, tenders, labourers as well as additional medical staff. Some were found locally while others, particularly nursing staff, travelled from England. Lamb, who was responsible for recruiting and employing these people, was obviously exerting considerable influence in improving the overall situation. In addition to the base hospitals, further facilities were opened during the course of the ensuing campaign at Dixmude, Liège and Namur as the situation demanded.

These medical units were sorely needed as, despite the failure of either side to force their opponents into a decisive battle, another enemy was on hand to devastate the troops. A widespread epidemic of smallpox raged throughout Europe, even claiming the life of Queen Mary in London. During the months from July to October 1694, when the smallpox epidemic was at its height, the hospitals in Ghent, Brussels and Mecklin opened additional isolation wards specifically to accommodate infected patients where their special needs could be addressed. Extra nurses were recruited, as usual on the basis of one nurse to sixteen patients. Fires were constantly lit, not simply to keep the rooms warm but also to heat water for the daily baths that formed part of their treatment. As a result a larger labour force was required to service the demand for the increased quantities of water needed, not just for the patients' baths but also for washing their 'sweaty linen, bedclothes, towels and bandages every day'. In addition, the cost of heating water for tisanes and other warm drinks for these men was a further significant expenditure. At the Bijloke Hospital, every day for 62 days during July and August, when the epidemic was at its worst, 40 pots of milk and half a barrel of beer over and above the normal supply were delivered specifically for the preparation of posset drinks as well as additional supplies of sugar, eggs, bread, brandy and vinegar. The last was used by the nurses as a mild oral disinfectant in cleansing and soothing mouthwashes. Equally, more than 30 guilders (£3) was expended on providing the pound and a half of candles that were required every night to provide sufficient lighting for the work of the surgeons and apothecaries. Similar provisions had to be made at the other hospitals and, in all, the additional costs imposed by the measures taken to counter the epidemic added some 1,500 guilders (£150) to Lamb's budget.[39]

Thus far in the war, each successive year had seen the French move from success to success. The 1695 campaign was to change that and provide a turning point. The internal French economy was severely depressed as resources began to dry up. Taxation had been increased, including the introduction of a new poll tax. Conversely, the allies were reaping the benefits of increased mutual co-operation, as demonstrated by their combined investment and re-capture of the fortress of Namur.

After a month-long siege, a successful attack by the English Guards on the outer defences during the evening of 8 July cost them between 2,000 and 4,000 men – reports vary.[40] The town eventually fell on 16 July with the further loss of 700–800 men and, finally, after a failed first attempt, Namur's citadel was stormed on 20 August. Although the troops gained an entry into the main works, it was a further two days before the French garrison finally surrendered.

In the immediate aftermath of battle, contemporary casualty figures were seldom accurate. On 26 November, the Secretary at War, William Blathwayt, wrote to the Paymaster General, the Earl of Ranelagh, citing an initial figure for the siege and storming of Namur of 55 wounded officers and 790 soldiers out of an overall casualty list of 1,349. A subsequent instruction required Ranelagh to pay a bounty of 20s to each of 1,253 wounded private soldiers, a difference of 463.[41] In his *History of the Army Medical Department*, Cantlie quotes 1,556 killed and 2,205 wounded but, as he fails to identify his source, his figures cannot be substantiated.[42] D'Auvergne fails to provide a complete casualty estimate but, in the light of the field hospital at Namur's overall admission total of 2,087, Blathwayt's second figure seems to be the most accurate available.[43]

Although a mobile hospital brought rapid assistance to the casualties at Namur in addition to regimental resources, it was also decided to establish a hospital at Liège where the casualties could be taken by river, down the Meuse, by *bijlander*, a local craft that was the most comfortable form of transportation available.[44]

The hospital was divided between two separate establishments, identified in the records as 'the Academy' and 'the Cornolian', which were requisitioned for the purpose. Some idea of the care taken to prepare these buildings to receive the casualties transferred from the field hospital at Namur can be deduced from a list of additional expenses totalling 1,878 guilders, roughly £190, subsequently submitted by Mr Evans, the hospitals' Clerk of the Kitchen, for the period 1 to 31 August 1695.[45]

While carpenters, thatchers and others worked speedily to build additional ward accommodation and lavatories, other workers were hired to clean and prepare the requisitioned buildings, twelve at the Academy and seven at the Cornolian, at the rate of 18 styvers (15s) a day, with several barrels of beer being supplied for their liquid refreshment. Additional local labour also unloaded beds and equipment and disposed of rubbish while three women were kept busy for 28 days making, repairing and filling straw mattresses and making up beds. Many items, including needles and thread, pots and porringers, weights and scales had to be bought locally, the erection of a copper boiler for the provision of constant hot water for making tisanes and barley gruel as well as for heating bread and milk poultices was equally essential.

The casualties from Namur arrived at Liège in batches that varied from 152 in one party to just 12 in another and, although the wounded were accompanied on their journey down the river Meuse by several 'carers', further local labour was needed to assist in carrying them from the boats into the hospital using barrows and hand carts. Eventually, once the situation at Namur had stabilized and all of the patients had been transferred to Liège, transport was hired to convey the field hospital's goods and equipment to the hospitals at Liège to augment the facilities there.

Monthly bed occupancy statements for the Liège hospitals from 11 July to 19 October 1695 (excluding the 21 days from 20 August to 10 September), compiled by Lamb's staff to support his claim for reimbursement from the funds deducted from patients' subsistence allowances, record the number of soldier/days spent in hospital and the number of deaths, regiment by regiment.[46] Although they do not quote the actual numbers admitted over the stated period, they do facilitate the calculation of average bed occupancy.

Table 4.2 Average bed occupancy and numbers of deaths at Liège hospital, 11 July –19 October 1695

Period	*Average no. patients*	*Deaths*
11 July–10 August	764	127
11 August–10 September	823	120
11 September–10 October	647	76
11–19 October	421	9

Source: SCRO, 112/1/327, 2379 and 2330.

Between 11 July and 10 August, the hospitals at Liège recorded 22,920 soldier/days in hospital. Similarly, between 11 August and 10 September there were 3,294, from 11 September to 10 October 19,406 and 3,789 between 10 October and the hospital's closure on the 19th of that month. During the whole period 332 deaths in hospital were recorded. The flow of casualties into Liège from the field hospital and regiments increased during the month immediately following the fighting at Namur until admissions reached a peak in August and then tapered off as patients either recovered and were discharged to their units or died. The numbers of in-patients had almost halved by the end of the campaign season in October and the hospital closed. This is clearly shown in Table 4.2

Meanwhile, the army's main base hospital, the Bijloke Hospital in Ghent, had been working under pressure from the moment that it opened in March until it closed on 16 October. During the busiest time of the 1695 campaign, from 9 May to 20 September, the Bijloke Hospital's work-load rose steadily. During May and June its average bed occupancy was 370 but the fighting at Namur was reflected in a sudden rise in admissions during July and August. These reached a high of 1,573 in September. There were 335 deaths in this hospital during the same period.

The hospital in Brussels experienced a similar influx of patients during the campaign season, particularly during the final two to three weeks before the army entered winter quarters as regimental hospitals closed. The average bed occupancy rose from only 172 between June and July through 410 in August and September to a high of 610 in the three weeks before closure on 20 October. There was a total of 126 deaths during the same period.

Table 4.3 Average bed occupancy and numbers of deaths at the Bijloke Hospital, Ghent, 10 May – 20 September 1695

Period	Average bed occupancy	Deaths
9 May–10 June	370	54
11 June–10 August	989	98
11 August–10 September	933	114
11–20 September	1,573	69

Source: SCRO, 112/1/322–4.

Table 4.4 Average bed occupancy and numbers of deaths at the hospital in Brussels, 24 June – 20 October 1695

Period	Average no. admissions	Deaths
24 June–2 August	172	3
3 August–24 September	410	67
25 September–20 October	610	56

Source: SCRO, 112/1/291–3.

At Dixmude, even though the hospital only functioned from 1 to 26 July, the average bed occupancy was 419 patients including, unusually, six local Flemish labourers and two wounded women. There were 32 deaths. When all of these statistics are consolidated, as tabulated in Table 4.5, it becomes obvious that the army hospitals' workload during the 1695 campaign season was very heavy.

Table 4.5 Hospital usage for the year 1695

Hospital	Total no. admissions	Days in hospital.
Ghent	3,351	125,884
Dixmude	1,061	25,597
Brussels	2,800	42,344
Liège	3,232	84,369
Sub-total	*10,444*	*278,194*
Bruges	985	3,427
Namur	2,087	8,007
Totals	13,516	289,638

Source: TNA, SP 8/15, fol. 240.

The field hospitals at Bruges and Namur admitted 2,087 patients between them during the year but, regrettably, their morbidity figures have not survived. Nevertheless, excluding the hospitals at Bruges and Namur, of the 10,444 admissions recorded in the four main hospitals, only 823 died, representing a surprisingly low death rate of 7.89 per cent. Of this total a considerable number would have resulted from factors other than combat, such as work injuries and the host of diseases that haunted contemporary armies on campaign. Regular reports on the state of the army's fitness were presented to the King during September and October 1695. These provide a glimpse of the general state of health among the English army's 28 regiments.

Table 4.6 Army statements of fitness, 4 September to 4 October 1695

Category	4 Sept.	24 Sept.	1 Oct.	4 Oct.
Effective	18,722	24,645	21,724	17,887
Fit for service	14,446	19,065	16,610	13,765
Sick in camp	282	346	231	169
In hospital	3,005	3,547	3,373	2,889
Missing or prisoners	73	77	61	51
Dead	11	15	24	18
Deserters	8	30	13	3

Source: TNA, WO 8/15.

The figures in Tables 4.5 and 4.6 provide ample evidence of the enormous workload of the army's hospitals throughout the 1695 campaign season. It is also evident from Table 4.5 that, given that the maximum strength of William's army in

Flanders that year was nominally 31,500, although it probably never exceeded an effective level of 25,000 men, somewhere between 42.5 per cent and 54 per cent of the army spent some time in hospital through sickness or relatively minor injury. The average stay in hospital was around 21 days.

At the end of October, in line with established practice, the hospitals were again closed. At least part of the significant rise in bed occupancy at the Bijloke Hospital during the last few weeks immediately before seasonal closure must be a reflection of the desire by individual regimental hospitals to transfer their patients to the base hospital in order to free themselves of an encumbrance during their preparations for the coming months, especially in the case of units earmarked for redeployment to England.

Those sick and wounded patients who could be repatriated were transferred to the port hospital at Rotterdam to await repatriation. As usual, this operation was expensive and on 21 February 1696 Lamb was presented with a bill in excess of 4,339 guilders (almost £450) in respect of the transportation of the patients who were fit to be moved from Liège to Rotterdam.[47] Inevitably, many others could not be moved and therefore additional arrangements had to be made for them to remain and be cared for in Liège.

The involvement of local Flemish civilians in the care of sick or wounded British soldiers can be gauged by various account entries. For example, on 1 January M. Bricquell, a priest in Louvain, was paid for work undertaken on behalf of soldiers at his local hospital and, over the next six weeks, similar payments were also made to the nursing staff of religious establishments who cared for soldiers in Mecklin, Bruges and Liège. Soldiers were also cared for by the local townsfolk of Liège, as is evident from a payment made to M. Smettaise, Adjutant to the Prince of Vaudemont, who was reimbursed for care provided to a group of sick English soldiers' wives left behind in that city when their husbands' regiments withdrew.

Hospital goods and equipment were stored over the winter months in hired buildings in Brussels until, in March, they were recovered, checked, the linen laundered and repaired, defective items replaced and everything generally made ready for further use. At the end of April the hospitals' senior staff returned from England to Flanders, and it is significant that many were accompanied by a variety of personal servants. The party consisted of Herbert Pike, Clerk of the Hospitals, who took two servants with him, while James d'Ayrolle, Patrick Lamb's Deputy Controller, was accompanied by his wife, his nephew, a manservant and a maidservant.[48] The Physician General, Dr Thomas Lawrence, also travelled with his personal servant while Isaac Teale, the Apothecary General, and his servant were accompanied by twelve apothecary's mates. Interestingly, included in the group was a lady by the name of Joan Hedley, described as a 'nurse to the hospitals in Flanders'. As the only 'nurse' listed in a group of relatively senior staff, Hedley may well have been the hospitals' senior nurse or matron.[49] Thirteen surgeons, James Chambers, John Fairly, James Crawford, George Dundas, William Deas, Thomas Wilson, Levi Ball, Samuel Camlin, Alexander Garshore, Cornelius Vandike, John Kirkwood, George Ramsey and Samuel Westwood, completed the party.[50]

During the campaign of 1696, both armies marched and counter-marched incessantly but, in the end, neither succeeded in forcing a decisive engagement upon their enemy. William returned to England on 16 August leaving his army to enter winter quarters in early September. The campaign of 1697 was equally devoid of action despite the French having retained three armies in the field with a total of 156,000 men under arms. The medical staff list remained much the same as the previous year except that even more personal servants accompanied them. For example, Isaac Teale, who was accompanied by his daughter, Elizabeth, also took two servants. This time the presence of three nurses in the party, Elizabeth Grey, Mary Harvey and Petronell Porter, is of note as it clearly demonstrates that the employment of nurses in the hospitals included women brought from England as well as those recruited locally in Flanders. It may be, however, using the same argument as that given for Joan Hedley above in the previous year, that these ladies were intended for a senior position in the various hospitals established throughout the area of operations.

By this time, however, the opponents, both France and the allies, were financially and physically exhausted. Negotiations for a settlement were commenced and peace was finally declared following the signing of the Treaty of Ryswick on 11 September 1697. As part of this agreement, Louis formally recognized William as King of England, at least for the time being. Once again, the many in-patients who remained unfit to be returned to England were, whenever possible, transferred to local civilian establishments for continued care in Ghent, Mecklin, Louvain, Tirlemont and Asch.

It is appropriate at this point to examine the situation regarding the sick and wounded who were repatriated to England. Patients who were capable of being moved were repatriated, those who were mobile and capable of making their own way being paid passage money. For example, on 11 March 1694, some 85 guilders were paid to disabled soldiers to enable them to return to London. Less mobile stretcher cases were initially transferred to the casualty collection hospital in Rotterdam where Commissary James Morrison controlled arrangements for their onward journeys.[51] Again, for example, during the spring of 1696 some 420 invalids were taken to Rotterdam, of whom 220 were returned to England, the remainder being retained until later in the year when they were fit to travel onwards.[52] A regular packet-boat service plied between Flanders and East Anglia, bringing a continuous flow of casualties to the East Anglian ports but, regrettably, when the evacuated soldiers reached England their problems were far from being resolved. As had so often been the case during earlier campaigns abroad, scant attention had been paid to providing an efficient system of ongoing care for those casualties returned from overseas. Inevitably, the local authorities in the coastal towns of Kent and East Anglia again bore the brunt of the problem.

As early in the war as November 1690, frequent complaints were registered by both local authorities and individuals concerning the unheralded and unexpected arrival of large numbers of sick and wounded soldiers and sailors on their doorsteps in a repeat of the scenes that had been so common during the earlier Dutch Wars.[53] Predictably, at Harwich, several townsfolk refused to offer accommodation and, within days, a few evacuated casualties had died in the streets from exposure and lack of care. Many more would have died if the local mayor had not lodged them in the Town Hall on straw, and arranged for private charity to assist them.[54] Soon, up to 700 casualties were found begging from house to house as a result of governmental parsimony. Robert Seaman, a local Harwich surgeon, had to wait until February 1695 to receive payment for work that he had undertaken in treating wounded soldiers and burying others between 15 September 1691 and 13 October 1692.[55]

On 17 January 1694, Harwich's Mayor, Simon Sandford, was paid £22 3s 1d so that he could reimburse those who had accommodated sick and wounded evacuees during the previous winter. Nevertheless, casualties continued to arrive in the port throughout the remainder of that year. Eventually, in February 1696, Sandford's successor, Thomas Langley, received a further payment, this time of £26 15s 6d, for the ongoing care and treatment provided to sick and disabled soldiers landed in the town between August and December 1694.[56]

Similar situations were common elsewhere in coastal towns. Jacobus Vereeche and William Long, two surgeons on the Isle of Wight, received £19 15s 2d and £28 12s 6d respectively for their services in treating soldiers evacuated to the island between 17 June and 6 August 1694. On 2 August 1694 the accounts of the 2nd Guards recorded that three carts were hired at a cost of £6 10s, calculated at 8d per mile, for the transportation of sick and wounded men from their landing at Portsmouth to hospital in London. In addition, the entire battalion of 528 men was subsequently given a course of an unidentified 'physick' between 1 January 1693 to 31 December 1695 for which £69 4s was claimed as reimbursement.[57]

The mass disbandments that were enacted following the end of hostilities would, once again, leave the army in a parlous state. For some of those who were incapable of further service, or of earning their living at a trade, long-term accommodation was found in the Royal Hospital at Chelsea, but for many others theft was the ultimate resort in a time that saw an unprecedented rise in highway robbery. It was indeed fortunate that, with the outbreak of the War of the Spanish Succession in 1702, Marlborough and Peterborough were available to bring the army once again to a state of effective readiness.

In comparison with the mismanagement and fraud that characterized Venner's time as Governor, the general rise in standards seen throughout the hospital service under the King's former master chef provides clear evidence of his considerable personal commitment to his work. Lamb succeeded in his appointment, confounded the sceptics and retained his post until the end of the war. His reputation was enhanced by an ability to set up new hospitals quickly and remove them when the centre of operations shifted, or when the army went into winter quarters. On one occasion he boasted that, given two days' notice, he had set up a hospital in Louvain, where 500 patients were subsequently treated. He even managed to secure a payment of £472 9s 6d in belated reimbursement for the medical stores that had been seized in 1692 by the French during the raid on Dixmude.

The significant improvements made in hospital provision in the Low Countries were not matched by an equivalent improvement in reception and continuing care facilities in England. In the absence of an acute receiving hospital for military casualties on the English mainland, it was inevitable that some of the more serious cases eventually arriving in London were seen and treated at St Thomas' and St Bartholomew's Hospitals. The role played by these hospitals in the care of military sick and wounded is examined in detail in the next chapter.

Notes

[1] E. D'Auvergne, *A History of the Campaign in the Low Countries for the Year 1696* (London, 1697), p. 3.
[2] J. Childs, *The Nine Years' War and the English Army, 1688–1697* (Manchester: Manchester University Press, 1991), p. 60.
[3] L.M. Waddell, 'The Administration of the English Army in Flanders and Brabant, 1689–1697' (unpublished PhD thesis, University of North Carolina, 1971), p. 428.
[4] E. D'Auvergne, *The History of the Campaigne in Flanders for the year 1691* (London, 1735), *passim*.
[5] *Cal. S.P. Dom., 1690–1*, pp. 549–50.
[6] Ibid., p. 550.
[7] BL Add. Mss, 61330, fols 63–4; TNA WO 25/3138, fol. 208.
[8] TNA, WO 25/3138, fol. 196.
[9] *Cal. Treas. Books, 1693–4*, vol. 10, part 4, p. 292: Henry Guy to the Earl of Ranelagh, 24 July 1693 – 'To insert in his next memorial for money, £25 17s 6d for John Flower for so much due to him and his wife as belonging to the Marching Hospital in Flanders on the descent in 1692'.
[10] Sir N. Cantlie, *History of the Army Medical Department* (2 vols, Edinburgh: Churchill Livingstone, 1974), I, pp. 52–3.
[11] BL Add. Mss, 34,096, fol. 88.
[12] Ibid.; D'Auvergne, *A Relation of the Most Remarkable Transactions of the Last Campaigne in the Confederate Army, 1692* (London, 1693), p. 50.
[13] A percentage of all non-military items captured from the enemy, known as prize goods, was either given to the hospital for issue to the patients or auctioned and the profits used for the benefit of the sick and injured.
[14] BL Add. Mss, 34,096, fols 208, 213 and 221: Warrants dated 2 July 1692, 2 August 1692 and 21 August 1692.
[15] BL Add. Mss, 9724, fol. 54.
[16] Ibid.
[17] Ibid.
[18] Ibid., fol. 94.
[19] Ibid.
[20] The Cell Brothers, otherwise known as Cellites or Alexians, formed a religious congregation in Mecklin in the fifteenth century during the ravages of the Black Death when they tended the plague-stricken and buried the dead. The order spread rapidly throughout Flanders, Brabant and Germany. They remain active today, caring for and providing accommodation for the aged and infirm: *Catholic Encyclopaedia*, http:// www.newadvent.org.
[21] Gutmann, pp. 151–66.

22 For example, on 7 December 1693, Peter Kruger paid 183 florins for fat from the hospital kitchen at Ghent and Peeter de Potter paid 665 florins for returned unused butter and cheese: BL Harl. MSS, 7435, fol. 23v.
23 For a discussion on nurse-to-patient staff ratios during the English Civil War and Interregnum see Gruber von Arni, pp. 144–70.
24 SCRO, 112/1/354.
25 Dalton, *Army Lists*, III, p. 152.
26 E. D'Auvergne, *The History of the Last Campaign in the Spanish Netherlands, 1693* (London, 1693), p. 89
27 Walton, p. 269.
28 BL Add. Mss, 38,697, fols 141a and b.
29 BL Add. Mss, 9731.
30 Bouille, 'Histoire de la ville et pays de Liège', vol. 3, p. 500, quoted in Gutmann, p. 165.
31 J. Daris, 'Histoire du diocèse et de la principauté de Liège pendant le XVIIe siècle', vol. 2, p. 231, quoted in Gutmann, p. 165.
32 BL Add. Mss, 38,697, fols 141a and b; HMC *Bath Mss*, vol. 3, p. 14.
33 Ibid.
34 BL Add. Mss, 38698, fols 99–100.
35 BL Add. Mss, 38698, fol. 1.
36 TNA, WO 25/3139, fol. 30.
37 *Cal. S.P. Dom., 1693*, p. 141 and *Cal. S.P. Dom., 1694–5*, p. 89.
38 BL Add. Mss, 38698, fol. 115. The contents of Regimental Surgeons' Chests are tabulated in Appendix D.
39 SCRO, 112/1/287, 420 and 421.
40 Fortescue, vol. 1, pp. 378–9; Walton, p. 295.
41 TNA, WO 25/ 3139, fols 377, 389 and 408–9.
42 Cantlie, vol. 1, p. 54.
43 TNA, SP 8/15, fol. 240; E. D'Auvergne, *The History of the Campagne in Flanders for the year 1695* (London, 1696), pp. 153–5.
44 The *bijlander* was a two-masted Walloon vessel used mainly on the larger rivers, such as the Meuse and the Waal, as well as on the canals of Flanders. These vessels ranged from 34 to 38.5 metres in length and were about 5 metres wide. They carried a cabin amidships and had a large carrying capacity: P.J.V.M. Sopers, *Schepen die Verdwijnen* (Amsterdam, 1971), p. 153; H.B. Culver, *The Book of Old Ships* (New York: Doubleday, 1924 reprinted 1992), p. 145.
45 SCRO, 112/1/357.
46 SCRO, 112/1/327, 2379 and 2330.
47 SCRO, 112/1A/1.
48 *Cal. S.P. Dom., 1696*, p. 149. The travel warrants quoted here were issued on 28 April 1696. They provide a useful insight into the life-style of the people employed on hospital business.
49 Ibid., pp. 151–2.
50 Ibid.
51 TNA, WO 25/3139, fol. 381. Morrison was paid £200 on 12 December 1695 for charges at this hospital.
52 TNA, AO/1504/203.

[53] For a description of the casualty situation in East Anglia during the First Dutch War see Gruber von Arni, *Justice to the Maimed Soldier*, pp. 113–39.
[54] *Cal. S.P. Dom., 1691.*
[55] TNA, WO 25/3139.
[56] Ibid.
[57] Ibid., fol. 437.

Chapter 5

Soldier-Patients in the London Hospitals

As has been shown in the preceding chapters, during the Nine Years' War a variety of military hospitals were established in overseas theatres of operations staffed and equipped for the care and treatment of soldiers falling sick or suffering injuries. Those who were unfit to return to their units were subsequently repatriated to England via an evacuation chain that initially conveyed them to a port of embarkation where they came under the control of an agent of the Commissioners for Sick and Wounded Seamen. The agent was normally responsible for their supervision and maintenance while awaiting transportation and for securing their passage in naval vessels, packet boats or hired merchant vessels. On their arrival in any of the ports along the south and east coast of England, another agent assumed responsibility for their accommodation while a locally retained surgeon, paid at the rate of £1 per patient by the Admiralty Commissioners, continued or carried out any treatment required. Accommodation was normally found in local inns or boarding houses for which a government allowance of 6s a day was payable for each soldier's quarters. In due course, those who could not either be returned to duty, or discharged from the service to their home parishes, and who required long-term care, were transferred to either the Royal Hospital, Chelsea or the London hospitals under arrangements made by the Commissioners for Sick and Wounded Seamen. This chapter analyses the nature and extent of the contribution made to contemporary military health by the London Poor Hospitals, using financial records as well as surviving admission and discharge statistics.

In following an old but ill-defined tradition, and in compliance with several vague agreements with various monarchs and governments, the great London Poor Hospitals of St Bartholomew's and St Thomas' had provided hospital care for soldiers and seamen for centuries. During the Civil Wars they contributed a significant service to the sick and wounded of Parliament's army and their involvement in such work did not cease with the Restoration. Indeed, the admission and care of sick and wounded seamen and soldiers became a major element of their day-to-day work.

The first significant move towards regulating the hospitals' position as regards service patients was initiated on 25 September 1666 when, at a meeting with the Commissioners for Sick and Wounded Seamen and Prisoners of War, the Court of Governors of St Thomas' Hospital formally agreed to continue to accept sick and wounded soldiers and seamen for admission and, with the memory of the frequent disciplinary problems experienced during the Commonwealth fresh in their minds, promulgated a set of additional rules specifically for service patients; see Table 5.1.[1]

Table 5.1 St Thomas' Hospital additional rules for service patients.

They take the diet of the house or the house allowance
They lodge in the house
They keep within the house and frequent the chapel on the Lord's Day and other times when required
They be in bed at the time, 8 or a little after
They take not tobacco in their beds to the endangering of the house by fire

Source: LMA, H1/ST/A1/5, St Thomas' Hospital, Minutes of the Court of Governors, fol. 140.

At times, whole wards were given over completely to the admission of service patients, especially during periods of high demand in time of war. For example, on 18 March 1672 the Governors of St Bartholomew's Hospital decreed that Martha Ward, formerly known as the King's Ward, was to be set aside and prepared for the admission of sick soldiers and seamen. Again, on 4 April 1674 it was recorded that Lady Mary Harvey had made a bequest of £50 to St Bartholomew's Hospital in which she referred to the hospital as 'the wounded hospital' and also, for three weeks in September 1678, at the specific request of the Duke of Monmouth, the hospital closed its doors to all new admissions except sick or wounded soldiers and sailors.[2] Meanwhile the routine care of syphilitic patients was also catered for by their separate admission to 'The Lock' in Kent Street, Southwark, if male, and the 'Outhouse' in Kingsland Road, Shoreditch, if female relatives, both being former leper hospitals and out-stations of, and administered by, St Bartholomew's Hospital.[3]

The two large hospitals were not, however, the only London establishments to receive service patients. The Surgeon General's suggestions for the day-to-day running of the camp hospital on Hounslow Heath in 1686, mentioned in Chapter 2 above, included a recommendation that the patients' food should be funded by the same method as that employed at both St Katherine's Hospital and another small hospital, both adjacent to the Tower of London.[4] St Katherine's Hospital was a medieval foundation established in 1148 by Queen Matilda as a hospital for sick travellers, women, children and poor scholars. It was adopted as a Royal Peculiar[*] in the fifteenth century with its own ecclesiastical court and survived the sixteenth-century Dissolution of the Monasteries although, by the end of the seventeenth century, it was in somewhat reduced financial circumstances. The identity of the second, smaller establishment is unclear but was probably the same as that referred to in a warrant issued to Lord Dartmouth, Master General of the Ordnance, on 19

---

[*] Royal Peculiar: an establishment exempt from the normal forms of administration and coming under the direct jurisdiction of the Crown.

February 1686 in which he was instructed to convert three nonconformist meeting houses in the City of London, one in Broad street, near Old Gravel Lane, another at the uppermost part of Old Gravel Lane and a third in Nightingale Lane:

> to be fitted up and used as barracks for soldiers belonging to the Tower of London, and one at least of them to be employed constantly as a hospital and a house adjoining it in Broad Street, near Old Gravel Lane, to be a house for the surgeon and tenders of sick soldiers to live in, the rent to be paid by the Ordnance office, likewise all necessaries found wanting for the benefit of the said soldiers.[5]

This would seem to indicate that the hospital referred to was contained within three separate buildings all in the neighbourhood of St Katherine's. The proximity of St Katherine's to the Tower of London rendered it an ideal location for the routine care and treatment of men from both the garrison of the Tower and, possibly, the Royal Guards stationed elsewhere in London. Indeed, as noted in the previous chapter, when Tangier was evacuated three years earlier, St Katherine's Hospital was one of the establishments identified by Lord Dartmouth as a potential reception facility for repatriated sick and wounded soldiers. Regrettably, the hospital's admission records do not appear to have survived but, nevertheless, it is significant that in the spring of 1686 the Surgeon General should choose to quote the service and methods employed there as models in his proposals for the camp hospital at Hounslow Heath. Presumably the extra facilities requested in Lord Dartmouth's instructions of 19 February, transcribed above, were required to cater for the combined effects of the increasing size of the army and the aftermath of the Monmouth campaign six months earlier.

The hospitals had suffered a considerable drop in their income from rents as a result of the Great Fire of 1666 and, as the years passed, the increasing demands placed upon them by the steady influx of service patients contributed in no small way to their straitened financial circumstances. Eventually, in 1686, the Governors of both St Bartholomew's and St Thomas' appealed to the King for assistance in recouping their costs. In response, they were granted greater recognition for the role they played in caring for sick and wounded soldiers when, on 28 May 1686, James II issued a royal warrant acknowledging their situation and authorized a payment to them of 4d per day for every soldier or seaman admitted.[6] This sum, intended to offset the cost of both food and treatment, was later recouped by an equivalent deduction from the individual soldiers' subsistence allowance. A week earlier, in preparation for the implementation of these new arrangments, William Blathwayt, the Secretary at War, had written to the Paymaster General, Lord Ranelagh, instructing him to pay the appropriate funds directly to the hospitals as soon as the necessary certificate had been received from the Surgeon General.

The food supplied to patients was similar in all of the hospitals discussed. Although the catering services came under the general supervision of the steward in the larger hospitals, in the St Katherine's group the matrons were responsible for purchasing and preparing the patients' diet. In return for this work they personally received the 4d a day deduction from the soldiers' subsistence allowance. Apparently, this had also been the system employed by regimental surgeons during the military expedition to Flanders under the Duke of Monmouth some seven years earlier, a practice that probably served as a model for the newly introduced regulations at home. If the recommendations made by the Surgeon General were indeed followed in the hospital at Hounslow Heath, it is likely that the food provided to soldier patients in all of the London hospitals was of similar quality to that at St Katherine's. There a pound of beef, a quart of porridge and a penny loaf were provided on four days of the week with milk porridge, water, gruel, panadoe (another cereal mixture), cheese and butter and the same allowance of bread on the remaining three days. Additionally, patients received a quart of beer daily in the winter, increasing to three pints in the summer.[7] This arrangement also provided a potentially significant financial benefit for the matrons for, when recommending the system for use at Hounslow, the Surgeon General added a comment that they 'may well afford to fund the sick such diet ... and diet themselves and servants out of the profit thereof'.[8]

For administrative matters affecting service patients the hospitals liaised with the offices of the Committee for Sick and Wounded Seamen and Prisoners of War, newly reformed on 2 September 1689, with Thomas Addison, Edward Leigh, Anthony Shepard and John Starkey as members. On assuming their duties the new Commissioners were given a specific brief that instructed them to 'require St Thomas' Hospital to make room for such sick and wounded soldiers and seamen as were sent to them'.[9]

In the aftermath of the 'Great Revolution' of 1688 there was widespread confusion and, with the new King's inherent mistrust of English troops, the Dutch Guards who had accompanied him from Holland were granted significant preferential treatment. This included extending to them the facilities of the Royal Hospital, Chelsea, sometimes to the detriment of English veterans, as well as the more reasonable access to London's hospitals. Inevitably, a widespread resentment of Dutch servicemen spread throughout the capital and the prevalent atmosphere of mistrust and aggression seems to have spilled over into the London hospitals, as is evident in correspondence that passed between the Committee for Sick and Wounded Seamen and the Governors of St Thomas' Hospital in August 1690. The Dutch Ambassador complained to Queen Mary that Dutch seamen recently admitted to that hospital had been fed on nothing but small portions of bread and cheese and that the surgeons were 'very negligent in healing their wounds'.[10] In instructing the Governors to ensure that, in future, there should be no differentiation between the English and Dutch as regards both food and treatment, the Commissioners also passed on a directive from the Queen, that arrived via the Secretary of State, Lord Nottingham, that, in future, the Steward was to provide the Commissioners every Monday with the names of any Dutchmen who were fit to be discharged from hospital during the coming week in order that money could be sent to them and transport arranged to convey them to a naval vessel in readiness for their return to Holland. The Governors were also asked to forward a copy of the hospital's diet sheet for patients to Lord Nottingham for his personal information. The warning seems to have been effective as there does not appear to have been any repeat of this incident.

In an era when public accounting was at a very elementary stage of development and graft, misappropriation and fraud were rife at every level of society, from Parliament down to the lowliest member of staff and was almost expected as part of normal, everyday behaviour. Hospital administration and that of the Committee for Sick and Wounded Seamen were no exceptions to the rule. The archives of the London hospitals offer a rich area of research for the student of military health care in the seventeenth and early eighteenth centuries and indicate that the hospitals' finances were ready-made and lucrative potential targets for inventive accountants. Although only £8 3s 4d was received by St Bartholomew's Hospital during 1685–6, the first relevant year after the regulations for payments of 4d per day for every soldier admitted was introduced, that same hospital's income from later payments rose to £312 10s in 1686–7 and £211 6s 1d in 1687–8. Similar amounts became a permanent feature of the hospital's income for the next 76 years, with notable rises during times of war until, in 1762–3, a final payment of £8 6s was recorded.[11]

Nevertheless, accounting methods at St Bartholomew's Hospital were remarkably efficient for the period. One particular document entitled *'Soldiers Received into St Bartholomew's Hospital – An accompt of His Majesty's Forces sent to St Bartholomew's Hospital'* throws considerable light upon the hospital's involvement in admitting and treating soldiers during the entire span of the Nine Years' War from 1 January 1689 to 31 December 1697.[12] This item was compiled by the Surgeon General, James Pearce, with the aim of accurately recording each admission in order to calculate the debt owed to the hospital in respect of the regulation 4d per day allowance. Details of every soldier admitted are recorded showing the date he entered, his company and regiment, the date of his discharge and the total number of days spent in hospital. Some 818 admissions were recorded of which 16 have an unclear admission date. Of these, six relate to 1691, eight to 1692, one to 1693 and one more to 1694. There were 96 patients listed as admitted on 1 January 1689, the date that the record was started, although, as some of their regiments of origin were of the pre-Revolution army of James II, many were probably admitted earlier. For the purposes of statistical analysis, it has been decided to exclude these from this study.

No details of diagnoses are known. The average time spent in hospital by these patients was 83 days although the maximum period that any soldier remained in hospital during the period covered was, in one extraordinary case, 857 days, almost two and a half years. Surprisingly there were only four recorded deaths of soldiers during the entire eight years. It is particularly noticeable that the highest admission figures, during 1689 and 1690, coincided with the traumatic experiences of the troops in Ireland at that time. In 1691, despite ongoing active operations in Ireland, only 62 soldiers were admitted and in 1692 a mere 40. This is a particularly significant observation as by then, although fighting in Ireland had more or less ceased, English troops were fighting in Flanders and suffered a severe setback with a defeat at Steenkirk on 3 August 1692. Equally, the following year, during which another defeat was suffered at Neerwinden on 19 July, there was only a modest rise to 98 in the number of soldier admissions for that year, 59 of which had arrived by the end of June. This would seem to indicate that the care received by sick and wounded soldiers treated by regimental surgeons in the field and in the army's hospitals in Flanders was sufficiently satisfactory that ongoing hospital care on return to England was unnecessary for the majority of casualties.

A similar picture is seen with regard to discharges. Of the 818 patients admitted, five have no recorded discharge details and probably remained resident in the hospital at the end of the period in question. Six are shown has having left the hospital on unspecified dates in 1691, eight in 1692 and one each in 1693 and 1694. Although there were 76 admissions in 1694, the distribution of admissions month by month does not appear to relate directly to any significant military event. In particular, the successful but costly siege and storming of Namur lasted from June to the end of August 1695 but there were only 49 admissions in the whole of that year, evenly spread at intervals across every month. When this information is combined with identification of the regiments to which the admitted patients belonged, it may be determined that, despite 87 different regiments, including seven Dutch units, being represented in the admission list, most sent only a few soldiers to the hospital. For a list of regimental totals see Appendix D.

Table 5.2 Admissions and discharges of soldiers to St Bartholomew's Hospital, 1689–1697

Admissions

	Jan	Feb	Mar	Apr	May	Jun	Jul	Aug	Sep	Oct	Nov	Dec
1689	109	19	29	19	28	12	20	17	26	2	7	19
1690	15	33	10	5	7	12	4	4	12	8	11	1
1691	5	2	5	1	9	8	5	2	7	5	5	8
1692	2	4	1	6	6	2	3	3	1	7	1	4
1693	7	15	12	10	6	9	8	7	4	9	10	1
1694	5	8	9	9	5	5	13	5	7	5	2	3
1695	3	1	1	5	6	4	3	4	4	5	8	5
1696	3	5	5	6	3	5	4	2	1	1	2	1
1697	2	3	2	1	0	0	0	0	1	1	0	0

Discharges.

	Jan	Feb	Mar	Apr	May	Jun	Jul	Aug	Sep	Oct	Nov	Dec
1689	22	38	38	26	20	21	27	16	14	20	10	8
1690	18	18	28	18	12	15	13	5	2	12	6	8
1691	4	4	4	1	9	6	8	3	4	6	3	4
1692	5	6	3	7	8	3	3	5	0	3	2	1
1693	4	7	6	9	9	7	8	5	7	2	10	3
1694	12	2	6	12	9	9	6	7	7	5	10	3
1695	5	5	4	9	4	1	4	0	5	3	2	4
1696	7	8	2	5	5	7	4	3	4	2	1	2
1697	3	2	3	3	1	1	0	0	0	0	1	1

Source: St Bartholomew's Hospital Archives, Ha/20/36.

It should be noted that Table 5.2 omits sixteen soldiers whose admission dates are unclear and excludes five entries without a recorded discharge date and sixteen that only provide the year of admission: six in 1691, eight in 1692, one in 1693 and one in 1694. The figures for May and November 1695, July 1696 and April 1697 each include one death.

Table 5.3 St Bartholomew's Hospital: soldier admissions and discharges, 1689–1697

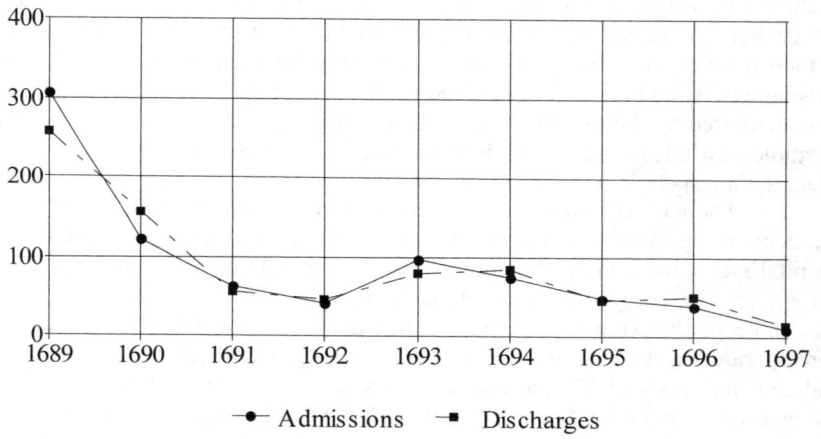

Source: St Bartholomew's Hospital Archives, Ha/20/36.

By far the largest group of soldier admissions, as might be expected, came from the units most commonly quartered in London, that is to say the relatively small number of Household troops, particularly the three regiments of Foot Guards. For example, of the 818 entries recorded, including those admitted before 1 January 1689, over half, 403, were from the five troops of Life Guards and three regiments of Foot Guards as opposed to 396 from all of the remaining regiments of the line (and including 19 Dutch soldiers). Similar factors affected the number of troops admitted from line regiments. For example, Colonel Babington's (later 6th Foot) and Lord Cutt's Regiments, units from which jointly some 108 soldiers were admitted, had both served on the Dutch establishment prior to accompanying William of Orange on his journey to England in 1688. As a result, they were highly favoured by the new king and, from May 1689, Babington's were billeted in and around London, initially at Hounslow and, later, at Tower Hamlets in the immediate vicinity of St Bartholomew's; Lord Cutts's troops were possibly also based in the same neighbourhood.[13]

Apart from the Household troops and the two regiments just mentioned, no more than five units, one of which was the Royal Hospital, Chelsea, sent more than ten soldiers to St Bartholomew's Hospital during the entire recorded eight-year period. The majority are only recorded on two or three occasions and it is therefore tempting to speculate that, although St Bartholomew's Hospital received significant numbers of ill soldiers during 1689–90 (probably repatriated casualties from King William's war in Ireland, once that war had been concluded) the London Poor Hospitals' work involvement with soldier patients was more to do with the treatment of routine sickness among London's garrison troops rather than the direct reception and treatment of evacuated battle injuries. Those battle injuries that were admitted probably arrived as referrals from the surgeons working in the ports of disembarkation. Such patients would probably have spent a reasonable time in military hospitals close to the field of battle, been repatriated through the chain of evacuation to England and subsequently cared for at their port of arrival. As has been suggested earlier, having survived most of the life-threatening aspects of their injuries, only the permanently disabled with conditions requiring long-term nursing care would have been referred to the London hospitals. Such a scenario is also supported by the fact that the deaths of only four soldiers were recorded in St Bartholomew's Hospital during the eight years from 1689 to 1697, coupled with an average time spent in hospital of less than three months.

At St Thomas' Hospital matters were conducted somewhat differently and, as the accounting system in use there left much to be desired, the extent of the hospital's involvement in the care of service patients is much more difficult to determine. The hospital accounts indicate that no payments were received during the whole of the Nine Years' War, a fact that is corroborated by contemporary correspondence. As early as 17 July 1691, the hospital's surgeons claimed that they had, thus far, treated 1,771 patients, mostly seamen, since the beginning of the war, but their petition fell on deaf ears.[14] The following year English troops were sent to Flanders and, between 19 to 20 May 1692, the Royal Navy gained a decisive but bloody victory against the French Fleet at Cap La Hogue. After this latter battle, St Thomas' Hospital admitted 150 seamen and, in order to make sufficient room for the influx, an equal number of pre-existing in-patients had to be found alternative accommodation in nearby houses, a situation that became commonplace for the duration of the war. In due course, the Governors of both St Bartholomew's and St Thomas' Hospitals were spurred into submitting an appeal to the Commissioners for Sick and Wounded Seamen for payment of the monies due to them in respect of soldiers admitted since the beginning of the war. Unfortunately, at St Thomas', their request remained unanswered.[15]

Surprisingly, after this one, unsuccessful, half-hearted petition in 1692 the hospital's Governors failed to pursue the matter for another ten years, during which time soldiers and seamen continued to be admitted to their hospital. The Nine Years' War ended in 1697 without St Thomas' Hospital receiving any payment whatsoever in respect of the work undertaken in caring for sick and wounded soldiers and seamen throughout the war. It is only as a result of peculation by members of the hospital's staff that anything is known of the contemporary situation regarding the admission of service personnel. Making the most of his trusted position, the hospital steward decided that one of the benefits of his office allowed him to demand 5d from each soldier discharged from hospital in return for the necessary certificate required for presentation by the soldier to his unit on rejoining the ranks.[16] In due course, some 50 soldiers took exception to this imposition and refused to pay the charge but, despite the questionable legality of the steward's actions, the system seems to have been condoned by the hospital's Governors, who agreed to offset the steward's losses by paying him the equivalent amount out of hospital funds. In the event, the steward died prematurely but, nevertheless, the Governors abided by their decision and paid 25s to Elizabeth Whitehill, his widow, in respect of the 50 certificates issued to the soldiers who had refused to pay.[17]

More seriously, on 25 March 1702, Dr Richard Torlesse, the hospital's principal physician, and Thomas Elton, the senior surgeon, took it upon themselves without the prior knowledge of the Governors, to write to the Commissioners for Sick and Wounded Seamen in an attempt to acquire some personal financial reimbursement for their work with service personnel. They argued that even if the Commissioners agreed to settle for a single payment of £200 per annum, a total of £2,000 for the ten years in question, that figure would only provide £40 for each member of the medical staff when divided between all of them. In the event the petitioners pressed for a sum equivalent to the regulation allowance of 6s 8d per head.

In their reply, the Commissioners tried to bargain with the medical staff by offering to pay them 5s per patient but, on 16 April, when Torlesse and Elton responded to this offer, they held out resolutely for their 6s 8d per-patient fee and listed three major elements in their defence. First, they claimed that their work was undervalued in comparison with the rates paid to contracted surgeons working in the major ports of Deal, Portsmouth and Rochester, for whom the Lords of the Admiralty had authorized a salary of £400 per annum plus £20 for each amputation performed. Second, they pointed out that most of the patients sent to them for treatment were suffering from conditions that required long-term care and, in many cases, were referred by the port surgeons who, in any case, 'always sent the worst of their patients to this house'.[18] Their third point was a reminder to the Commissioners that the patients admitted to St Thomas' Hospital were accommodated and fed without charge whereas those treated in the ports were paid an accommodation allowance of 6s a day.[19]

Torlesse and Elton then went on to claim that the huge total of some 4,146 soldiers and seamen had been treated in St Thomas' between 1689 and 30 June 1698 but no indication was given as to how that figure had been arrived at, nor was any indication given regarding how many were seamen, soldiers or prisoners of war. Eventually, it was agreed that they would be paid at the regulation rate of 6s 8d per head as originally requested, 'considering what great service the Government would have in future from the said hospital'.[20] Their award, which significantly made no mention of the other surgeons and members of staff, translated into a total sum due of £1,382 but, although that figure was agreed, they had to settle for payment in three instalments. The first third was paid to Torlesse on 1 May and the second to Elton on 22 June but, in the event, instead of the £460 13s 4d due to each, they only received 300 guineas apiece, the remainder being swallowed up by intermediaries for 'services rendered' during the negotiations.[21] Torlesse and Elton, however, had failed to inform either their hospital Governors or their colleagues of their dealings with the Commissioners.

On 7 October, in response to an order from the Lord High Admiral, the Commissioners for Sick and Wounded Seamen were summoned to a meeting of the Court of Governors with the express intention of establishing how many seamen the hospital could receive in case of emergency. The Commissioners were reminded not only that the foundation was for 'the relief of all poor, sick and diseased persons in general without [particular] regard to the soldiers and seamen', but also that the Governors of the hospital had hitherto always demonstrated their willingness to do whatever they could in emergency situations. The hospital would continue to accept as many sick and wounded seamen as could be conveniently accommodated providing as much notice as possible was received on each occasion. The meeting concluded with a request for the usual allowances to be continued.[22] Four months later, on 12 February 1703, the Governors received a letter from Mr King, Secretary to the Committee for Sick and Wounded Seamen, asking for an account of what seamen were taken into and discharged from this hospital during the Nine Years' War and also of what monies had been paid to the hospital or any of its officers by that Committee.

In discussion with the Committee for Public Accounts, Mr King was told that although large sums of money had been issued by the Committee for Sick and Wounded Seamen for medicines and patient care in the London hospitals, strangely no sum whatsoever appeared to have been received by St Thomas' Hospital. The Committee immediately summoned the physicians, surgeons and apothecaries and questioned them, both collectively and separately, as a result of which the activities of Dr Torlesse and Mr Elton during the previous year came to light. The two officers claimed that once they had received the final payment they would have distributed the money between themselves and their colleagues in proportionate amounts but, when the other hospital doctors and surgeons declared that they were in no way privy to this arrangement or to the receipt of any money, the Committee decided that Dr Torlesse and Mr Elton had acted illegally in both soliciting for and receiving the money without proper approval and ordered their suspension and, pending further investigations, confiscated the monies they had received.[23] It is surprising that, despite, or indeed as a result of, the furore caused by the Torlesse and Elton incident, there is no evidence of any further payments being made to the hospital for soldiers admitted during the Nine Years' War.[24]

Torlesse and Elton's figures remain the only accessible information relating to service admissions to St Thomas' but, given that the personalities involved were doubtless anxious to provide the highest possible total of service admissions to suit their own material ends, their figures must be regarded with scepticism.[25] Their figure of 4,146 service admissions is remarkably high in comparison with that of St Bartholomew's Hospital, and refers to seamen rather than to soldiers.[26] It is currently impossible to make accurate comparisons with the known figures for St Bartholomew's Hospital although it might appear, superficially, that St Bartholomew's Hospital received redominantly soldier patients and St Thomas' sailors. Any conclusions reached regarding the division of labour between the two hospitals as regards the admission of service personnel would be speculative.

Notes

1. For a description of the disturbances in the London hospitals during the First Dutch War see Gruber von Arni, Ch. 6.
2. Moore, II, p. 333; Sir D'Arcy Powers, *A Short History of St Bartholomew's Hospital, 1123–1903* (London, 1923), p. 83. James Pearce, the army's Surgeon-General, was appointed one of the Governors of St Thomas' Hospital on 28 May 1686: F.G. Parsons, vol. 2, pp. 116–7.
3. Powers, p. 48.
4. St Katherine's Hospital was demolished in 1825 to make way for the construction of St Katherine's Dock.
5. TNA, SP 44/164, fol. 297: Broad Street, Old Gravel Lane (later renamed Wapping Lane) and Nightingale Lane were adjacent to St Katherine's Hospital.
6. LMA, H1/ST/A91/1; Parsons, vol. 2, pp. 116–17; Powers, p. 48.
7. Powers, p. 48.
8. HMC *Dartmouth Mss*, p. 143.
9. LMA, H1/ST/A91, fol. 2.
10. Ibid., fol. 4.
11. St Bartholomew's Hospital Archives, Hb/1/9–13 and Hb2/1–2, *passim*.
12. St Bartholomew's Hospital Archives, Ha/20/36.
13. R. Cannon, *Regimental Records of the Sixth or Royal First Warwickshire Regiment of Foot* (London: Longman, Orme & Co, 1893), p. 20.
14. LMA, H1/ST/A91, fol. 9.
15. LMA, H1/ST/A16, fol. 42.
16. Ibid.
17. Ibid.
18. Ibid., fol. 99.
19. Ibid.
20. Ibid., fol. 100.
21. Ibid.
22. LMA, H1/ST/A6/4, fol. 81.
23. Ibid., fol. 83.
24. Ibid., fol. 97.
25. LMA, HO1/ST/B/001/001. Admission register of wounded seamen; Letter Archivist to Author of 12 June 2003. As a result of the scandal, a register of wounded seamen, including the names of their respective ships as well as the Dutch prisoners admitted to St Thomas' Hospital between August 1672 and October 1692, was made available to the Governors. Whether soldiers are included cannot, at present, be determined as, although this document has survived, its condition renders it unavailable for scrutiny until conservation techniques have rendered it suitable for public access.
26. In an undated draft, now lying among the hospital's papers in London's Metropolitan Archives, a former archivist of St Thomas' Hospital has commented that he could find no surviving evidence that soldiers from the guards and garrisons of London had been admitted.

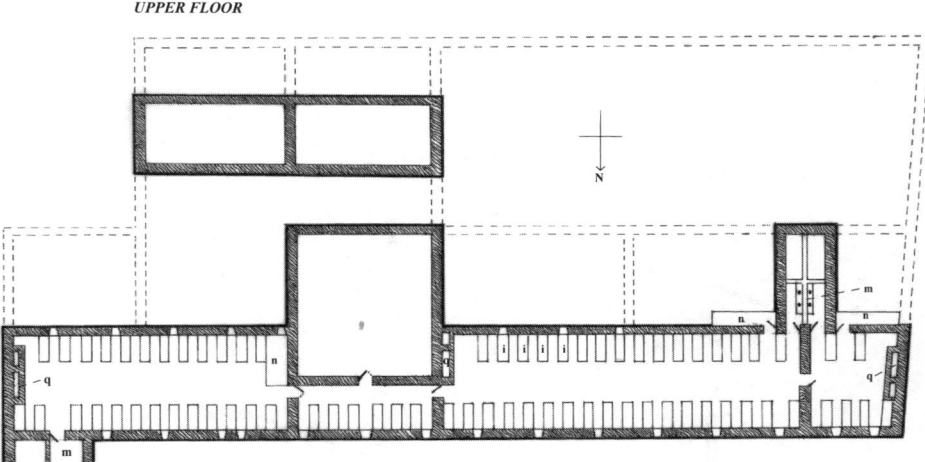

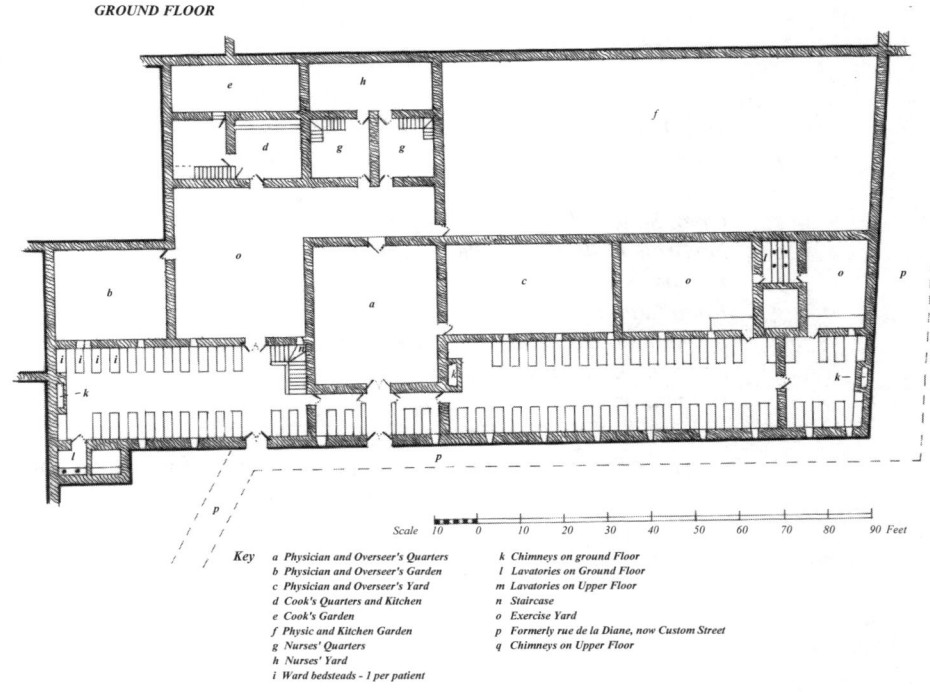

Key
a Physician and Overseer's Quarters
b Physician and Overseer's Garden
c Physician and Overseer's Yard
d Cook's Quarters and Kitchen
e Cook's Garden
f Physic and Kitchen Garden
g Nurses' Quarters
h Nurses' Yard
i Ward bedsteads - 1 per patient
k Chimneys on ground Floor
l Lavatories on Ground Floor
m Lavatories on Upper Floor
n Staircase
o Exercise Yard
p Formerly rue de la Diane, now Custom Street
q Chimneys on Upper Floor

1 Plan of the garrison hospital in Tangier, 1662–1683

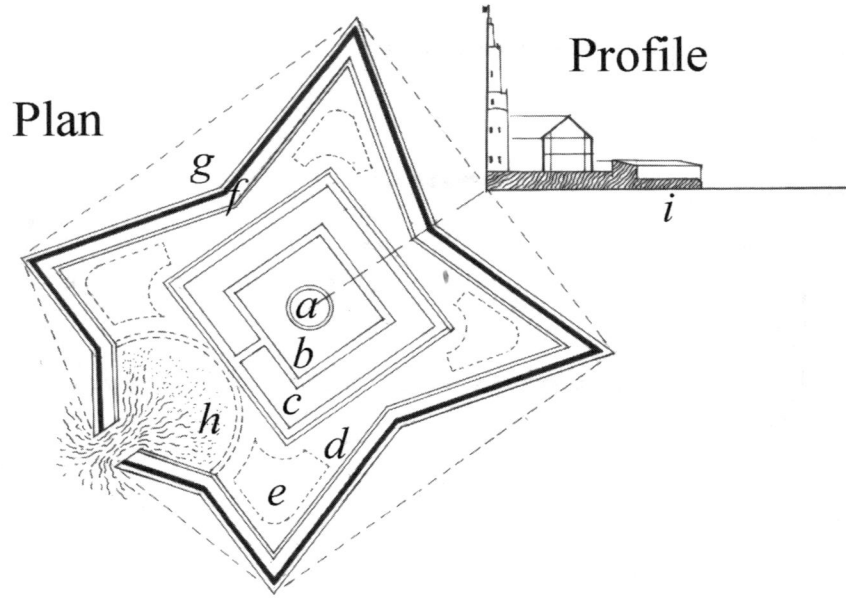

Key
a   Lighthouse
b   Courtyard
c   Buildings
d   Open Space
e   Separate buildings for the quarantine of infected goods or people
f   Ramparts
g   Foundations
h   A small mole and harbour for securing boats in foul weather and for the convenient landing of goods
i   Ground level

2   Plan of Sir Hugh Cholmley's proposed lazarette for the port and town of Tangier, April 1675

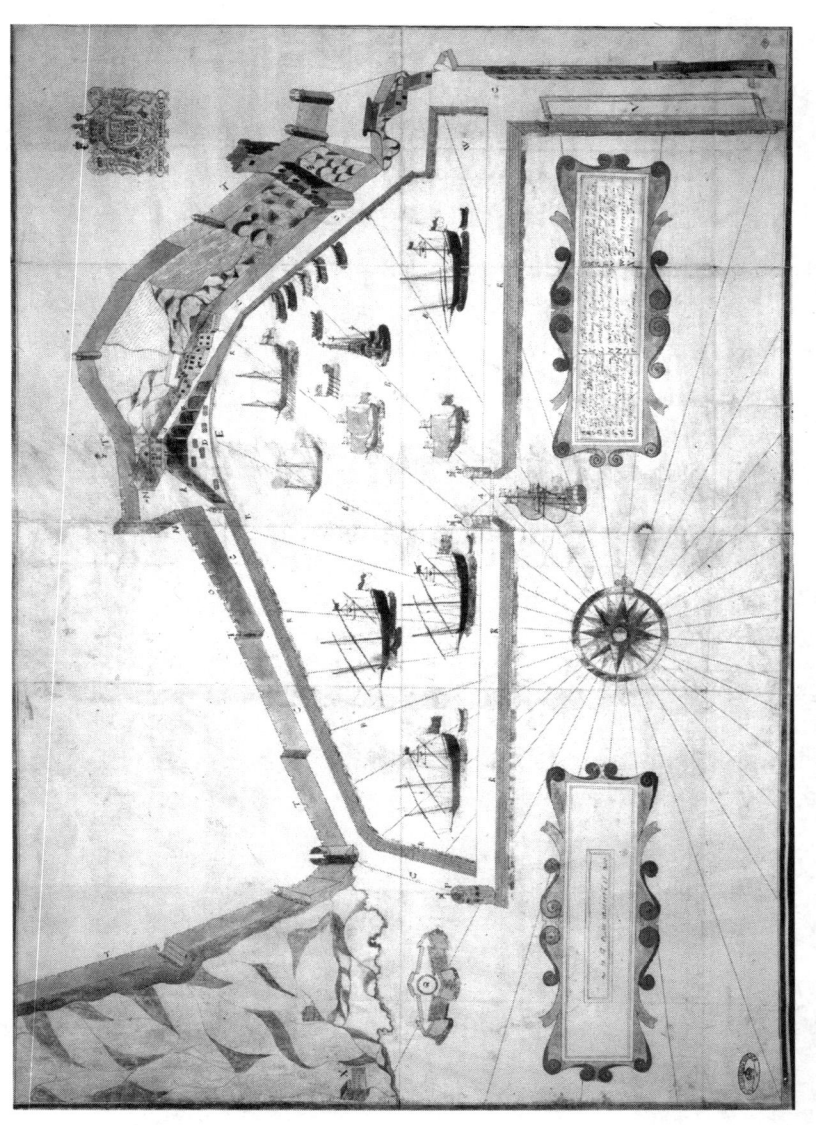

3 Sir Hugh Cholmley's design for the proposed mole, showing the intended site for the lazarette to the south of the mole and harbour (the cruciform structure on the extreme left of the drawing)

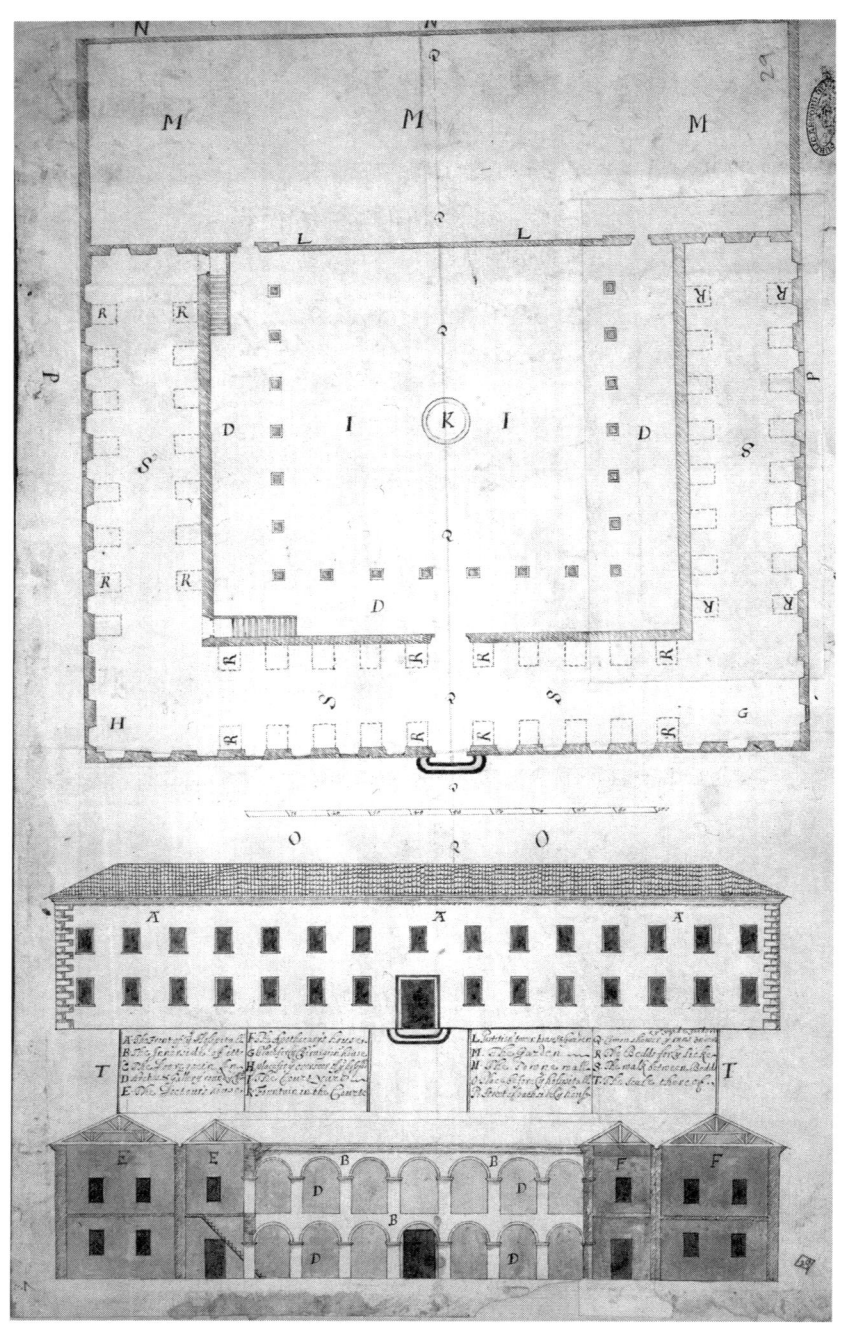

4 Sir Hugh Cholmley's proposal for a garrison hospital for Tangier, 1677

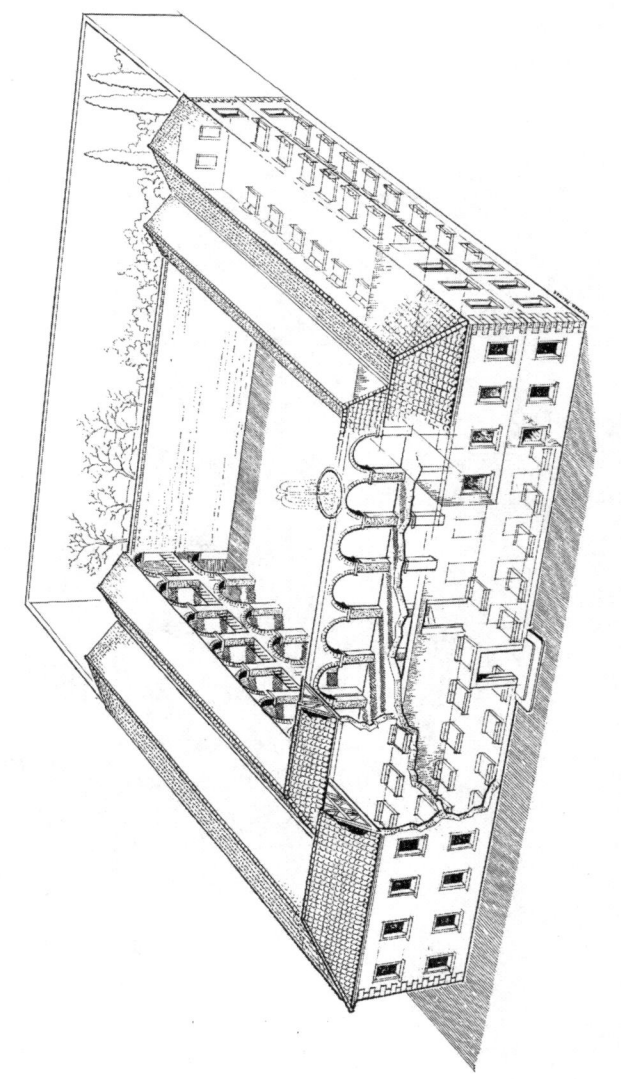

5 Artist's impression of Sir Hugh Cholmley's proposed garrison hospital for Tangier 1677

6 Artist's impression of the Hospital built for the encampments on Hounslow Heath, 1685–1688

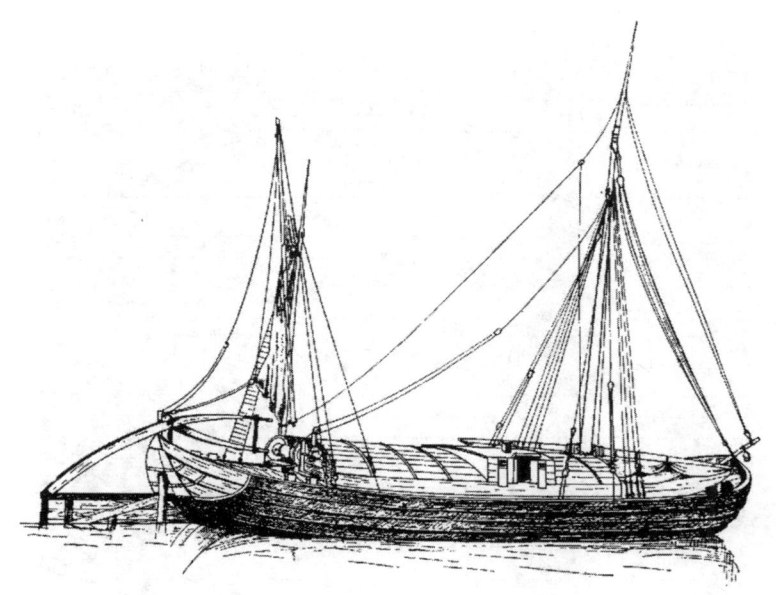

7 A bijlander (or walenmajohl)

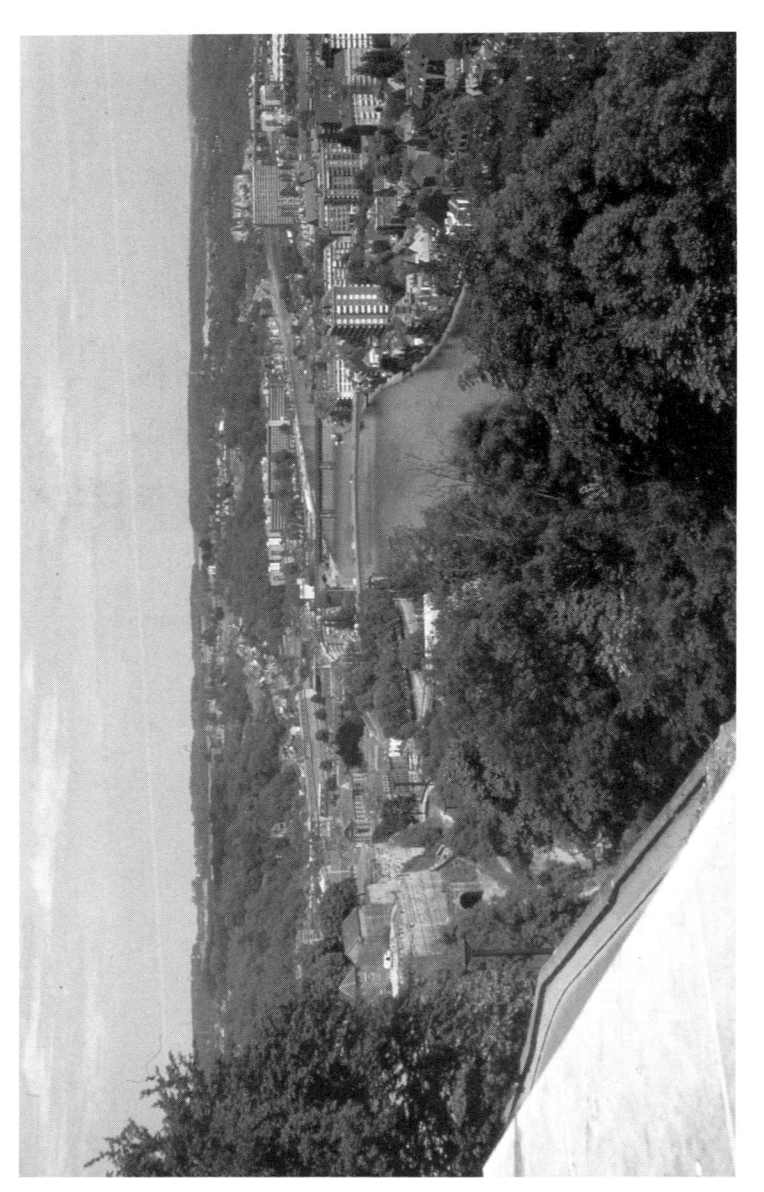

8 The River Maas looking east from the Citadel of Namur

This is the direction taken by the transports carrying the wounded to Liège after the capture of the fortress in 1695

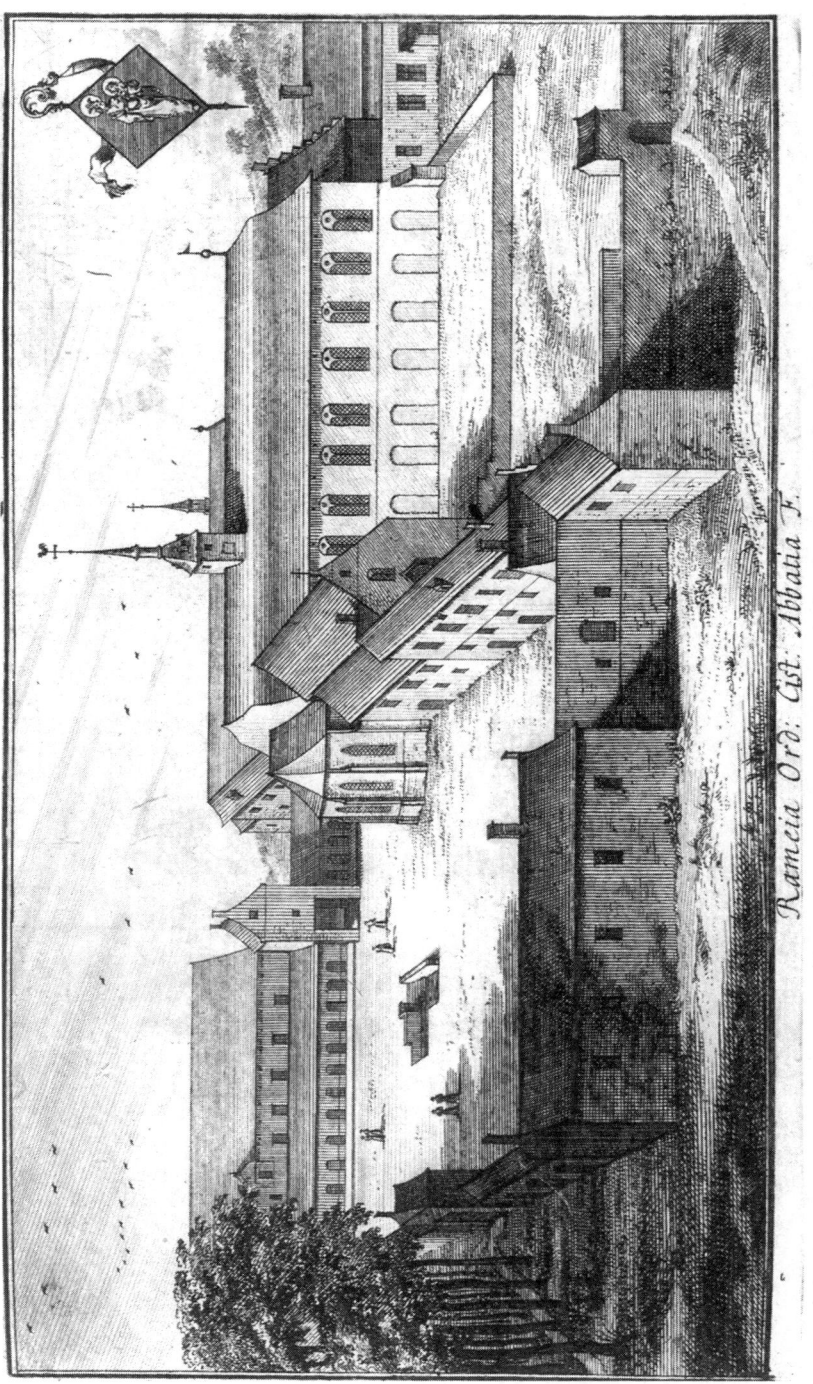

9 An engraving of 1696 showing the Abbey of La Ramée
The abbey would have looked very similar to this at the time of the battle of Ramillies in 1706 when it was used as a field hospital

10 The Bijloke Hospital: Main gate looking north

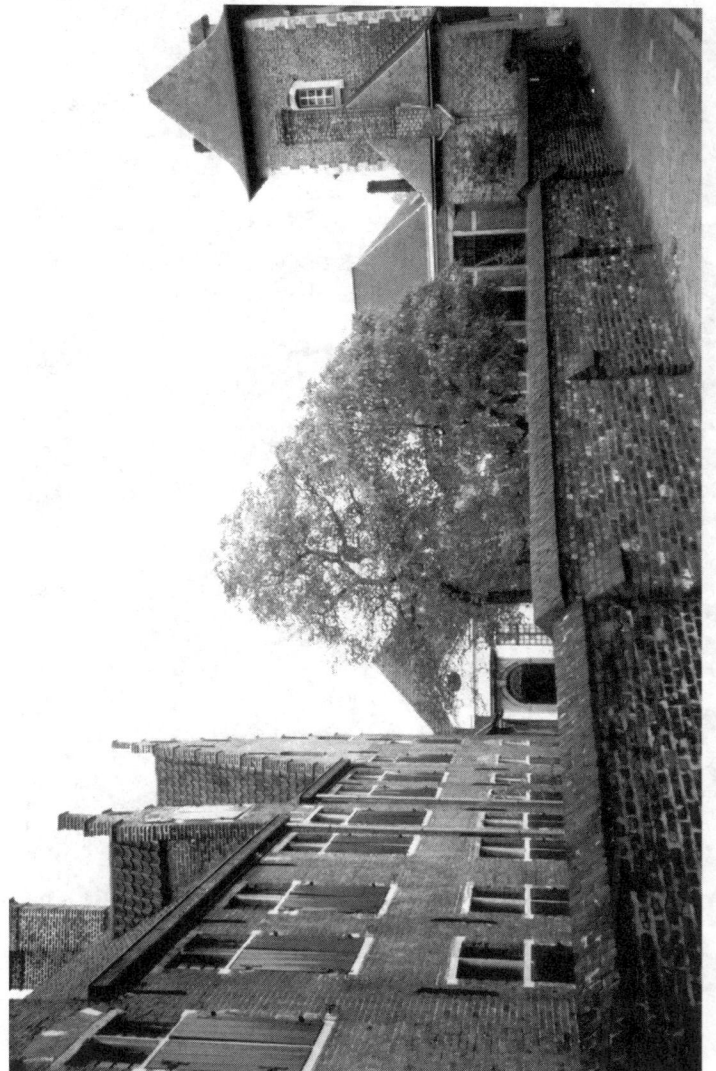

11 The Bijloke Hospital: Main gate looking south

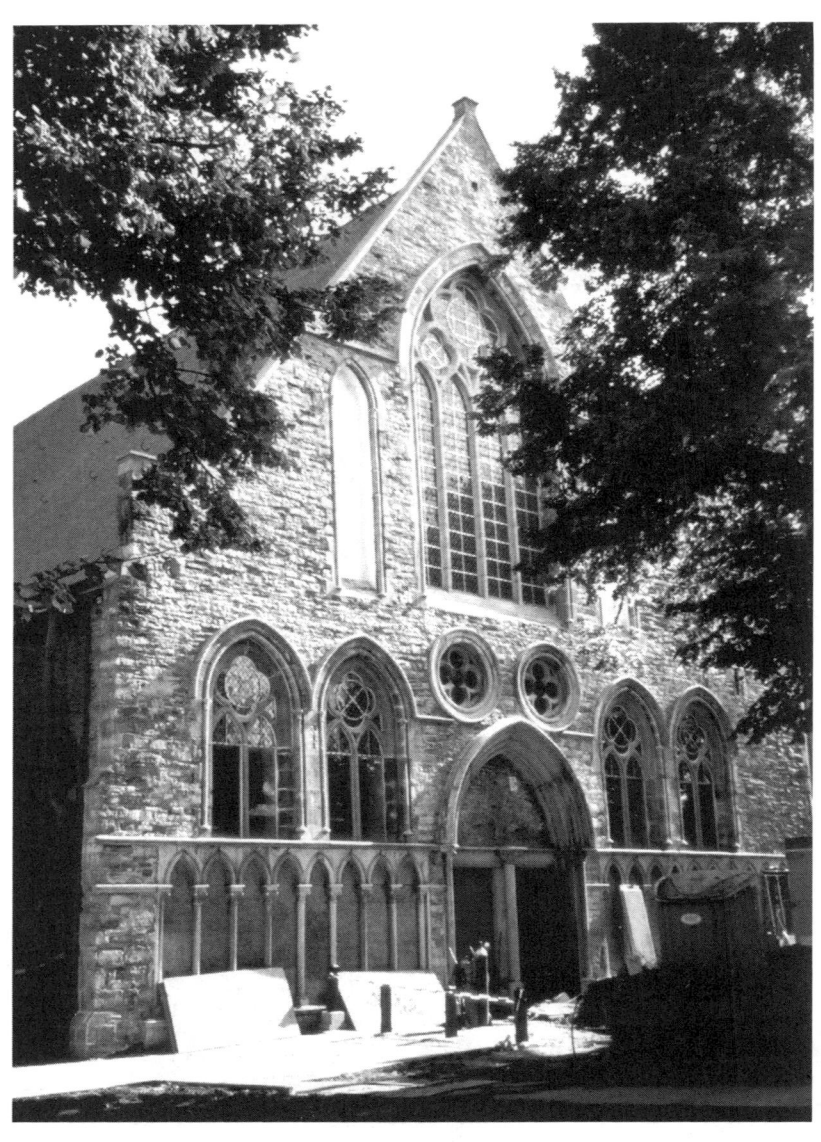

12 The Bijloke Hospital: Entrance to the Main Ward

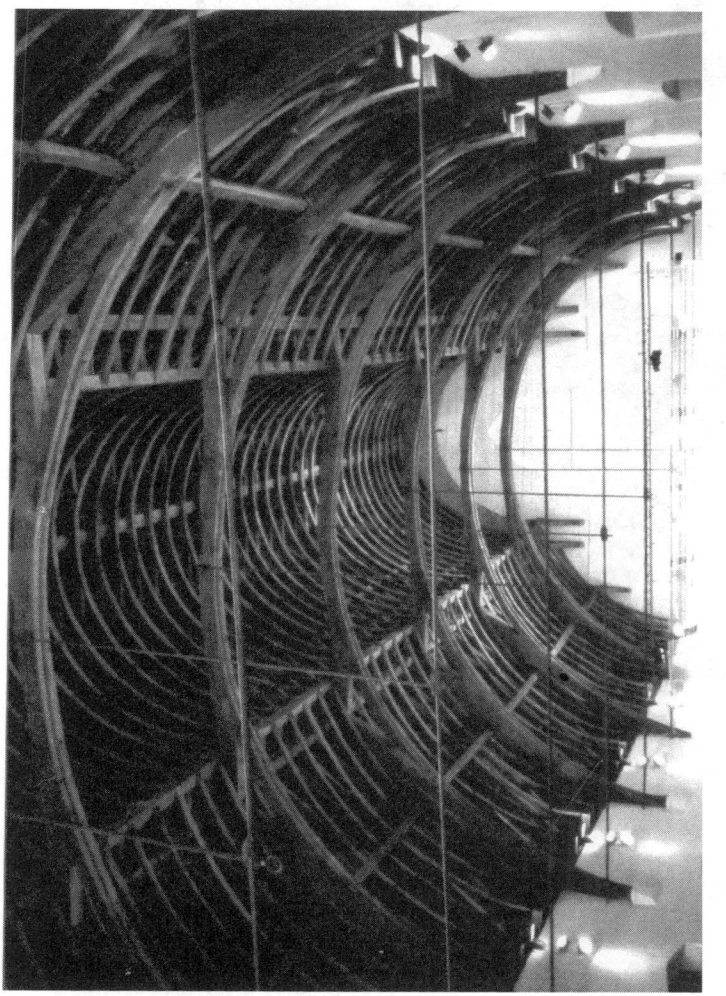

13 The Bijloke Hospital: Roof beams of the Main Ward
(now a Concert Hall)
Note the high ceiling typical of medieval hospital wards

14 St John's Hospital, Bruges, showing proximity to canal access

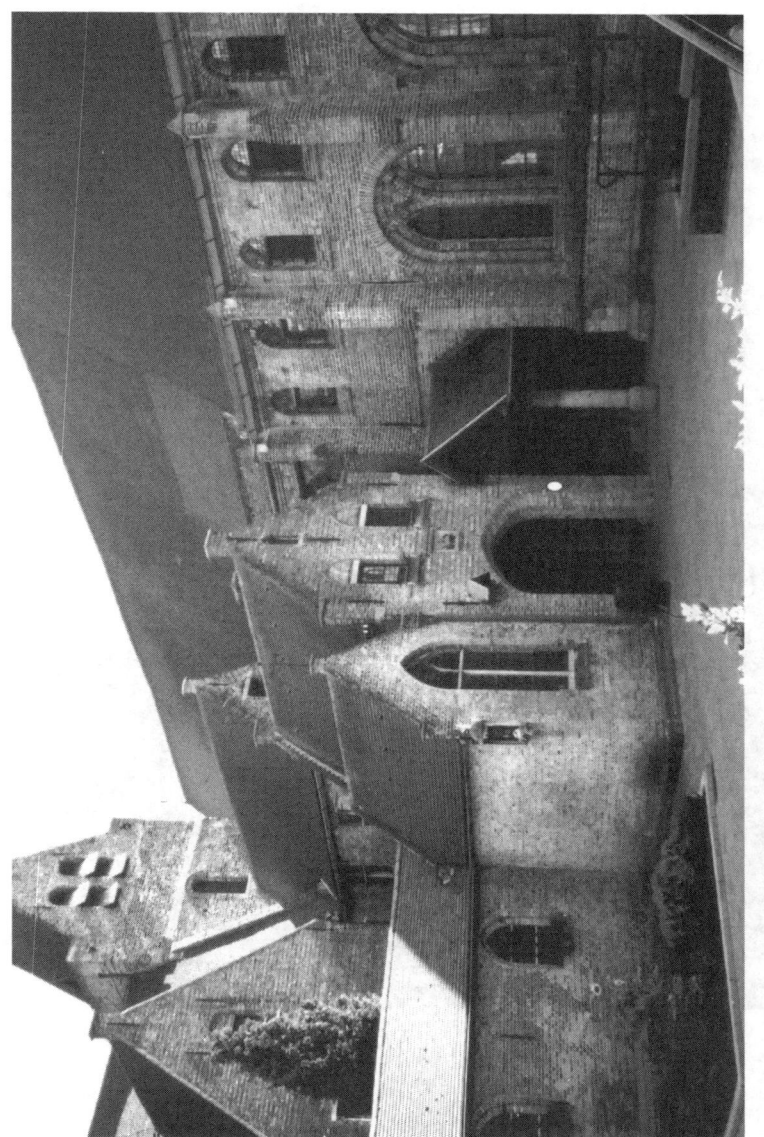

15 St John's Hospital, Bruges: Inner courtyard with main ward building on the right

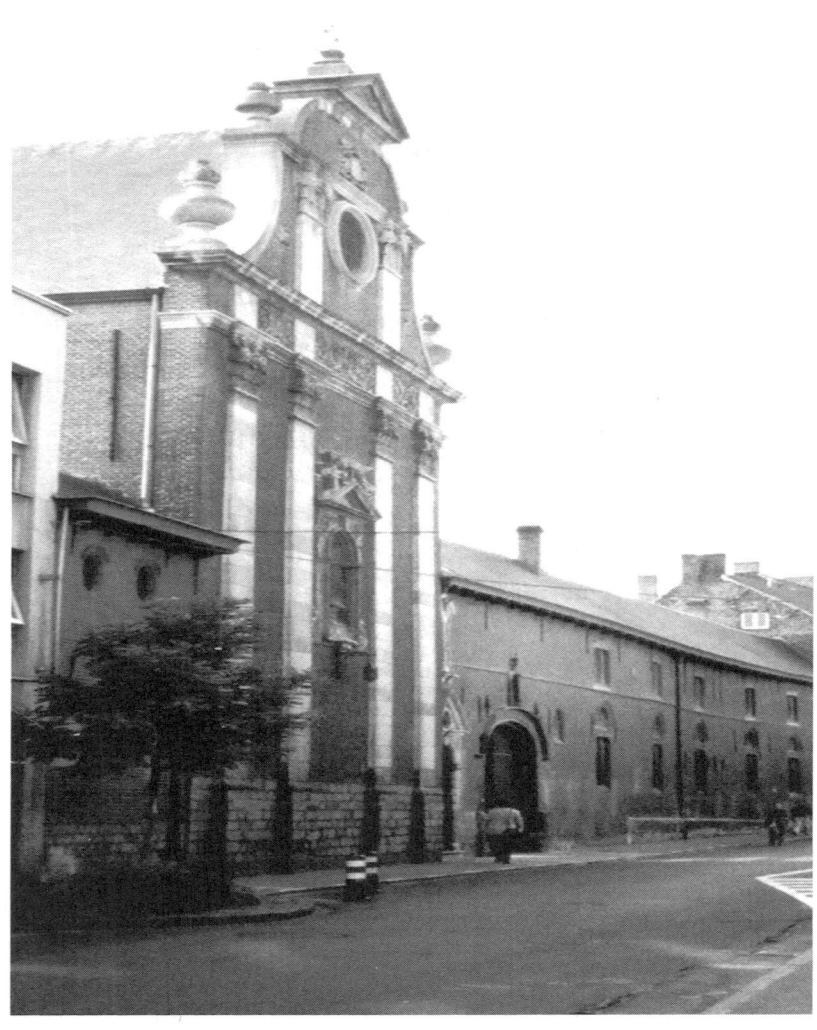

16 The Hospital of Our Lady, Courtrai

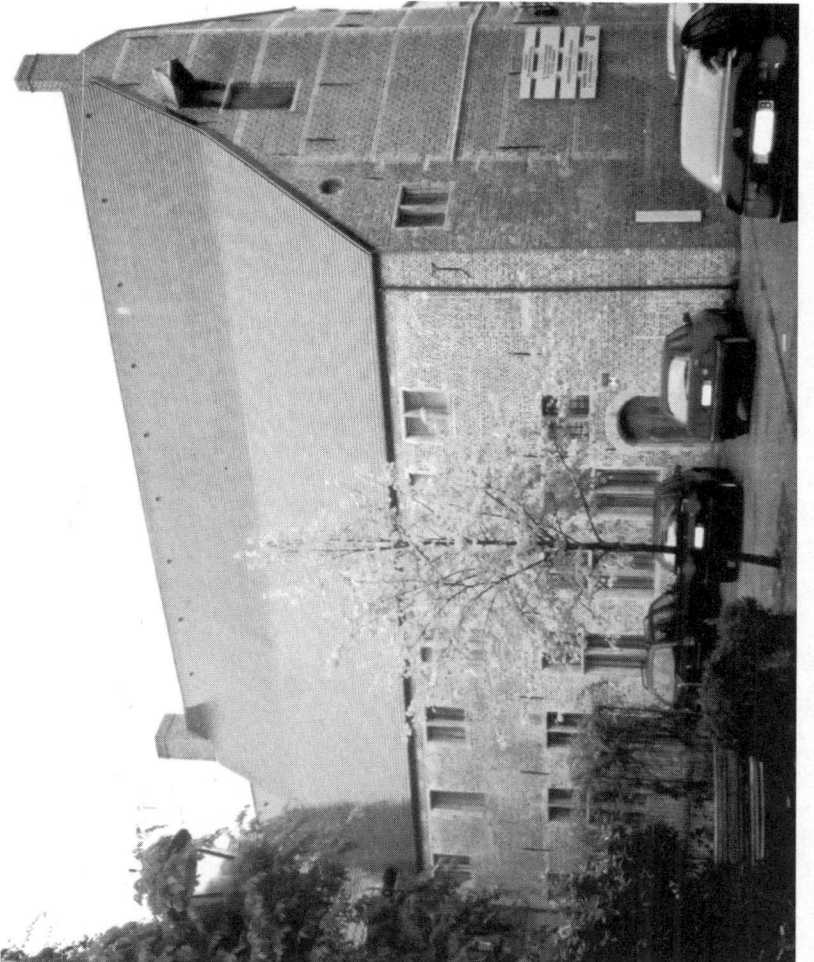

17 The house of the Cell Brothers, Mecklin

Chapter 6

Hospital Provision during Marlborough's Campaigns

In his classic work *The Armies of Queen Anne*, a highly respected description of the organization and function of Marlborough's army, Scouller claims that:

> while the Physician General and Apothecary General exercised a vague supervision over the provision of medicines ... any central [medical] organization or arrangement in a campaign area was purely *ad hoc* and had to be staffed within the existing theatre establishment.[1]

He then proceeds to emphasize his assertion by adding that it was 'doubtful how many of the staff were military, and our figures will not be far wrong if we ignore them completely' and later 'it is safe to say that the medical services of Anne's armies were remarkable for mismanagement, brutality, inhumanity and, possibly, corruption'.[2] Obviously, Scouller does not rate the medical services of Queen Anne's armies very highly although, in his research, he does not appear to have looked too deeply into Marlborough's surviving papers and associated documents, now held by the British Library, when compiling his work. The following two chapters will provide a more balanced and, perhaps, more accurate assessment.

The War of the Spanish Succession was fought to maintain a balance of power in Europe. By 1700, in the eyes of William III and others, Louis XIV of France had threatened the equilibrium of European politics by agreeing to his grandson, Philip, Duke of Anjou, succeeding to the throne of Spain following the death of the Spanish King Charles II. For the rest of Europe it required no great leap of imagination to appreciate that a merger of the thrones of France and Spain was a very real possibility. Apart from the potential loss of maritime trade with Spanish territories, particularly in the Americas, a joint Franco-Spanish military policy became a very real danger.

Under the terms of the Peace of Ryswick, the frontier fortresses of the Spanish Netherlands had been garrisoned by Dutch troops as a barrier to any future French aggression. Early in February 1701, with the connivance of the Elector of Bavaria, the governor of the Spanish Netherlands, a French army under Marshall Boufflers crossed the border, surprised the garrisons of the border fortresses, known collectively as 'the Dutch barrier', and almost overnight 15,000 Dutch troops became prisoners of the French. By this *coup de main*, Louis's northern border, which had formerly stretched from Calais to Metz, was realigned to run from

Antwerp and the Scheldt estuary in the west through Liège to the hills of Luxembourg in the east.

On 6 September 1701 James II died in exile at St Germaine. At his bedside, Louis of France, in denial of his agreement at the Peace of Ryswick four years earlier, promised to recognize the former monarch's son, James Francis Edward, as King of England and, amidst pomp and pageantry, the pretender to the throne was proclaimed King of England on French soil by French heralds. As far as the British were concerned, this insult was the final straw.

The health of William III was deteriorating rapidly but, ever conscious of the threat posed by Louis against both the United Provinces and England, he began the process of repairing the damage to his army caused by the wholesale reduction of forces that had followed the Peace of Ryswick. One of his earliest actions in this regard was to seek advice regarding the provision of military medical care. A contractor, John Hudson, was invited to submit an estimate of the costs involved in providing hospital care should a force be deployed to the Continent in the near future.[3] Hudson based his figures on earlier experience gained during the Nine Years' War, and worked on the premise that, 'one month with another, there will be not less than a thousand sick in an army of 18,000 men', but qualified this with an optimistic assumption that any future campaign season would last no longer than 200 days. The submission was also based on the correct assumption that the former practice of closing the hospitals when the army went into winter quarters would continue.

Hudson gained the contract having agreed that, in return for receiving 'into his hospital any soldier who is in the pay of the United Provinces or of England or Denmark', he would receive 12 styvers per day for each soldier admitted. In return, each sick or wounded soldier would be provided with bread, bedding, clothing and medical attention.[4] As regards the staff, Hudson proposed that his medical personnel should consist of three physicians, three master surgeons, eight surgeons' mates, one master apothecary and four apothecaries' mates. He also suggested that the hospital's stock of medicines and utensils should be valued at £400, the contents of which were to be viewed and approved by both the Physician General and the Surgeon General.

On campaign, the decision when and where to establish a hospital lay in the hands of the Commander in Chief or his sub-commanders, who identified the town or location nominated to receive the army's sick and wounded and then informed the Contractor accordingly. Hudson's personal description of his appointment as 'Comptroller of His Majesty's Town and Field Hospitals in Flanders' indicates that, from the start, he intended to repeat the earlier formula of maintaining both static and mobile hospitals. Even so, as Hudson pointed out, due to lack of available accommodation and adequate staff, it was unlikely that the English hospitals could accept all the sick and wounded that occurred during the campaign. In the light of experience gained ten years earlier it was recognized that, if casualties were to receive treatment as soon as possible, it would be necessary for patients to be routinely admitted to whatever Dutch hospitals were available and willing to receive them. To ensure that, under such arrangements, anyone so admitted received appropriate treatment, the radical concept was introduced whereby patients would receive an extra 5½ styvers daily, over and above their normal remuneration of just over 5 styvers a day, thereby, theoretically, doubling their income. From this sum they would be expected to pay for their food, accommodation, the services of a physician or surgeon and any additional treatment that they received. This extra payment was to be reduced to 3½ styvers if the patient was very ill, presumably because he would then require less food. An additional hospital was to be provided for garrison troops. Regardless of where the casualties were sent, Hudson was required to provide the Commander in Chief with an up-to-date statement, every one or two weeks, of the numbers admitted, died, discharged or remaining in the hospitals throughout the army.[5]

King William III died on 8 March 1702 and was succeeded by his sister-in-law, Anne, who ascended the throne on a wave of public loyalty and Protestant fervour. Eight weeks later, on 4 May, England, allied to Austria and the United Provinces, declared war against France and Spain. The Earl of Marlborough was created Captain General of the British forces as well as Anne's plenipotentiary to the States General of the United Provinces. He left London on 23 May and, following his arrival at The Hague, he undertook the mammoth task of organizing his British troops while engaging in protracted negotiations with his Dutch Allies. In due course he was accepted by the other allied nations as the Captain General of all allied troops in the Low Countries and, on 2 July, moved his joint army headquarters to Nijmegen where he concentrated a force of some 60,000 men. As the town chosen for the Commander in Chief's headquarters, Nijmegen would have been a logical site for the establishment of base hospital facilities but Hudson's accounts, which recorded a payment of 30 guilders for 'making clean the hospital at the Bosch ... with presents to obtain the same', indicate that it was actually deployed adjacent to an existing Dutch hospital at 'sHertogenbosch, commonly referred to as 'den Bosch'.[6]

The British medical staff in Flanders at that time included the Physician General, Dr Thomas Lawrence, who for four months was assisted by Dr Oliphant, another physician who had seen considerable previous service in Flanders. Isaac Teale remained as Apothecary General while the master surgeons' vacancies were filled by Claudius Amyand and Messrs Wilson and Inglish, all of whom served throughout the ensuing campaign, assisted by Mr Gowdy, a surgeon's mate.[7]

From the outset the hospital admitted a steady trickle of patients suffering from the various diseases that inevitably occur in any large concentration of troops – but it wasn't long before battle casualties began to arrive and, through July, the hospital at 'sHertogenbosch contained an average of 306 in-patients, as shown in Table 6.1.

Table 6.1 Sick and wounded in the British hospital at 'sHertogenbosch, 27 June–20 July 1702

	27 June–1 July	1–5 July	5–12 July	13–20 July
Bed Occupancy	316	294	292	321
Admissions	0	66	41	46
Discharges	2	90	43	17
Deaths	0	1	3	4

Source: BL Add. Mss 61318, fols 233–4.

From 5 to 25 September Fort St Michael and the Citadel at Venlo were besieged and captured by allied forces, followed shortly afterwards by the town of Roermond. Of the more than 400 sick and wounded allied soldiers resulting from these actions, some 297 British were brought the short distance down the river Rhine by horse-drawn barges to the hospital where an average of over 300 beds had been continually occupied since June.[8]

In addition to the figures quoted above, the Dutch hospitals were paid nearly 7,000 guilders for the 6,940 soldier-days (a daily average of 56 patients) spent by British soldiers in their establishments between 27 June and 1 October 1702.[9] Later, in a letter written on 9 November, Marlborough's secretary, Adam Cardonnell, informed Hudson that the Duke had approved his leaving 30 sick men in the care of the Dutch Hospital when the British unit was closed at the end of the campaign season.[10] Reciprocal arrangements were also offered to the Dutch. During August another base hospital had been opened in Maastricht where Hudson was instructed to accept soldiers of the United Provinces under the same financial arrangements as offered by the Dutch for their treatment of British soldiers.

During that first campaign season of 1702, the sick and wounded British and allied troops in British pay were also cared for in a variety of hastily formed locations where the flying hospitals set up their facilities. For example, on 23 October, an order was issued for two houses to be made available for use as a hospital for the army in Bourgue and, on the same day, Marlborough wrote from Liège to the Mayor of the village of Herstal requesting him to provide two houses in his village for use as a hospital for the army's sick and wounded.[11] The Duke also showed concern for the allied troops in British pay and, seven days later, he wrote to the magistrates of the town of Visse, asking them to furnish four houses for the sick and wounded of the allied troops from Luneburg and to furnish the officers who accompanied them with rations and forage.[12]

As Director of Hospitals throughout the years that Marlborough fought in Flanders, John Hudson maintained meticulous accounts that were submitted for audit on a monthly and annual basis. These documents, which form a treasure trove of information on the various hospitals' day-to-day transactions, were each laid out in an identical fashion starting with the tasks necessary to secure a safe environment when first setting up a hospital. These included the cleaning rooms and windows, mending leaking roofs and generally putting the building in acceptable order. An initial stock of stores and equipment was dispatched from England each spring but this was seldom sufficient to satisfy demand. Beds in particular were either hired or constructed by local carpenters. Bedding, including 'coverlids', palliasses and pillows, was also made on the spot. Large quantities of straw were needed to fill the mattresses and also to renew the same from time to time.

Old linen, in significant quantities, was required for use as wound dressings and bandages and, as many soldiers arrived almost naked, clothing for the patients, especially shirts and nightcaps, was in constant demand. Local assistance was recruited to wash the soldiers' clothes, linen and woollens as well as for digging graves and burying the dead. Wood, turf and charcoal were also in constant demand for the kitchens as well as for heating the rooms, especially those containing patients suffering from 'the bloody flux' (dysentery). Chairs, earthenware drinking mugs, chamber pots, porringers, jugs and cans, lamps, candles and oil, wash tubs 'for the convenience of the men' and also kettles and utensils, such as ladles and spoons, for the kitchen were all acquired locally. Food purchases, which were many and various, included meat, either mutton, beef or veal, bread, beer, cheese, rice, milk 'to mix with the water for drinking posset drinks or to mix with flour', oatmeal, sugar, salt, wine and brandy, eggs, butter and nutmeg, cinnamon and the various other herbs and spices used in the preparation of cordials and tisanes (herbal teas). Gruel, and milk 'to burn with the wine and brandy', were all cited as were candles, and soap to wash the men's linen. Naturally, the hospital clerks were in constant need of books, paper, ink and the payment of postal charges.

Next came lists of payments to hospital 'servants', a term that included the wages, at 8 styvers per head, paid to nurses 'that attended the sick and wounded men with a head nurse to oversee the rest', the butler, cook, washerwomen, various assistants and a porter who 'ran errands and drew water'. It is this figure of 8 styvers per nurse, per day, that has been used later in this chapter to calculate the number of nurses employed in hospitals. The accounts concluded with entries detailing receipts, including the deductions taken from the pay of soldiers admitted to hospital, a statement of amounts spent on burying the dead and, finally, a list of extraordinary expenses particular to the period in question.

Any qualitative assessment of the standards of care offered must attempt to establish norms as regards contemporary expectations and, to this end, it is necessary to compare British arrangements with those of the enemy. During the War of the Spanish Succession the French army was supported by 50 military hospitals, the provision of which was arranged by contracting out to private entrepreneurs whose actions were subject to regular inspection. As late as 1708, an ordinance was passed that determined the permanent establishment of military hospital staff – although it is more than likely that the ordinance merely recognized existing practices. The combined total of medical staff consisted of 50 médecins-major (physicians), 50 chirurgiens-major (surgeons), plus 22 other superior doctors and surgeons charged with inspecting the hospitals and advising their physicians and surgeons.[13]

The provision of nurses in French hospitals was based on a standard allocation of one nurse to every ward of 15 beds although, if the work-load increased, more could be employed up to a maximum of three when patient numbers rose above 30. They were paid in local currency at the equivalent of 1¼d in contemporary English money per day plus about 5d for their food. In total, each nurse was paid 9 guilders (18s) per month. If they became sick they received care in the same manner as if they were soldiers.

The heating of the wards and the washing of patients' nightshirts and caps was also the entrepreneur's responsibility and, although a basic issue of shirts and caps was made at government expense, the contractor was authorized to sell shirts to patients who were admitted to the hospital without sufficient clothing. Food, medicines and equipment were also purchased from private contractors. In 1701, at a French military hospital in Antwerp, a local contractor, Monsieur DeLuke, had assumed responsibility for supplying food items to the hospital.[14] His contract, dated 7 September, stipulated that, in return for a basic payment of 7 sols, 6 deniers per day for every sick or wounded soldier, he was required to provide each soldier admitted to the hospital with a pound of meat per day, in the ratio of two-thirds beef and one-third veal or mutton, with the quantities of veal and mutton dictated by the physician or surgeons according to the needs of specific patients. Bread was also supplied to each patient according to the individual's condition. Convalescent patients each received a daily ration of 21 ounces divided through the day as 10½ ounces for breakfast, 6½ ounces for lunch and 5 ounces for supper. Alternative diets were provided according to the patient's condition and included either a half-portion of 10½ ounces of bread daily or, for those on quarter-rations, 5¼ ounces. Only white bread was to be supplied to hospital patients.

DeLuke's contract also required him to supply 'small' beer, 'of a quality mid-way between strong and weak beer', white or red wine and hot milk in such quantities as were stipulated by the hospital physician or surgeon. Eggs were also provided in large quantities, both for consumption by the patients and for use by the surgeons and apothecaries in compounding various topical applications. Although DeLuke's contract exempted him from paying tax or duty on the bread, beer, meat, utensils and coal that he supplied to the hospital, it was also made very clear to him that he was to make appropriate allowances for variations in patient numbers and that he should take steps to avoid waste wherever possible. It was hardly necessary to remind the contractor of this as excessive costs for purchases and over-stocking would, inevitably, have reduced his personal profits.

When a soldier was declared fit for discharge from hospital the contractor was required to ensure that he was correctly equipped and provided with the necessary accoutrements so that he could report to his unit fit for duty in all respects. In addition, he was to be issued with 1½ days' rations for the return journey to his unit. When soldiers died in the French hospital, DeLuke was entitled to claim payment of 3 guilders for each suit of clothing subsequently returned to the regiment concerned. In comparison, the British system entitled Hudson to a rebate of only 1 guilder for each suit of clothing returned.

It is evident that apart from the number of hospitals provided, the French system of hospital care contained many similarities to the British equivalent and vice versa. Much of this may be due to the fact that, some years earlier, during the second and third Dutch Wars, English personnel working with the French army gained first-hand practical experience of continental methods and subsequently carried the knowledge home with them. As noted earlier in this work, King William III had introduced the Dutch military medical system into the English army with considerable success during his Irish campaign and later, as the wars progressed, contact with the French, even as enemies, may well have added further refinements, especially through contacts made via the channels of prisoner exchange.

When Isaac Teale, the British Apothecary General, submitted his pre-deployment estimate for field units, he stipulated that each of the twelve regiments nominated for the campaign would receive a pair of medicine chests valued at £24 5s.[15] These were to be augmented by a reserve stock valued at £30, an amount that Teale believed would be adequate to provide for the needs of patients who remained in regimental lines or billeted in civilian houses as well as those in the hospital. As might be expected, he paid particular attention to the provision of medicines for the use of the General or other officers, despite the fact that the cost of these was included in the overall supply of drugs covered by the ongoing system of deductions taken from soldiers' pay. Whether or not officers entered into private arrangements to pay Teale for drugs that he supplied to them is not known, but it seems likely and, if such were the case, Teale would have been paid twice for the same items at the expense of the soldiers. Teale proceeded to end his statement with a request that, should his submission be approved, he required as much notice as possible to allow him sufficient time to gather and pack the necessary items.[16]

The contents of regimental surgeons' chests had not changed over the previous ten years and were, therefore, identical to those supplied to King William's army (as listed in Appendix E). In the event, matters were taken out of Teale's hands. An undated comment written by Hudson in 1702 refers to 22 pairs of surgeons' chests costing between £17 8s and £20 each that were delivered to the deployed regiments having been packed locally in a hired building in Rotterdam. This represented a saving of £3 10s per pair of chests on the normal London price, a saving that was made without any loss of quality as, in Hudson's opinion, the quality of goods supplied was 'extraordinarily good'.[17] This was a unique arrangement that flew in the face of the normal monopoly whereby drugs were supplied by contract through the Apothecary General and Apothecaries' Hall in London. It more closely resembled the French system for drug supply whereby, rather than centrally ordering medicines and materials through an Apothecary General, they preferred to place individual orders for these items with local tradesmen, such as in Antwerp where this was arranged through a master apothecary and burger of Mecklin, Monsieur Jean Albert van Meurt. Van Meurt was required to supply everything needed in the way of drugs, external applications, brandy, wine, beer and vinegar for fomentations, his own linen, pottery wares, the receptacles necessary to contain and distribute medicines and the coal needed to heat his apparatus. The main exceptions were surgical instruments, which were furnished by each individual hospital surgeon, and herbal drinks which were supplied by the Commissary of Provisions.

In the British service, apothecaries received a statutory rate of pay regardless of their work. Under the French system, van Meurt's pay depended upon the accuracy of his accounts, which listed the actual amounts issued and consumed each month by the chief surgeon. His relationships with the surgeons were fraught with opportunities for conflict as van Meurt's instructions required him to maintain strict supervision over the conduct of the surgeons and their mates in order to prevent them 'misbehaving whether by passion, mischievousness or other means, with the wine or linen or other articles'. Equally, he was advised to maintain his own records of the numbers of wounded who have 'unbalanced humours, sciatica, paralysis and others who require external remedies' and cautioned not to permit unnecessary or exorbitant use of commodities, particularly those ordered as a result of the personal preferences of surgeons for expensive items.

Marlborough's attitude towards the health and welfare of his troops was also tempered by measures introduced to prevent abuse of the system. Elements of the Duke's standing orders stipulated that regimental adjutants were required to ensure that their sick were sent promptly to the hospital and also to maintain a daily record of all who had reported sick, were admitted to or discharged from hospital.[18] As a means of reducing the risk of patients absconding in transit to the hospital, a nominated individual was to accompany the sick and return with a receipt for the number delivered. Meanwhile, regimental surgeons recorded every sick man's name, along with their illness and date of attendance, and specified whether the patient was sent to the regimental or another hospital. They were expected to visit their sick twice daily and report on their progress each morning to the Commanding Officer. If a regimental sub-unit with a strength in excess of 200 men were deployed, either the surgeon or his mate was expected to accompany the detachment. Partly for this reason, surgeons maintained their own independent personal transport and carried their medicine chests and instruments on a packhorse.

One wagon was allowed to each regiment for the movement of sick soldiers unable to march. These would travel in the rear of the regiment while additional transport could also be requested prior to a march and would be provided, one per regiment, in the form of bread wagons. These would subsequently be returned to the commissariat wagon park as soon as possible after a halt was called. Women, children and baggage were specifically excluded from travelling in these vehicles.

With regard to the spiritual and welfare needs of the patients, chaplains were required to visit the sick in hospital on a shared rotational basis. The wives of wounded English soldiers who had been captured and admitted into the enemy's hospitals were able to apply to their husbands' commanding officers for travel passes and approval to visit them but, when such permission was granted, for security reasons they would not be permitted to return to their own lines until their husbands were exchanged and could return with them.

Soon after the deployment of British troops to Flanders in 1702, an additional set of rules for the 'better government of Her Majesty's land-forces in the Low

Countries and parts beyond the Seas' was issued covering a wide variety of aspects of service life.[19] In contrast with the proprietorial vagaries of the army's management systems in former years, a firmer grip, possibly Marlborough's, is evident amidst the minutely detailed instructions that covered and improved a broad spectrum of the soldiers' social condition. Officers were to ensure that the men's quarters were kept clean and tidy. If a soldier died, his personal belongings were to be protected and, if anyone misappropriated them, the offenders would be liable to trial by court martial and face penalties that included a fine of twice the value of the stolen items. The officer in charge of the deceased's company was required to take such property into safekeeping and dispose of it in payment of any outstanding debts that the soldier may have incurred. Any surplus would then be held and made available to the next of kin, who could claim the same within three months of the soldier's death. After a victorious battle, captured enemy ordnance, ammunition and victuals were to be secured for general use by the army but one-tenth of any spoils were to be set aside for the relief of the casualties. The sick and wounded continued to receive their pay until it became apparent that they would never regain their fitness for further service. In such cases arrangements were made for them to return to their homes with sufficient money for their journey.

Once they were back in England there was no single authority nominated to assume responsibility for their immediate care. Inevitably, as had happened so often in the past, when soldiers began to arrive in the east coast ports the local citizens began, with justification, to protest. In one instance at Harwich deserters entered the town masquerading as disabled soldiers recently evacuated from Holland. This led to the Lord Treasurer instructing the Mayor of Harwich that, in future, he was to ensure that checks were made so that relief was only offered to servicemen who carried appropriate certificates signed by a regimental officer and to arrest deserters.[20] The captains of the packet-boats that plied between the east coast and Flanders also received orders to carry only those soldiers who could produce a certificate showing the true nature of their situation.[21]

As has been mentioned earlier, it was accepted military practice that fighting was normally confined to the summer months and hospitals closed when the troops went into winter quarters. The campaigns of Marlborough were no exception. At the end of each campaign season patients who were fit enough to move were usually repatriated to England while those whose condition precluded them from making the journey were admitted to local civilian hospitals. Some were even discharged from the service while still in Flanders in accordance with a set of published instructions whereby officers in command of garrisons, acting on the advice of their medical staff, were the ultimate authority for determining which soldiers were unfit for service.[22] In such cases instructions would be passed to the soldiers' company commanders or commanding officers to pay each soldier his dues up to the day of his discharge. Subsequently, when the disabled soldiers were ready to leave and everyone had been issued with the appropriate passes and paperwork, a commissioned officer conducted them in a group to their port of embarkation, taking care that they had adequate warm clothing. The nominated officer carried sufficient money to pay for all their meals and accommodation until his charges were embarked. The amount issued was based on a set rate of 2 styvers per day for every private foot soldier, 7 for dragoons and 10 for each trooper of Horse. In addition, immediately prior to their sailing, the officer was to pay each soldier 14 days' subsistence money at the same rate to cover their journey home after landing.

Once they had sailed, the conducting officer was required to remain in the port of embarkation for two or three days in case the ship was forced back by contrary winds, in which case he was to continue his supervision of the men and provide them with food and lodging allowances for as long as they remained in port and then make good their 14 days' subsistence allowance from the time of their re-embarkation and final departure, presumably out of his own pocket until he, in turn, could be reimbursed.

Rather than enter winter quarters at the end of a campaign, some regiments returned to England. Frequently the sick men of these regiments travelled with them and were subsequently deposited in naval hospitals at Deal or Portsmouth, whichever was closest to the port of disembarkation. Such was the case when Brigadier Livesey, with six regiments under his command, arrived at Ostend for embarkation with orders to land at Deal where he left the sick men of his regiments in the local hospital.[23] Meanwhile a proportion of the physicians and surgeons accompanying Livesey's brigade remained in Ostend caring for any sick who were unable to make the channel crossing until they, in turn, were fit to complete their journey.[24]

Once they had arrived home, those who were certified unfit for further service could apply for admission as pensioners to the Royal Hospital at Chelsea and there, as elsewhere in society at that time, it helped if a prominent patron was willing to support their application. For example, on 6 January 1703, the Duke of Marlborough wrote to David Crawford, the current Governor, with a request for him to admit 27 wounded soldiers who had recently returned from Flanders.[25] This was by no means exceptional. Indeed, most of the candidates who presented themselves for admission after service in Flanders and Germany during the remaining years of the war were accompanied by a personal recommendation from the Duke. Others carried letters of introduction signed by the Secretary at War on behalf of the Queen's husband, Prince George of Denmark, nominal Commander in Chief of the army.[26] For example, as late as 5 November 1711, George Granville, then Secretary at War, replied to the Governor of the Royal Hospital after presenting a letter from the latter to the Queen:

> concerning the miserable condition of the invalid soldiers discharged and sent home from the army abroad, for want of having some suitable subsistence or pension money issued to them and for want of quarters. Her Majesty has been pleased to represent the same to the Lord Treasurer in an especial manner, to the end that some further provision and better care may be taken of those poor people for the future. At the same time I am to desire that you will let me know that quarters are already allotted to all those invalids for whom there is no room in the hospital, what enlargement would be suitable for you and what else you may have to propose ...[27]

This letter was copied to the Treasury with an added footnote stating that, if the current funds allotted to Chelsea were insufficient, a review was to be instigated and, subsequently, appropriate demands were to be submitted during the next session of Parliament. In due course, on 24 October 1712, it was eventually agreed that men who had been discharged unfit for further service, for whom there was no vacant place in Chelsea, were to be retained on the books of their regiments until such vacancies should occur. During this time the men to whom the arrangement applied retained their entitlement to their army pay. Similar improvements had been instigated in increased grants and pension payments to officers' widows and the plight of soldiers' widows had, at least, been recognized.

Meanwhile, as the war progressed and the number of casualties mounted, the burden on the east coast towns increased accordingly until, as late as 18 July 1709, after receiving a begging letter from the Justices of the Peace at Chelmsford, the Lord Treasurer, Godolphin, was forced to write to the Secretary at War, Walpole, requesting him to

> prepare a royal warrant for making a like allowance for the future for the cure and lodging of every disabled soldier brought from the Low Countries to Harwich as is made for disabled soldiers brought from Portugal to Falmouth; as likewise 5s for conduct money for each man from Harwich to Bow being 60 miles at a penny a mile.[28]

Godolphin's letter was prefixed by a report written earlier by Walpole in which the latter was forced to concede that no official provision had been made for conveying disabled soldiers from Harwich to London.[29] This admission was made in reply to a petition from Chelmsford's Justices of the Peace complaining that the Constables on the road between Harwich and Bow had spent £1,000 in relief and transport for 'the many poor sick, lame, maimed and disabled soldiers that have been weekly brought over in the packet boats from Holland'. These funds had been provided out of the parish rates and, in order to realize the necessary cash, the magistrates had been forced to raise local taxes to double, treble or in some cases quadruple the normal amount throughout the county of Essex. Naturally, this had brought forth widespread complaints from many communities situated some distance away from the Harwich Road who had rightly claimed that the situation was unreasonable, contrary to law and would very likely prove to be the cause of several future law suits.

Eventually, this correspondence brought about the creation of a new appointment with a specific officer assuming responsibility for the provision of care and transportation for sick and wounded soldiers landed at Harwich from Holland. Although the Committee for Sick and Wounded Seamen was henceforth no longer directly involved in the hands-on treatment and movement of such soldiers, its officials would still be required to certify the correctness of any accounts submitted by the new post holder. The army's Paymaster General would then make payment of the associated bills. Although these arrangements took time to implement, nine months later, in April 1710, Robert Hazlefoot was appointed to the office.[30]

At the end of the 1702 season, Hudson was particularly complimentary in his praise of the work carried out by his medical staff when he remarked that, without their assistance, 'the sick and wounded must have suffered greatly for want of those helps which their distressed condition did absolutely require'.[31] Some attention must have been paid to his comments as, at the beginning of 1703, the medical staff of the British hospital was expanded to include a third physician, Dr Nathaniel Ogle.[32] Isaac Teale, the Apothecary General, was to be assisted by three mates, James MacCartney, William Ore and Robert Puzey. Claudius Amyand and Alexander Inglish remained as master surgeons but were now joined by a third surgeon in the person of Richard Pear – although the number of surgeons' mates remained at only six, namely Robert Thomas, Simon Shoade, John Lynn, David Cockburn, Robert Rodham and John Goldy.[33] A warrant for the transportation of sixteen hospital officers and servants to the Low Countries, together with fifty chests, cases and hampers of medicines, was signed by Secretary Blathwayt on 11 March.[34]

From the outset of the 1703 campaign season, frustrating differences between the allied leaders emerged. A plan by Marlborough to capture the ports of Antwerp and Ostend was compromised by the Dutch withholding their support for any direct action other than the siege and capture of Bonn. The latter objective was captured after a siege lasting from 25 April to 15 May, but movements and counter-movements by both the Allied and French armies, without any significant gain by either side, took up most of the mid-summer. Eventually, Marlborough stormed and captured Huy on 25 August and the Dutch took Limbourg on 23 September, but by then the campaign season was coming to an end and no further significant action occurred that year.

The 1703 campaign had brought little change to the medical scene. In January 1704, Isaac Teale was ordered to supply 23 regimental surgeons' chests, followed by a demand for a further three in June.[35] In July a hospital was established in a church in Breda, alongside a Dutch facility, where Mr Inglish, the chief surgeon, was told to 'be as sparing as maybe' when fitting out the building. At the time, worries about the costs involved in providing hospitals for the army appear as a constant theme in Secretary Cardonnel's correspondence with Hudson and Teale. Cardonnel was a personal friend of Isaac Teale and, in a letter sent by him to the Apothecary General on 15 June 1703, he had confided to him that the Duke regarded many of the current charges as extravagant:

> you know only too well that the opinion His Grace has of the Physick and therefore may guess how displeased he will be to find that each man ... costs seven to eight styvers a day. If the numbers get more you would get nothing at all so consult the physicians and take measure accordingly.[36]

In due course Cardonnel announced the imposition of a limitation of the daily expenditure on each hospital patient's food to 3 styvers, a sum that he claimed would provide the prescribed daily ration for hospital patients. This consisted of three-quarters of a pound of meat, one-quarter pound of cheese and one and a half loaves of bread together with broth, water gruel, butter and eggs – 'at which rate', he added, 'one would think they should have little want of physick'. As a final comment, he added 'I have said 3 styvers a day as last year the men were well taken care of at the Dutch hospital at the Bosch for 2 styvers a day above deductions'.[37] Strangely, when shortly afterwards the 1703 rate for treating British soldiers in Dutch hospitals was raised to 8 styvers per man per day, an increase of 6 styvers on the rate of the previous year, it seems to have passed unnoticed.[38]

Three weeks later, on 5 July, Cardonnel sent yet another letter to Teale advising him that 'if you have any extraordinaries, surgeons' instruments, old linen etc., put it in an article apart from the account of the physick'. In other words Cardonnel was suggesting that his friend Teale should attempt to soften the impact of his true costs by splitting his consolidated bills into their component parts, thereby lessening the impact of a large overall figure. Teale was then informed that, in arrangements reminiscent of the hospital auditors established by William III during the Nine Years' War, it had been decided to nominate certain regimental officers to examine both Teale and Dr Lawrence's accounts every two or three days. Cardonnel's letter ended with the comment that 'If I were in Mr Hudson's place I should have no rest without it [as] I am sure his accounts will never be allowed in England'.[39]

Naturally, despite these financial difficulties, casualties continued to arise and the following day Lawrence, who was at the Duke's headquarters in Maastricht, was told that several sick soldiers were being sent to him for care as the army was moving forward and there were 'no officers nearer to care for them'.[40] When subsequently Hudson received orders to move forward to Maastricht, there were 63 patients in the buildings at Breda, with a further 93 men dispersed in local billets. However, almost a month had passed when, on 1 August, with the hospital still not having moved, Cardonnel hastened Hudson by repeating the Duke's orders, adding that, upon his arrival at Maastricht, further orders would be issued. Eventually, leaving one or two members of staff at Breda to care for the few patients left behind in 'private quarters', and carrying over 50 patients in hired wagons, the unit set out on its circuitous march to Maastricht, via Grave, Venlo and Roermond.[41] This longer route had been chosen due to the absence of an adequate escort, much to the annoyance of Marlborough, who complained that, had the hospital moved when first ordered, this would not have been necessary as it would have been screened from the enemy by the main body of his army. The hospital's progress was very slow and on 16 August Cardonnel wrote another highly critical letter to Hudson informing him of the Duke's displeasure that they had not even reached Maastricht where Dr Lawrence had been awaiting them with instructions for an onward journey to Liège.[42] The hospital subsequently remained in Liège until October when it was ordered to return to Maastricht prior to the winter closure.

Meanwhile, regarding the soldiers' spiritual welfare, Marlborough had noticed that, during both the 1702 and 1703 campaigns, several regimental chaplains had been absent from their place of duty without prior authority. The situation was deemed sufficiently serious to merit the publication, on 28 October 1703, of regulations that clearly laid down the chaplains' responsibilities. Henceforth, no chaplain was allowed to be absent from duty unless personally authorized by the

Duke of Marlborough himself. Even when a chaplain was fortunate enough to receive such an authority, he was personally required to ensure that his duties were performed by the chaplain of the adjoining regiment when in the field, or by a chaplain of the same garrison if in quarters. The Chaplain General, or the commander of the regiment concerned, had to certify that these duties had indeed been performed regularly during such absences. If the period of absence lasted for more than six months, the individual concerned would forfeit the whole of his subsistence allowance and the forfeited monies would be retained by the Paymaster for charitable use. In normal times, the Commissary General was required to certify that each chaplain was present with his unit when it was mustered on parade and note any who were absent.[43]

The following year, 1704, was remarkable in the history of the British army and one in which the medical services had to face greater challenges than any heretofore experienced. Having decided to take the war to the Elector of Bavaria's own territory by an audacious march from Flanders to the Danube, the Allies subsequently achieved two outstanding victories: the successful storming of the Schellenburg on 2 July and the almost total defeat of their French and Bavarian enemies at Blenheim on 13 August. Throughout these manoeuvres a hospital service was maintained as close to the fighting troops as was physically and tactically possible.

Numerically, few changes were evident in the medical establishment at the beginning of the year. The physicians, apothecaries and surgeons remained unchanged with the exception of surgeon Thomas Wilson, who took the place of Richard Pear, but there was a major turnover among the surgeons' mates, with only John Goldy and Robert Rodham remaining from the previous year. For whatever reason, possibly promotion to regimental surgeons' posts or as a result of personal career moves, the others had been replaced by Andrew Greyerson, Robert Lee and William Nelson while John Paulet (or Pawlet) had been promoted as assistant surgeon to the Artillery Train.[44]

As usual, when the campaign season opened, hospital equipment was recovered from warehouses in Rotterdam, assembled, sorted, washed and repaired while additional replacement and supplementary items were dispatched from England.[45] With the assistance of a local notary, two large *bijlanders* were hired for the campaign season together with another smaller craft for temporary use during the coming deployment. By 2 May Marlborough had completed his plans and Hudson received orders to load his boats, 'with beds, medicaments and other provisions for the hospitals'. These included 760 bedsteads, 650 pairs of sheets 'made from 14 ells* of material', 820 single blankets, 520 palliasse mattresses and bolsters, 2 large copper boilers for the kitchen and 11 smaller ones for surgical use, earthenware pots, jugs, pans, jars, mugs, washing tubs and buckets as well as 1,020 pairs of crutches.[46] The total value of these stores exceeded 9,000 guilders, approximately £900, a sum more than double the value of the reserve stock that had been proposed by Teale in 1702.

---

* An ell was a cloth measure that, in England, represented 45 inches (114 cm).

When everything was ready the three boats set off along the Rhine, forming a small flotilla in company with the transports carrying the artillery munitions. Unfortunately, they had not progressed very far when it was discovered that the smaller vessel was inadequate for its task and had to be replaced. As official military convoys on duty were not exempt from paying standard river tolls, there was considerable additional incidental expenditure associated with such a journey. Some 65 guilders were remitted in tolls at Bommel and at Arnhem, where a pass had to be purchased from the local representative of the States General. At Tiel another 25 guilders were expended on 'presents and gifts to the poor' while at Nijmegen a further pass required an extra 12 guilders.

Once again, Marlborough expressed his impatience over the slow progress of the hospital when, on 26 May, Cardonnel wrote to inform Hudson that he

> may well guess that we take you to be very dilatory in getting up to us and that the artillery boats were not yet reached Nijmegen on the 16th when you wrote to me from there. I acknowledged it yesterday and sent my letter to the Postmaster at Cologne to be delivered to you when you arrived there. I opened it again to give you warning that there were French parties roaming on this side of the river. His Excellency commands you not to stop at this place [Cologne] but hasten up with the rest of the boats as fast as possible to Mayence [Mainz] where you will receive further orders and inform yourself whether there be any sick left here and, if so, to bring them with you.[47]

After passing through Wesel, Düsseldorf and Cologne, the convoy arrived at Coblenz where, due to the increasingly dangerous, rocky nature of the river, Hudson was forced to stop and purchase ropes and a horse in order to continue the journey. Under tow from the river bank, the party eventually arrived at Mainz and, on 24 May, established a transit hospital in Kassel, a small village on the right bank of the Rhine above the city, for those who had fallen sick or been injured along the lines of communication. This hospital, led by Dr Oliphant, remained in use as a casualty collecting and medical staging post throughout the campaign season until 22 October.

On 6 June Hudson received instructions to proceed to Mannheim, where he was to acquire sufficient wagons for the carriage of his 'medicines and provisions and for such stores for the artillery as might be immediately necessary'. He was then to march with them, at all speed, to Gislingen via Heilbronn, leaving a sergeant and ten men as a guard on the artillery and hospital boats that were to remain at Mannheim.[48] However, a week later, on 14 June, these instructions were countermanded as the Duke's intelligence services had identified a French presence in the Mannheim area. Instead, Hudson was ordered to continue his journey by taking the boats up the river Maine via Frankfurt to Wertheim.

At Wertheim, the hospital and staff transferred to road transport for the final part of the journey to the village of Heidenheim, where a small transit hospital was formed. The weather had deteriorated, rain had fallen for several days and an unidentified sickness had broken out among the troops. On 22 June, Marlborough, who had ridden ahead with the cavalry, wrote to his brother General Charles Churchill who was further back along the line of march with the infantry:

> I received yesterday yours of the 20th at Blockingen, and having informed myself of the most proper place for sending your sick men, I am assured they will be best at Heidenheim, which is not far from you (about 35 miles), and therefore desire you will forthwith send them thither in carts with an able chirurgeon and a mate or two to look after them, and such commission[ed] and non-commission[ed] officers as you shall think fit, giving them at the same time money for their subsistence ... the enclosed is the Duke of Wurtemberg's order for your sick to be received in the town of Heidenheim.[49]

Marlborough had decided to divide his support services between two locations – Heidenheim, situated roughly halfway between Stuttgart and Augsburg, and Nordlingen, some twenty miles to the northeast, the latter being the larger storage base. On 22 June Marlborough's army joined with that of Prince Louis of Baden and, during the evening of 1 July, the decision was taken to attack the Bavarian troops who were attempting to fortify the Schellenburg, a prominent hill on the outskirts of Donauworth. That same evening, having made his decision, Marlborough demonstrated his awareness of the need for close medical support and his concern for the welfare of his troops by ensuring that the hospital was in the best possible location to treat the casualties that would inevitably be suffered during the forthcoming battle. He sent a dispatch to Hudson waiting at Heidenheim 'to hasten him [with the hospital] away to Nordlingen and to march day and night till he had settled with it there'.[50] Two additional messages were sent summoning the surgeons and apothecaries to the same place and enclosing a copy of a letter from Prince Louis addressed to the magistrates of Nordlingen requiring them to provide every assistance to the hospital.

After leaving a detachment in Heidenheim under the command of a regimental officer, Lieutenant Blake, to care for the patients under treatment there, elements of the main hospital left that location on 1 July and arrived in Nordlingen, some twelve miles north of Donauworth, on the morning of the day of battle. They established themselves in whatever buildings were available although most were in a state of disrepair and, over the next few days, local craftsmen had to be employed to improve both the structures and the fittings. For example, a blacksmith made or repaired ironwork in the kitchen, a glazier replaced window glass and a mason constructed a brick furnace for heating the copper boilers used to heat water for making herbal medicines and tisanes. The number of blankets supplied was insufficient and more were purchased locally, together with straw for filling the mattresses and bolsters. A nearby hot water spa was available and patients who were sufficiently mobile could make use of the facilities at the army's expense.[51]

The attack on the Schellenburg took place in the afternoon of 2 July. According to Lediard, of the 1,423 allied troops that were killed and nearly 3,981 who were wounded, the British suffered a total of 1,589 casualties. These are identified in Table 6.2. As the action ended a torrential downpour exacerbated the plight of the wounded and Marlborough issued orders for them to 'be dressed with all possible haste, and to be forthwith sent to the hospitals'. Indeed, the Duke appears to have personally superintended many of the tasks associated with the work of organizing casualty care that would normally have been delegated to a quartermaster or other subordinate officer.

Table 6.2 Casualty list for the storming of the Schellenburg

Rank	Killed	Wounded	Total
Officers	28	88	116
Sergeants	21	47	68
Private Soldiers	397	1,006	1,405
Totals	446	1,141	1,589

Source: T. Lediard, *The Life of John, Duke of Marlborough* (London, 1736), pp. 333–4.

Three days after the battle, widows who had lost husbands at the Schellenburg were ordered to report to the hospital for food, accommodation and to work as nurses while they waited for passes and passage money to enable them to return home.[52] Gathering them together in one place also enabled the staff to determine their numbers while retaining an element of control over them. On 7 July Cardonnel wrote again to Hudson, this time expressing his hope that the hospital was well settled in Nordlingen and also to request a 'very exact account' of the number of wounded men listed by regiment. After the battle, Hudson's hospital staff had been augmented by the addition of several regimental surgeons and their mates who volunteered their assistance. For a time this was tolerated but Hudson was advised that he should return those that could be spared back to their units as soon as possible. It is also worthy of mention that Marlborough's attitude towards hospital expenditure noticeably improved at this time. Cardonnel sent credit notes drawn against bankers in Nuremburg to the value of 12,823 guilders to Hudson and arrangements were also made for the merchants of Nordlingen to grant him extended credit.[53]

It was further suggested to Hudson that, if he had the room, he should transfer the sick who had been left at Heidenheim, described not so much as 'sick but rather half-foundered by the long marches so they want rather rest than physick', to Nordlingen, 'where they might be better looked after'.[54] However, the time was not appropriate for such a move as, apart from the large numbers of battle casualties under care, the local inhabitants of Nordlingen had started to complain about the presence in their town of so many garrison troops and military casualties. On 8 July a deputation had approached Marlborough asking for their burden to be reduced and, in due course, Hudson was asked to select the most convenient villages in the surrounding countryside where casualties with relatively minor injuries could be dispersed. It was also acknowledged that, for the time being, the sick in Heidenheim would have to remain where they were despite pleas from Lieutenant Blake that he did not have access to the services of a surgeon.[55]

The significant degree of cooperation between the allied leaders at this time, especially in casualty care, is evident in the response that Blake received to his requests from the Duke of Wurtemburg, the local ruler. Blake was authorized to billet the sick in local houses and was also granted permission to employ the best civilian surgeon that could be found locally.[56] A few days later, Hudson was told to ensure that Blake was provided with the necessary funds and assistance so that he could pay the nurses that had been employed at Heidenheim, who, it appears, had demanded a higher rate of pay than those working in Nordlingen.

On 11 July, Hudson was reassured that the Duke was 'very pleased with the care being taken of the sick and wounded' and had expressed the hope that some of them would soon be fit to return to their regiments, thereby easing the hospital's workload and improving the care available to the more seriously injured.[57] As mentioned earlier, several regimental surgeons had left their units to go and work in the hospital. By doing so they had left their regiments without immediate medical support and, aware of the possibility that a further major action was imminent, the Duke now issued orders insisting that they return to their normal place of work, 'as there may be occasion for them any day'. He did, however, agree that local medical practitioners could be hired to work in the hospital while the 'great throng of business' continued.[58] These were sound decisions as, on 13 August, the battle of Blenheim was fought with the joint forces of Marlborough and Prince Eugene winning a remarkable victory against the combined armies of the French and Bavarians. During the engagement the English and Dutch forces lost some 190 officers and 3,102 soldiers killed, with 464 officers and 4,927 soldiers wounded.[59] Such figures, serious as they were, demonstrate that the ratio of killed to wounded was significantly improved in comparison with those suffered in the battles of the Nine Years' War fought ten years earlier, as discussed in Chapter 4 above.

Very little information survives regarding the situation of the hospital in Nordlingen during the immediate aftermath of the battle. With over 5,000 casualties to treat, no doubt the surgeons were far too busy to put pen to paper. To make room for the new admissions, existing patients who had recovered sufficiently were discharged from the hospital to be cared for by their own regimental surgeons.

As soon as it could be arranged, those who were unfit for further service, but who could travel, were evacuated rearwards along the lines of communication to Heidenheim and Kassel via the same route by which the hospital had deployed at the start of the campaign. In Kassel, patients were able to rest pending their transfer into boats for their onward journey down the Rhine to Nijmegen. Some indication of the work carried out at Kassel can be found in the hospital's bills summarized in Table 6.3. Although it is not possible to assess daily bed occupancy from these figures, a rough estimate of patient numbers can be determined by dividing the total amounts of meat purchased by the number of days in the month and dividing the result again by the standard daily allowance of three-quarters of a pound of meat per patient. This figure can only provide an approximate guide as the hospital staff would also have been fed from these food purchases. Nevertheless, using this calculation, it would appear that the hospital housed an average of approximately

168 patients in June, 132 in July, only 90 in August but increased again to 154 in September. A final figure of 381 for the 22 days that the hospital remained opened during October must reflect an influx of patients that occurred during the evacuation of patients from Nordlingen. These calculations do not, of course, take account of patients who were on 'low' or 'milk' diets and therefore did not eat meat.

Table 6.3 Food items purchased for the Hospital at Kassel, 24 May–22 October 1704

Commodity	Jun	Jul	Aug	Sep	Oct
Meat (lb)	6,711	5,292	3,582	6,154	11,198
Bread (loaves)	7,113	5,661	3,918	6,505	11,703
Beer (firkins)	98	88	63	87	143
Cheese (lb)	1,352	1,074	719	887	1,865
Rice (lb)	525	431	323	529	933
Oatmeal (bushels)	36	36	23	33	61
Sugar (lb)	431	425	284	317	557
Eggs (each)	5,100	3,825	2,108	3,650	7,350
Butter (lb)	64	60	56	75	147

Source : BL Add. Mss, 61370, fol. 367.

At Heidenheim, by the time the facilities there closed, in addition to those admitted directly from the lines of communication, some 1,710 sick and wounded had passed through the hospital en route to Flanders from Nordlingen. Once back in Flanders, on arrival at Nijmegen the evacuated patients were divided into two groups. Those who did not require further hospital care were taken to Dort, where they waited in a cantonment area pending the return of their regiments to Flanders. Those who needed continued hospital care were transferred to the Bijloke Hospital in Ghent where an English hospital was established within the grounds of the existing civilian hospital, in a similar manner as had been undertaken during the Nine Years' War ten years earlier. However, when the patients arrived, arrangements to receive them were incomplete. While they waited in the boats, the physician in charge ordered that they be supplied with bread, wine and brandy and additional local nurses were hired to provide ongoing care and attention.

In total the transportation costs for moving the casualties back to Flanders exceeded 3,000 guilders. Some 61 widows and 11 children who had been orphaned by the fighting were also provided with food and support amounting to 1,202 guilders while they waited for a local agent to arrange passage for them to England. Each of them was given 5 guilders to cover their onward travel after they had been repatriated although, exceptionally, two unattached orphan children, possibly the orphans of a British soldier and a Flemish mother, both of whom had died, were deposited in the Bijloke Hospital and were maintained and clothed there by the Purveyor at a cost of 180 guilders.

In due course the sick and wounded who had been returned to Ghent were repatriated to England. Some were landed at Portsmouth whence, on 24 October, the physicians and surgeons who had accompanied them wrote to the Commissioners for Sick and Wounded Seamen, in the absence of any other responsible body, informing them that several of their patients were fit to be moved to St Bartholomew's and St Thomas' hospitals in London and requested to know how many they could send forward.[60] In response the London hospitals pleaded that they were already almost full, having recently received an influx of wounded seamen from both Portsmouth and Rochester. The medical officers in Portsmouth were asked not to dispatch any more patients until they were told to do so by the Commissioners, but it seems that this request passed unheeded.[61] On 9 November the Governors of the London hospitals registered further specific complaints about the officers of the ports who, it was claimed, were forwarding 'many patients whose condition was so bad as to make their removal dangerous while others were not in need of relief'. This prompted the Secretary at War to issue an instruction to the port medical officers to send only those whose condition really merited transfer to London.[62] Nevertheless, the situation remained unresolved until, on 19 December, Marlborough himself intervened by writing to the Stewards of the London hospitals requesting them to

> use their utmost endeavours that the sick and wounded men lately sent up from out-ports may be admitted into their hospitals before the holy days [Christmas] for that the keeping of them in out-quarters will not only be to the prejudice of their health but a hindrance to the service as well as an extra expense for Her Majesty.[63]

On 17 March 1705, the Secretary of State wrote to the Commissioners of Chelsea Hospital informing them that 300 invalids had just arrived in London from Flanders and would require accommodation in Chelsea 'and places adjacent'.[64] Marlborough had already directed that the Commissioners were to examine each man to determine whether they should be admitted into the Royal Hospital, accommodated locally in lodgings or discharged the service with a pension. Two senior officers, General Withers and Brigadier Cadogan, were to assist the Commissioners in assessing the worthiness of each candidate but, regardless of the board's findings, all who had been disabled during their service in Germany, with certain exceptions, were to be provided for with sums of money from a bounty fund of £4,000 that had been allocated for just such a purpose. Those whose service was 'less than a year or two' were deemed not entitled to participate in the bounty money. In their case, the Duke urged compassion and suggested that the Commissioners should 'give them a small allowance and a pass to convey them home'.[65]

The Duke of Marlborough provided a further demonstration of his close concern for the welfare of his soldiers when, on 20 March, he sent a direct order to the Commissioners at Chelsea instructing them to ensure that priority was given to such of the invalids as being wounded in the last campaign in Germany are in the worst condition and want more than ordinary care to be taken of them. For the remainder of those invalids who, having likewise served in Germany, are entitled to the benefit of the hospital, and for whom there is no room at present, His Grace does think fit that you appoint a person upon the most reasonable terms to take care of quartering them. And of the due payment of their quarters until vacancies shall happen. If any are found willing to return home and to quit their pretensions to the hospital ... for their encouragement £3 a man is to be paid them out of the £4,000.[66]

The bounty was to be distributed according to a set formula asshown in Table 6.4

Table 6.4 The Blenheim Bounty allocation to sick and injured by rank as pensions

Horse	
Corporal	1s 6d per day
Trooper	1s per day
Dragoons	
Sergeant	1s per day
Corporal	9d per day
Trooper	7d per day
Foot	
Sergeant	9d per day
Corporal	7d per day
Private Soldier	5d per day

Source: TNA, WO 4/3, fol. 186.

Surgeons' mates, who were not regarded as being of officer status, also retained the right to apply for admission to the Royal Hospital Chelsea. One such person, Samuel Gash, had served for 30 years as a surgeon's mate with the Royal Regiment of Foot when he was granted the pension appropriate to a Corporal of Horse 'to keep him from want' on his retirement in January 1712.[67] In due course the Duke requested that a list of patients' names and their ultimate placement – either into the hospital, to out-pension or otherwise – was to be sent to him annotated to show, additionally, what arrangements had been made for those whose limited service excluded them from a share in the bounty. In due course this was done and, on 26 March, the Commissioners were informed that the Duke had expressed his approval of their arrangements, particularly those made for men 'whose wounds were running'.[68] These patients had been admitted directly into the hospital while others, for whom no immediate beds were available, had been found quarters locally.

By April 1705 it was obvious that it was impossible to provide everything that was needed for the 'invalids lately arrived from Holland' out of the £4,000 allocated for that purpose, especially as the widows of soldiers killed in Germany were also entitled to benefit from the Blenheim Bounty fund. One such recipient was Eleanor Brown who, in November 1705, received £60 along with other widows who had also lost their husbands the previous year. By the time that these women came to be paid, the fund was exhausted but the Duke of Marlborough personally ensured that they received their entitlement 'having been pleased to apply the £600 accrued by him as his share of the bounty as Captain General for the use of the widows who lost husbands in Germany'.[69]

The absence of a specific general fund from which routine payments could be made to the widows of officers and soldiers who were killed or died on duty became the topic of increasing debate in official circles over the following months. During August 1706, in response to an enquiry by the Secretary of State, St John admitted that the only provision for officers' widows relied upon funds collected by a semi-private arrangement whereby deductions were taken from the officers' pay but, even then, this only applied to those serving under the Duke of Marlborough in Flanders. There were no similar arrangements applicable to the pay of officers serving elsewhere.[70] Another year was to pass before official provision for officers' widows became available when, on 31 October 1708, the Lord Treasurer was authorized to issue them with pensions according to an official scale relative to the dead husband's rank from ensign to lieutenant colonel.

The fund from which these payments were to be made was to be financed by deductions of a day's pay per year taken from the salaries of officers serving in Flanders and also by adding a premium to payments made when an officer's commission status changed. The equivalent of ten days' pay was to be credited to the fund from the amount paid when an officer purchased a promotion. Similarly, when officers sold or purchased new commissions, twelve days' pay would be transferred to the fund but, if an officer lost his commission as a result of a decision by a court marshal, he would be expected to contribute 30 days' pay. An official, Theophilus Parsons, was appointed to administer the fund and receive these various amounts.

For the first time, arrangements were also made for pensions to be paid to the widows of officers killed while serving in Spain, Portugal and the West Indies. The authorized rates for widows' pensions relative to the rank of the husband are listed in Table 6.5. These figures were equivalent to those previously allowed except that, henceforth, entitlements were extended to the widows of full colonels, surgeons and chaplains. The financial arrangements for this fund differed in that money would be made available by allowing each troop or company of every regiment serving in these areas to draw the pay of a fictitious soldier whose name would be added to their muster lists. The Secretary of State would then forward the sums received to the fund manager, in this case James Taylor, who worked in parallel with his colleague Theophilus Parsons. These arrangements related only to officers' widows and there were still no specific funds put aside for the relieving the plight of the widows of ordinary soldiers, but early in July 1708, Walpole commented that the Queen was considering 'enlarging the fund to provide for other widows'.[71]

Table 6.5 Annual pension allowance authorized October 1708 for the widows of officers killed on duty

Rank	Flanders	Spain, Portugal and West Indies
Colonel	N/A	£50
Lt. Colonel	£40	£40
Major	£30	£30
Captain	£26	£26
Lieutenant	£20	£20
Cornet	£16	£16
Ensign	£16	£16
Quartermaster	£16	£16
Surgeon	N/A	£16
Chaplain	N/A	£16

N/A: No pension available from this fund

Source: TNA, WO 4/8, fol. 28.

As the war continued, the cash crisis relating to soldiers' pensions at the Royal Hospital grew worse. Among those who sought redress for their situation were James Savage, Walter Butler and Daniel Palmer, three soldiers who failed to receive benefits as a result of this crisis despite being qualified for an out-pension of 12d a day. They were told that the hospital had run out of money but, in their cases, exceptions were made after recourse to the Duke of Marlborough for advice. Permission was duly given for them to be paid out of other funds released for the purpose.[72] It was a further four months before the financial shortages were finally resolved. On 28 March 1706 the Paymaster General was issued with a warrant permitting him to charge £1,909 2s 0d to the accounts of Chelsea Royal Hospital for the benefit of soldiers wounded at the Schellenburg and Blenheim who remained 'alive and not otherwise provided for'. Authority was also granted for the appointment of an office holder to assume responsibility for paying an accommodation allowance to such veterans up to a maximum of 2s a day.[73]

Meanwhile, back in Nordlingen, the Duke's original intention had been to move everyone back to Flanders before winter set in, but the condition of some patients precluded this. It was left to Hudson to make the decision to retain a small hospital in the town over the winter and, in due course, the physician Nathaniel Ogle volunteered to remain behind along with a surgeon, Claudius Amyand, plus three surgeons' mates, William Nelson, William Genest and Edward Lee. In addition one of Hudson's clerks was detailed to stay and assume administrative responsibility for the hospital.[74]

Once the majority of casualties had been evacuated and in-patient numbers had been reduced to more manageable proportions, leaving between 200 and 250 remaining, it was decided to transfer the hospital into a smaller building nearby that was rented for the coming winter. Additional local surgeons, nurses and servants were employed to assist the permanent staff, tend the sick and wash the linen in an adjacent washhouse. Inevitably, the move into smaller premises was accompanied by further expense as some basic refurbishment work was needed, such as the repair of windows, the construction of water boilers and the services of a smith to fit iron doors onto the kitchen stoves. Even the process of transferring the beds and bedding from one building to the other was a major undertaking.

During the winter, food supplies for the patients were bought locally; Table 6.6 lists the quantities purchased between 26 June and 28 March 1705 when the hospital closed. Unfortunately the figures for the period between 21 August and 19 October, during the chaotic weeks immediately after the battle of Blenheim, have not been traced. Using the calculation methods used earlier in this chapter, it is possible to determine that the hospital's meat consumption indicates an average number of 350–450 patients at any one time through June and July. By October this figure has risen to over 700 and it is likely that in the weeks immediately following the battle, during the period for which figures are not available, this total would have been even higher.

Table 6.6 Food items purchased for the Hospital at Nordlingen, 26 June 1704–28 March 1705

Commodity	*Jun/Jul*	*Jul/Aug*	*Oct/Dec*	*Dec/Mar*
Meat (lb)	13,978	29,759	8,326	10,490
Bread (loaves)	16,043	3,160	8,805	10,917
Beer (firkins)	647	899	150	1,551
Cheese (lb)	5,932	10,606	1,726	1,652
Rice (lb)	1,266	2,093	1,167	1,092
Oatmeal (bushels)	104	163	163	63
Sugar (lb)	1,068	1,410	547	562
Eggs (each)	5,150	8,500	6,025	4,260
Butter (lb)	115	135	93	84

Source: BL Add. Mss, 61370, fol. 407.

Maintaining the hospital in Nordlingen over the winter was an expensive but unavoidable addition to Hudson's annual budget. The cost of providing medicines and dressings alone amounted to 20,043 guilders, while officers' pay came to 4,521 guilders. When the hospital finally closed in March 1705, the bill for transporting the remaining patients and staff back to Flanders added a further 2,118 guilders to the account. Over that winter of 1704–5, in addition to nurses, the hospital staff included a butler, cooks, washerwomen, various assistant personnel and 'several men and women who daily emptied the excremental tubs out of the several hospitals'. While the number of nurses employed to attend patients in the British military hospitals was variable, their continued presence in significant numbers, as well as cooks, clerks and other 'servants', is indicated by their total wage bill, which amounted to 42,800 guilders – ten times the cost of the medical staff over the same period.[75] By comparing the recorded wage payments made to nurses against the standard rate of pay, it is assessed that, during the winter of 1704–5, an average of 20 nurses were employed on a day-to-day basis in the Nordlingen hospital. Obviously, nurses were regarded as a common and essential component of patient care.[76]

As the following year's campaign season approached, 35 officers and servants crossed from England to Flanders on 2 March 1705, accompanied by baggage that included 260 casks, barrels, packs, boxes and hampers containing stores of provisions, medicines and other equipment.[77] Three days later, however, Dr Lawrence, the Physician General, supported by two surgeons, Gardiner and Tiguell, and three surgeons' mates, Eeles, Danvers and Fabricious, wrote to the Duke of Marlborough to express their concern over perceived shortages in the previous year's medical establishment.

> That whereas last year there was a great want of surgeons to assist the sick and wounded in the hospital in Germany, and very few surgeons fit to be employed that are to be purchased in these parts, it is humbly offered to your Grace's consideration that there may be an additional allowance of one master-surgeon and three able mates as absolutely necessary for Her Majesty's hospital.[78]

As the medical staff list included a fourth master surgeon but lacked an equivalent complement of surgeons' mates, it appears that their request was only partially met.[79]

The allied campaign for 1705 began with a plan to invade France from the east along the course of the Mosel River. By adopting this course of action, Marlborough hoped to circumvent the imposing defences, known as the 'Lines of Brabant', that the French had constructed across the Low Countries from Namur to Antwerp. As events were to prove, the small increase in hospital staff numbers granted at the beginning of the year's campaign was amply justified. Once the hospital stores and equipment had been recovered from the warehouse in Rotterdam, cleaned and checked, and replacement items received from England, they were loaded into Dutch ships that had been hired for the duration of the campaign. It seems that the 1702 experiment of purchasing surgeons' chests on the Continent noted earlier had not attracted long-term approval and was not repeated in subsequent years as the Apothecary General was allocated £542 16s 7d for 27 chests of medicines, equivalent to approximately £20 per pair of chests in England, intended to cater for the needs of some 40,000 men. Another £7,598 17s 7d was allotted for the annual provision of drugs for the Hospital.[80]

A decision was taken to establish an advanced marching or field hospital at Triers where the army's main storage magazine was located. As has been noted earlier, in time of war, the movement of traffic on rivers continued to attract unabated tolls and the field hospital's journey to its deployment location entailed the payment of the statutory duty at each of the toll stations of Bommel, Arnhem, Tiel and Nijmegen. From Nijmegen onwards to Coblenz, the journey necessitated the hire of extra towing horses and harness plus pilot's fees and, at Coblenz, in order to 'oil the wheels of commerce', a bribe of 175 guilders had to be paid to the

Burgomaster before the boats could be unloaded. The stores were then transferred into six smaller vessels for the remainder of the journey up the river Mosel.[81]

When the convoy finally arrived at Triers, after a journey lasting almost six weeks, the usual task of unloading the stores into wagons and warehouses began, as did the collection of sufficient quantities of straw for mattresses, bolsters and palliasses, cleansing the designated buildings, constructing lavatories and setting up stoves as well as dealing with many other routine maintenance requirements. The hospital opened on 17 May and functioned until 13 June when it was suddenly ordered to retire to Neuwied, on the river Rhine a few miles downstream from Coblenz. Marlborough's plans had been obstructed by the failure of his allies to provide sufficient numbers of troops and artillery. Meanwhile, a French and Bavarian army had advanced northwards to threaten the Dutch borders. They recaptured the town of Huy on 13 June, the same day that the hospital received its orders to move, thereby forcing Marlborough to issue an order for his forces to retire. The hospital was hurriedly packed up and, once again, everything, including the patients, was loaded into a convoy of 16 boats and transported back down the Mosel to Coblenz.

This time the vessels used to convey the sick and wounded had been specially converted with the addition of deal boards and straw for the patients to lie on with overhead shelter for the most severely ill. Whn they arrived in Neuwied the hospital reopened and remained stationary in that location, collecting and caring for soldiers who fell sick along the army's line of march, for a month, from 14 June to 11 July. Eventually, it was ordered to redeploy, via Maastricht, to Liège alongside the base hospital that had again been established in the neighbourhood of a Dutch medical facility. Some 200 patients were subsequently moved, initially by boat to Coblenz, and thence by wagon to Maastricht. The bulk of the stores were transported separately and returned to 'sHertogenbosch for storage.[82]

While Dr LeCaan had been caring for 'great numbers of men in miserable condition' at the Dutch hospital in Liège, the Dutch hospitals in both Maastricht and at 'sHertogenbosch had also received sick and wounded allied soldiers. Between 12 July and 5 September, a fourth Dutch hospital at Breda was also utilized with a British apothecary being detached there to supervise the provision of drugs to British patients. Of course, this entire system was only made possible by the ability of the British army to pay for the additional medical care, despite Cardonnel's constant reminders to Hudson of the need to be 'sparing in the expense of the hospital'.[83]

Bombarded with messages from the States General, who were naturally anxious to secure their southern border, Marlborough marched his troops as quickly as possible through the Eifel region in an attempt to place himself between the French and the Dutch frontier. By the time that Marlborough reached Maastricht on 27 June, the French commander Villeroi, who was by now aware of Marlborough's march across his right flank, had ordered a full-scale retirement behind his defensive lines. Huy was retaken by allied troops on 12 July and, overnight on 17/18 July, Marlborough forced his way through the French defensive lines and captured the town of Tirlemont.

It is interesting to note at this point how both Marlborough and his secretary often used Hudson for private 'extra-mural services'. Cardonnel's correspondence records how Hudson frequently received luxury goods such as spirits, chocolate and other foodstuffs that had been presented to the headquarters staff into his warehouse for safe storage. It was not, therefore, regarded as anything but routine when, on 10 August, the enemy colours that had been captured at Tirlemont were sent to Hudson in a large wooden box for safe keeping at the hospital. They arrived along with a note containing a casual request for a surgeon and his mate to be sent to that town to provide care for the wounded.[84]

Casualties among the British troops had been relatively light. Taylor quotes a figure for this action of 'somewhere below 200'.[85] However, an undated bill compiled later referring to the British troops admitted to hospital at Tirlemont recorded a total of 3,454 soldier/days spent in hospital, a figure that would appear to reflect the ravages of disease rather than battle injuries.[86] A tally made some six weeks later, on 21 August, listed 746 British soldiers present in the Dutch hospital at Liège.[87] For some reason, Hudson was unwilling at this time to reimburse the Dutch hospital authorities without the specific approval of higher authority. This led to prolonged delays before the Dutch received their dues and, not surprisingly, they petitioned the Duke of Marlborough. In presenting a bill for food provided to soldier patients in Liège between 2 July and 22 July 1705, they demanded 646 guilders exclusive of payments due to the medical staff – such as the 21 Spanish ducats owed to the physician Dr Barthelemy and Surgeon Major Hingstman and the 408 guilders claimed by the apothecary for medicines.[88]

The French losses at Tirlemont were quoted as nearly a thousand killed and wounded but, when their hospital was captured, it was found to contain a mixed group of some 532 sick and wounded patients of whom only 130 were French, 40 were Spanish and 102 Bavarians who had been wounded during the recent fighting. Of the remainder, 110 had been admitted prior to the fighting and 150 were wounded British and Dutch soldiers who had been captured by the enemy.[89] Faced with such a large number of patients it was necessary to review their condition quickly in an attempt to establish how many, if any, could be safely discharged from hospital. Of the French and Bavarians, 91 convalescents were deemed fit for discharge, 31 of whom had been injured during the recent action. These were transferred to the main body of captured prisoners of war where they became eligible for return to their regiments when suitable exchanges could be arranged.[90]

Captured officers with serious wounds who were willing to give their parole were able to request leave of absence so that they could return to their homes for convalescence, having promised to return to their captors to await exchange when they had fully recovered. One such request came from a Swiss officer in the French service, Lieutenant de Stael of the Swiss Guards, who wrote to the Duke of Marlborough on 23 September 1706 requesting:

> very humbly, your Serene Highness will agree to look kindly upon my request for the favour of a passport for my journeying to Switzerland, my wounds have responded to the work of the surgeons and I now seek the succour of the climate of my country, as I

remain very susceptible to further damage. I hope, Monseigneur, that your Highness will not refuse my request which I have the honour to ask of him in the hope I can persuade him of the respect I hold for him and with which I remain, etc.[91]

Personal matters and domestic affairs were also put forward as reasons for seeking such permission. Samuel Weiss, a native of Berne in the Swiss Confederation, a Captain Lieutenant in Villars's Regiment captured during the Battle of Ramillies, applied for six months' leave of absence to go to Berne 'to sort out his domestic affairs'.[92] His request was granted.

Meanwhile, the field hospital that had retired from Triers and Neuwied arrived in Liège on 9 July. Having established itself in that city it remained there for a further two months, providing care and attention to soldiers wounded in action, as well as the routine sick of the forward units of Marlborough's troops. Some indication of the extent of the marching hospital's heavy work-load during the 1705 campaign may be obtained by examination of the list of food purchases made at that time as shown in Table 6.7.

Table 6.7 Marching hospital food purchases, 17 May–11 July 1705

Commodity	Triers	Neuwied	Liège
Meat* (lb)	3,168	14,745	8,736
Bread (loaves)	14,415	15,078	9,041
Beer (firkins)	175	134	115
Cheese (lb)	2,049	2,455	1,595
Rice (lb)	1,229	1,315	1,095
Oatmeal (bushels)	75	66	43
Sugar (lb)	650	588	942
Butter (lb)	49	66	53
* Mutton, beef and veal			

Source: BL Add. Mss, 61371.

In Flanders, the two base hospitals, at 'sHertogenbosch and Maastricht, received a constant flow of casualties throughout the campaign from 17 May until their closure on 18 October. By the very nature of their role as static receiving facilities, admitting patients sent rearwards from the field hospitals as well as casualties that arose in the rear base units – and as they remained open longer in the season than the forward units – their consumption of foodstuffs was, naturally, much higher.

Marlborough's standing orders specified that he was to be regularly informed of the fluctuating numbers of sick and wounded. Throughout the campaign, his British troops had been operating in three brigades and, on 24 July, following a long series of marches and the action of 'the Lines', his returns listed 1,869 men under care either by regimental surgeons or in hospital beds. Of these, 77 per cent were in the three main hospitals; 563 at 'sHertogenbosch and Breda, 425 in Maastricht and

454 in Liège. Of the remaining 23 per cent, only 19 were sick in camp while the rest were scattered among Dutch facilities in Hurdon, Workorn, Venlo, Roermond, Durant and Tirlemont.[93]

By 21 August, however, this figure of 1,869 had been reduced by well over a half to 746.[94] Nevertheless, by the end of October when the hospitals closed, the numbers of sick men requiring repatriation in Maastricht alone had risen again to some 1,700. This was the number recorded as having been transported in two large vessels to Dort, where a collecting point had been established. At Marlborough's express order, army surgeons accompanied patients during the journey across the North Sea and three were with the large group sent from Maastricht.

Strangely, there was no significant increase in the number of nurses employed at either Maastricht or 'sHertogenbosch during the transfer of patients rearwards from the field hospitals at Triers, Neuwied or Liège during July and August. Nevertheless, it is tempting to infer that the subsequent significant increases recorded during the weeks immediately prior to the closure of the hospitals were, once again, due to the regiments transferring sick men from within their lines to ease the process of entering winter quarters. For example, during the final six weeks at Maastricht, the number of employed nurses rose significantly from a reasonably steady monthly average of 25 during July and August to 60 in late September and October. A similar situation was evident at 'sHertogenbosch, the other base hospital, where the average number of nurses employed during October rose to 37 from a previous total that varied from 15 to 17.

As usual, the 1706 season began for the medical services with a payment of another £6,000 to the Apothecary General for the provision of drugs for the hospitals in Flanders.[95] The normal regime of removing and checking the stores and equipment retained in Rotterdam over the winter was undertaken prior to packing them aboard vessels for deployment to Maastricht, together with additional supplies that had arrived from England on 4 March. These latter items included 65 casks of cheese, 40 casks of flour, 50 casks of oatmeal, 20 casks of soap, 2 casks of sugar and 120 casks, chests, baskets and trunks containing medicines and instruments.[96]

Some twenty officers and six servants belonging to the hospital had also travelled on the same day. The first part of their journey took them to the Bosch down the river Maas. Inconveniently, the Maas was unusually low at that time and, although the onward journey from Bosch to Grave, Mook and Gennep was uneventful, when the boats arrived at the last-mentioned town, the river was too low for them to proceed further. Draught horses had to be hired to carry the stores around the shallows to a stretch of the river where the equipment could be reloaded into boats for onward carriage to Venlo. There they came upon another shallow stretch of river that, once again, necessitated the stores being off-loaded and carried forward to a navigable part of the river further up stream. After reloading the hospital stores into two more boats and, having acquired more tow horses, they successfully negotiated the final leg of the journey to Maastricht where the work began to clean and establish the hospital prior to its reopening in readiness for the coming campaign.[97]

More of the hospital staff travelled to the Low Countries over a period of several weeks, and among the passes issued permitting them to cross to Holland was one signed on 13 May for Susannah Hughes, described as 'a member of the hospital staff', who was possibly travelling to assume the role of senior nurse.[98] Their arrival was none too soon as, on 12 May, the allied army fought a battle at Ramillies, north-west of Liège. This was a decisive victory for the allies, during which the opposing armies had each numbered around 80,000 men. A list of the allied casualties posted in The Hague after the battle recorded totals of 1,066 killed and 2,567 wounded, the majority having been suffered by the Dutch troops.[99] The regimental surgeon of the Scots Fusiliers, John Craig, was ordered to remain behind to dress and care for the wounded, including those of the enemy.

Craig was probably employed in a temporary field hospital known to have been established at the nearby Cistercian nunnery of La Ramée in the village of Jauchelette, about four miles north-west of the battlefield.[100] Some three months later Craig submitted a request for payment in respect of the drugs and dressings that he had been obliged to expend in performing this duty. The items for which he claimed, which reflect in some measure his treatment of battle wounds, are listed in Table 6.8.

Table 6.8 Mr John Craig's bill for drugs and materials used by him in treating the wounded on the field of Ramillies, 12 May 1706

Rectified Spirit of Wine 2 quarts
Tincture of Myrrh and Aloes 2 quarts
Oil of Turpentine 1 quart
Astringient Powder ½ lb
Plaister 3 lb
Cordial Waters 3 quarts
Six Sheets

Source: BL Add. Mss, 61335, fol. 181.

Spirits of wine, myrrh and aloes were used to cleanse wounds while astringent powder was applied in an attempt to arrest bleeding. Cordial waters could be employed either as stimulants or sedatives; plaister refers to wound dressings.

The defeat and subsequent flight of the French army was followed by an Allied advance that was so rapid that it threatened to cut off the French commander, Villeroi, from his communications with Paris. As a result of the battle of Ramillies, the French withdrew almost entirely from the Spanish Netherlands. The town of Ghent surrendered to the Allies on 1 June but the rapid advance of the army left the hospital at Maastricht sited too far behind the troops that it was designed to support. In response to the changing tactical situation it was decided to open an additional hospital in Liège, specifically to receive casualties from the Ramillies battlefield. Over the next few weeks further facilities were also opened in Brussels and at the Bijloke Hospital in Ghent, the same hospital that had been used by

William III's army ten years previously during the Nine Years' War. This became the army's primary base hospital for most of the remaining years of the war.

When the town fell to the Allies the hospital was found to contain 29 wounded French soldiers together with some of the French medical staff who had remained behind to care for them when their forces withdrew.[101] They included M. De Mare, a commissary, Surgeon Major la Roche, surgeons' mates De Mouline and L'Oke, a cook by the name of Cacan and three soldiers employed as 'tenders' or male nurses named as De Lantrelle, La Chene and L'Estrade.

The inhabitants of Ghent at this time entertained pro-French sympathies and, in an attempt to change their allegiance, Marlborough published an order that prohibited plundering by the troops and held regimental commanders responsible for making good any damage to property.[102] Nevertheless, fearful of the expense and effects that an uncontrolled influx of wounded soldiers might entail, the Abbess of the Bijloke Hospital wrote to the Duke of Marlborough requesting him to nominate a representative with whom she could negotiate and arrange appropriate reimbursement:

> Since the entry of your Highness to these parts with the troops of His Britannic Majesty, many sick and wounded soldiers have come to this hospital as patients who we have taken very particular care to return them to a state of service but nobody has come forward to provide maintenance for these soldiers. I therefore beg your Highness that it would be a service to nominate some person who can meet with us to agree on the steps to be taken, and other conditions which are regularly associated with occurrences of this nature. Such an agreement has been made with the Deputies of the United Provinces for their soldiers in their service admitted under comparable circumstances. We hope that your Highness will not decline to give us similar consideration.[103]

In terms of anticipated patient numbers alone her worries were well founded as, during the setting-up process 850 bedsteads were constructed and another 150 hired. In addition, 100 new palliasses and bolsters were purchased along with 50 pairs of sheets which, together, added more than 850 guilders to Hudson's bill.[104] The task of feeding and caring for such numbers must have been an awesome prospect but the Abbess may also have heard of events that took place at the hospital in Antwerp following the surrender of that city on 5 June, four days before she wrote her letter. There, Jean Albert van Meurt, the master apothecary of Mecklin mentioned earlier, who had held the French contract to supply medicines to that hospital, had complained to Marlborough that, following the surrender of the French garrison in Antwerp, all the medicaments in his pharmacy had been confiscated by the French when they departed under the pretext that it was the property of the King of France. Van Meurt requested that he be permitted to correspond with M. de Bagnole, the French army's Intendant (Commissary General), in an attempt to gain reimbursement of his losses:

> It is well known that the medicaments in the hospital were for the use of the local community. The establishment of a shop in the town would be a highly risky and

perilous undertaking as, if the contents were confiscated there, the costs would fall entirely on him and not upon the King.[105]

His petition for restitution of the confiscated material taken from the hospital eventually led to his reimbursement with 23 guilders.[106] But, with an eye to the future, Van Meurt then proceeded to describe how the French soldiers had shared the cost of medications by paying 'two patars'* per patient and suggested that a similar arrangement be agreed whereby every British soldier subsequently treated would also pay the same sum. At the rough equivalent of eight shillings this was possibly a one-off payment rather than a recurring charge.

Meanwhile, the campaign progressed with the capture of Ostend. In due course Courtrai, abandoned by the French, was entered by the Allies on 5 July and immediately established as a base for further advances towards Menin. On 8 August an order was issued for the hospital at Maastricht to close while a surgeon, with 'such other officers, people, necessaries and medicaments as judged requisite', was to be transferred to Courtrai.[107] The patients were to be moved to Ghent by water but, in the event, the Maastricht hospital remained open until 28 August. Most of the remaining in-patients were transferred over a few weeks to Ghent via Louvain and Brussels although not all were transported by water. Some were taken by road and, unfortunately, during one such journey, a convoy of hospital wagons was attacked near Louvain by a French raiding party. Hudson himself and various members of his medical and nursing staff were robbed and a hired draught horse was killed.[108] The hospital stores were forced to retrace the original tortuous journey undertaken during the initial deployment during the previous spring down the Maas via Venlo.

In due course the fortified towns of Dendermonde, Ath and Menin were besieged and, in order to provide close medical support, a 'flying' or field hospital was formed from a section of the staff at Ghent and moved into a building provided by Courtrai's mayor. The usual process of cleaning and repair began at once and, when completed, beds and bedding were begged and borrowed from the local population. The Courtrai unit remained open from 16 July for almost two months, closing on 9 September. During this time it was extremely busy, acting as both a hospital and an advanced dressing station. Contemporary accounts recorded that many convoys of boats were required to carry the large quantities of straw needed by the hospital for the renewal of bedding material as a result of the arrival of sick and wounded from the force besieging Menin. Patients who recovered to a point where they were fit to travel were arranged in groups and transferred to Ghent for ongoing care.

By 25 August the Bijloke Hospital contained 649 in-patients with a further 70 severely wounded men lying in Courtrai awaiting transfer to Ghent. Of the former figure, 110 were deemed fit for discharge back to their regiments but, as the season progressed, more and more nurses were employed to care for an increasing number

---

* 'Patar': probably a colloquialism for the 'Patagon', a silver coin issued by the Bishopric of Liège, equivalent to 4 guilders.

of patients, especially after the hospital in Maastricht closed and its patients were added to those in Ghent. The situation was further exacerbated when the 1706 campaign lasted longer than any preceding year. As a result, the hospital remained open until early November and the final month, from 8 October to 4 November, saw, once again, the seemingly inevitable end-of-campaign rise in patient admissions and a concomitant increase in nursing personnel to a total of 60.

Not surprisingly, some of the hospital staff also required treatment.[109] On Saturday 14 September, the apothecary visited and supplied drugs to 96 patients. These included Nurse Neale, who was prescribed three items; cinnabar, a form of mercury ointment, an extract of the herb *prunella* thought to be specific for diarrhoea, and a general sedative. Mrs Mackenzie, another nurse, received a plaster impregnated with galbanum, a resinous gum extract used as a stimulant when treating bronchitis. The following Monday, Mr Smallbones, surgeon to General Churchill's Regiment, was given various laxatives and two ounces of laudanum and, four days later, Nurse Trowman was provided with drugs and treated for a worm infestation.[110]

Due to the unusually prolonged campaign, the final closure of the hospitals and the dispatch of patients for repatriation were conducted with extreme haste in order to make the cross-channel journey before the winter gales caused further delay. Hudson had returned to England as soon as he could so that many of his contractors, who were owed money for goods supplied to the hospitals, were forced to wait until the following spring before their bills could be paid – a situation not conducive to future good business relationships.

The campaign of 1707 brought another frustrating series of marches and countermarches without any substantive gains. Marlborough's plans for another campaign on the Mosel were frustrated by continued reluctance on the part of the Dutch to permit their army to operate too far from their own frontier. The requirement for hospital support was not lessened, however, and, in March, some 15 surgeons and apothecaries crossed the channel to Flanders accompanied by a large consignment of hospital stores packed into 300 casks, chests and hampers containing medicines, oatmeal, cheese, flour and other items.[111]

Between 5 May and 21 October the Bijloke Hospital at Ghent functioned as the army's main base hospital employing an ever-increasing number of nurses while, during this period, hospital units were also opened in Brussels and at Courtrai.[112] At the same time a significant number of British troops continued to be admitted and treated in various allied hospitals including Dutch units in Liège, Louvain and Brussels.[113]

If 1707 was a year of frustrations, 1708 brought definitive action. Accompanied by 16 members of the staff, the annual stock of medical and foodstuffs for the hospital was dispatched from England on 11 March and in due course the hospitals reopened. However, the ongoing need to supply goods from England for the hospitals continued, of course, throughout the campaign season. The inventory of just one such shipment, in this instance that dispatched on 2 April is listed in Table 6.9.

Table 6.9 List of stores sent to the hospitals in Flanders on 2 April 1708

96 casks of flour
56 casks of cheese
46 casks of oatmeal
12 casks soap
4 casks of sugar
4 cases of glasses
4 boxes of candles
6 bundles of chairs
6 boxes and chests containing small necessaries
50 boxes and chests containing medicines
18 portmanteaux and trunks belonging to the officers of the hospital

Source: TNA, WO 4/7, fol. 16.

Affairs for the allies did not begin well. By a sudden bold stroke, the French under Marshal Vendome recaptured both Bruges and Ghent on 5 July. As a result, the facilities at the Bijloke Hospital, which had reopened on 9 May, were lost, although it appears that the hospital continued to function until 4 August. In the intervening weeks the enemy permitted the gradual transfer of the hospital stores and equipment, even including the beds, to Brussels, which then assumed the role of main base hospital.[114] As a magnanimous gesture, the French commander, Vendome, agreed to release all of the garrison, patients and staff remaining in Ghent and ordered boats to 'bring away not only the English but the whole army' by water to Brussels. In reciprocation, some of these boats returned carrying released French sick and wounded from Brussels to Ghent.[115]

Allied fortunes soon changed for the better when, at the battle of Oudenarde, fought on 11 July, they gained a spectacular victory over the French and, shortly afterwards, laid siege to Lille. As a result the work of the hospitals increased significantly. A detachment of medical personnel was dispatched to open a field hospital in Oudenarde which remained open until the end of the year. During this time casualties who had not recovered sufficiently to be repatriated to England and required long-term care were transferred to Brussels.[116] A few weeks later, in mid-August, the siege of the imposing fortified city of Lille was begun but, although the town surrendered on 25 October, the citadel held out until 9 December. During these operations some reports claimed that the Allies lost some 14,000 casualties although, as usual, such unsubstantiated figures cannot be relied upon. An official contemporary return of British losses quoted only 104 dead, and 204 wounded.[117] To care for these, another hospital was opened on 6 September at Menin to receive sick and wounded troops evacuated from the trenches. The workload of this unit was very high and, when the hospital at Lille eventually closed on 21 December, the staff of that hospital, including surgeon Claudius Amyand, were transferred to Menin, which unit remained open throughout the winter and into the following spring.[118]

On 8 September, Cardonnel wrote to Dr Wilson, who had been detached from Brussels to oversee the Menin hospital, ordering him to 'make haste making sure that a surgeon, three mates and whatever other staff accompanied [him] arrived as soon as possible'.[119] Two days later, having learned that the numbers of sick and wounded were increasing rapidly, Cardonnel wrote again to Wilson to let him know that some nurses 'had been ordered from the army' and advised him to ensure that Hudson was aware of the situation in case he required further help. He also pointed out that Wilson could order additional supplies from the hospital at Oudenarde which was regularly restocked from Brussels.

The fighting did not end with the capture of Lille, as Marlborough immediately turned his attention towards Ghent where, after a month-long siege, during which time a field hospital was provided in support of the besieging troops, the French and Spanish garrison capitulated on 2 January 1709. With the town once more under allied control, the Bijloke Hospital was re-established as the army's main base hospital. Subsequently, on 30 December, the hospital at Oudenarde closed having transferred its patients and staff to Ghent.

The 1708 campaign was unusual in that the troops were maintained in the field throughout the winter and hospital provision continued through until the early spring. Extra boats and wagons had to be hired to convey the wounded from the trenches surrounding the citadel at Lille to the hospital at Menin. When it was subsequently found that the field hospitals at Oudenarde, Menin and in the siege-lines of Ghent could not be manned efficiently from existing resources, a considerable number of additional surgeons was recruited locally on a temporary basis. The situation was not helped by the unauthorized absence of the physician Dr Ogle who had returned to England during the summer despite orders to the contrary. Cardonnel wrote to him saying that his absence would be overlooked if he returned to duty by 18 July while Hudson was instructed to withhold the doctor's pay if he failed to comply.[120]

There was also a shortage of bedding and a general lack of household equipment that necessitated the purchase of large amounts of mundane items such as kettles and copper boilers. These deficiencies were exacerbated when a consignment of stores intended for the hospital at Menin was dispatched from Brussels, but they were mistakenly routed via the river and the North Sea to the port of Ostend. As Bruges and Ghent were at that time still in enemy hands, the stores became isolated in Ostend. Eventually they ended their journey some months later when they were delivered to the Bijloke Hspital after the recapture of Ghent at the start of the new year.[121] The inevitable shortages that occurred as a result of this disaster forced the field hospital at Menin to make several local purchases of routine items, particularly replacement mattresses, sheets and bedspreads damaged 'by the extraordinary greatness of the men's' wounds'.[122] The forces of nature also contributed to the deteriorating situation as the onset of an extremely cold winter heralded a constant demand for large quantities of fuel for heating as well as extra wine and brandy, especially for the large number of patients suffering from dysentery.

The scourge of infectious diseases continued to produce many more casualties than the fighting, including freshly recruited soldiers who had not even reached the main theatre of operations. Between 12 August and 19 December, a transit hospital operated in Antwerp where large numbers of sick soldiers were deposited by regiments that had recently landed on the continent as reinforcements. As a result, extra medical staff had to be hired to care for these patients.

Some of the sick were sent back to England but the Secretary of State, Walpole, was annoyed to learn that, when a large group of casualties arrived in Dover on 17 August, the local agent of the Committee for Sick and Wounded Seamen demanded an allowance of 18d pery per man. This equated to three times the normal subsistence allowance. In response, Walpole was forced to negotiate terms with the Commissioners, eventually arriving at an arrangement whereby the officers of the sick men's parent regiments were to pay the standard 6d per man daily allowance, with the balance of 12d per man per day being paid by Whitehall after a completed, itemized invoice had been received. Shortly afterwards, a further 140 sick men were sent to Portsmouth under similar circumstances but in their case, although the soldiers had been accompanied by three officers, the Secretary at War had to spend several days attempting to identify the regiments whence they came in order to make the necessary financial arrangements for their care.[123]

As late summer turned into autumn the situation in Ostend deteriorated. On 14 October, there were 1,542 men lying sick in barracks and 268 in the local hospital.[124] The same picture was evident throughout Flanders where, as a result of that year's unusually extended period of continuous action, coupled with the frequent movement of large armies, many local civilian medical establishments were overwhelmed with sick and wounded soldiers. A similar problem arose on the other side of the North Sea among troops who were in the process of being mustered as reinforcements before travelling to Ostend, Many of these men fell sick while awaiting embarkation and 486 of them were sent to the Isle of Wight to recover. The island, which coincidentally afforded a deterrent against desertion, was in constant use as a convalescent depot and seems to have fulfilled that role admirably as, after a short interval, Captain Brooke, the officer deputed to supervise the group in question, was able to write to the Secretary at War to inform him that 186 of them had recovered sufficiently to continue their journey to the Low Countries, with many more likely to become so very soon.[125] Even so, there does not appear to have been any provision of permanent accommodation for the men on the island. Tented camps were the norm until two years later, in September 1710, when the Secretary at War wrote to Lord Shannon, who commanded a regiment of troops then encamped on the island awaiting overseas deployment, authorizing him to allow the soldiers to erect temporary huts as protection against the approaching winter weather:

> that for preventing the danger to which the soldiers under your lordship's command in the Isle of Wight might be otherwise exposed upon the approaching winter of falling sick, it might be proper that they should have leave to hutt. I can signify to your

Lordship Her Majesty's pleasure that you do accordingly cause the said troops to hutt when you shall judge it requisite for the service.[126]

It is clear that many lessons were being accumulated and learned regarding the problems to be encountered when conducting military operations during the winter months. In Flanders, out of necessity, frequent recourse was made to the services of a wide variety of civilian hospitals and religious communities in Bruges, Brussels, Courtrai, Lille, Mecklin, Menin and Tirlemont. The hospital at Menin finally closed on 9 March 1709 when the patients and stores were transferred to Ghent but, surprisingly, the hospitals at Ghent and Brussels were, themselves, also closed only three days later.

The status of the hospitals in Flanders during late March and early April 1709 is unclear. On 2 April the Secretary at War, Robert Walpole, instructed the Commissioner of Transportation to accept '55 parcels of medicines contained in chests, hogsheads and hampers' destined for the hospitals in Flanders.[127] These items are listed in Table 6.10.

Table 6.10 List of stores sent to the hospitals in Flanders on 2 April 1709

98 casks of flour
75 casks of cheese
68 casks of oatmeal
12 casks of sugar
4 cases of glasses
4 boxes of pewter, candles etc.
6 cases of books, a desk etc.
6 hampers

Source: TNA, WO 4/8, fol. 208.

There were significant increases in oatmeal and cheese but otherwise the quantities were similar to those of the previous year. Where these stores were sent is not known. Quite why it had been deemed necessary to close the Bijloke Hospital is difficult to understand as, only two months later, on 31 May, it was reopened in readiness for the next campaign. Brussels followed soon afterwards and, on 18 June, an additional hospital was also opened in Lille and operated there until 18 September.

There were two major actions during 1709. The first of these, the siege of Tournai, lasted from 1 July until the town capitulated on 27 July, although the citadel held out until 5 August. As usual a field hospital, manned by staff detached from both Ghent and Brussels, established itself immediately behind the trenches, where it remained for a month, from 2 July to 2 August. After the surrender of the town the hospital was moved into more substantial accommodation in the town, where it remained until it closed its doors on 2 September having transferred its patients to Brussels and Ghent.

The second action was the battle of Malplaquet which was fought on 11 September. In this action the Allies lost some 5,547 dead and 12,761 injured. By far the majority of these were Dutch soldiers although English losses totalled 575 dead and 1,281 injured.[128] When the field hospital had closed at Tournai it had redeployed on the following day to St Ghislain. The hospital had, therefore, a week to prepare, and it was there that the casualties were taken after the bloodiest combat of the entire war. Surprisingly, it appears that the local garrison commander at St Ghislain was reluctant to accept the hospital's presence until, on 13 September, two days after the battle, the officer in question received a letter from Cardonnel, requesting him to provide every assistance to John Hudson in ensuring that the hospital was able to function effectively. The unit continued to care for those injured in the battle for the next seven weeks until its closure on 25 October, when the patients were transferred to Brussels and Ghent for onward repatriation or dispersal to local civilian establishments.[129]

The following spring, before the start of the 1710 campaign, a revised hospital establishment was approved and remained unchanged for the final three years of the war as shown in Table 6.11.

Table 6.11 Establishment for the officers of the standing hospital for Her Majesty's Forces in the year 1710

Physician General: Thomas Lawrence
Physicians: Nathaniel Ogle, Dr Wilson and Alexander Sandilands
Director: John Hudson with two Clerks
Master Surgeons: Hosea Tiquet, Claudius Amyand and Thomas Danvers
Surgeons' Mates: 12
Apothecary General: Isaac Teale

Source: BL Add. Mss, 61372, fol. 390.

There was a fourth master surgeon's vacancy, for which Alexander Inglish was nominated but, in the event, the post remained vacant. When the field hospital was deployed, the base hospital retained this form with the single exception that one physician was transferred to the staff of the field hospital, making its establishment three physicians, a chaplain, a director and his clerk, three master surgeons, twelve surgeons' mates, a master apothecary with three mates, and a conductor for the wagons.[130]

On 18 February a consignment of hospital stores was loaded in London containing food items in quantities similar to the previous year. These included 60 casks of cheese, 75 of oatmeal, 3 of sugar, 12 firkins of soap, 8 cases of needles, 3 boxes of 'glasses' and a keg of oil.[131] As usual, at the beginning of the year the hospitals at Ghent and Brussels were reopened but, although the hospitals started the year occupying the same locations that had been used at the end of the previous year, by July, with the theatre of operations having moved much further south, it was deemed necessary to move the hospital from Brussels. The patients were transported in four shiploads to Tournai while a considerable number of casualties from the siege lines at Douai were taken to the Dutch and Hanoverian hospitals in Lille. In response, it was decided to open an additional base hospital in that town. This latter unit became the primary base hospital for the remainder of the campaign. A mobile field hospital, with Dr Ogle seconded to it as the senior officer, was also provided close to each of the besieged towns in support of the allied troops, and moved frequently as the situation demanded.[132] Between 3 and 31 May this facility was sited behind the siege lines at Douai until, following the capitulation, it moved into premises within the captured town, where it remained until 31 July.

Advance notice of this deployment had been issued with an order for Hudson to send a detachment to wait at Tournai, where it was to hold itself in readiness to move forward at an hour's notice with 'someone of discretion and understanding sent ahead to arrange matters before everything is seized or given out to other troops'.[133] Later, when the army transferred its attentions to Bethune, the field hospital moved with it, establishing itself outside that town between 27 July and 25 August. In due course, the sieges of Aire and St Venant required the field hospital to move again in support of the troops participating in those actions and, from 8 September, it operated from a site adjacent to the field works, where it remained until shortly after the final capitulation of Aire.

Not surprisingly, the frequent movement of hospitals caught the supply system wrong-footed at times. Hudson's accounts recall an incident that occurred early in the campaign when a wagon-load of medical supplies was sent from Ghent to Lille, 'we believing we had a hospital there', only to find that the hospital destined for that town had not yet opened and, as a result, the consignment had to be redirected to Tournai. In another episode a party of sick was sent from Lille to Ghent but, for some reason, was delayed at Courtrai and admitted to the local civilian hospital. This necessitated the dispatch of a surgeon from Ghent to care for them until they could complete their onward journey. While the actual number of sick and wounded admitted to hospital during this period is not recorded, some indication of the pressure under which the staff were working can be deduced by noting that, on more than one occasion, groups of around 150 patients arrived together for admission, having been evacuated from the field hospitals to Tournai and Lille, both by water and land. The latter part of their journey had been made in bread wagons from which they were off-loaded and taken into the hospital by hand carts.

The hospital at Tournai closed on 4 October when the staff and remaining patients were transferred to Lille, the latter continuing to function until 14 November, some five days after the final capitulation of the fortress of Aire. The last remaining field hospital at Aire finally closed on 20 November.

For Hudson, the 1710 campaign started on 7 March when an authority for a consignment of hospital stores from London for the coming year, consisting of 70 casks of flour, 50 of oatmeal and the same quantity of cheese, 20 casks of soap, 3 hogsheads of sugar, 2 bales of blankets, a chest of drawers, a table and four dozen chairs, together with 'ten bundles and baskets of necessaries', was sent to the Commissioner of Transportation.[134] The base hospital reopened in Ghent and a second facility was established at Douai, both opening their doors on 9 May. Marlborough's concerns regarding the expense occasioned by opening and maintaining hospitals now resurfaced and, on the same day that these units opened, Hudson, who was in Tournai arranging to set up a third hospital, received a letter from Cardonnel instructing him to desist as the Duke had decided that the contractor was opening hospitals too soon, thereby generating unnecessary expenditure.

In due course, a revised set of hospital instructions was issued from the army's headquarters. These clearly stated the expectation that the hospital staff were to provide a regulated, disciplined, hygienic and efficient service to the army.[135] It is also relevant at this juncture to record that Hudson's annual accounts confirm that a head nurse was employed to supervise the hospital nurses in their work and implement these standards.[136]

Meanwhile, during the preceding winter, following their loss of the fortified towns that had been captured by the Allies in 1710, the French had constructed yet another series of defensive fortifications that they now called their *'ne plus ultra'* lines. These became the target for the forthcoming allied war effort. During August 1711, Marlborough managed to out-manoeuvre his enemies and cross these lines, forcing the French to retire even deeper into their own territory, leaving the fortified town of Bouchain isolated. The subsequent siege of that town lasted for three weeks from 21 August until its final surrender on 12 September, during which time a field hospital was established in a house at Neuville 'near our bridges so that the wounded could be conveniently transported to Douai as soon as they were fit to be moved'.[137]

During the siege of Bouchain the army suffered more casualties as a result of disease than from any military action. The incidence of severe communicable diseases, such as plague and typhus, became so serious that an extra building situated adjacent to the waterways in Ghent and large enough to hold 200 beds, bedding and equipment was hired as a 'pest house' to accommodate infectious cases. Additional locks were fitted to the doors and the windows were sealed in accordance with standard contemporary practice in an attempt to limit the spread of infection. Inevitably, mortality was high and for two months a special boat was hired specifically to carry the bodies of the dead out to sea for burial.

The capture of Bouchain was the last victory of Marlborough's spectacular career. On 31 December 1711, his incredulous troops learned that, as a result of political changes and court intrigue in London, the Queen had dismissed the Duke from all of his public offices. He was superseded in overall command of the British army in Flanders by the Duke of Ormonde, whose inauspicious arrival was later described by one of his regimental commanders, Kane, who wrote: 'In the beginning of May the Duke of Ormonde, a good-natured, but a weak and ambitious man fit to be made [a] Tool by a Set of crafty Knaves, came over [as] Captain General'.[138] The new commander's orders effectively instructed him to abstain from actively pursuing the war while the British government sought a negotiated peace with France. In due course the British army was withdrawn to the coastal area of Western Flanders where, in cramped conditions, sickness among the troops increased. Hospitals were opened in Ghent, Lille, Douai and Bruges for varying periods from April onwards but, although the troops were confined to their cantonments, sickness and death rates among them continued to rise.

The units at Lille and Douai closed in July 1712 followed, at the end of October, by those at Bruges and Ghent. However, despite the continuing presence of transit hospitals to service the needs of returning troops at the embarkation ports of Dunkirk and Nieuport, six surgeons attached to the various regiments remaining billeted in Ghent and Bruges complained that, after the hospitals closed, they had been left poorly equipped.

The army was rapidly stood down from its state of warlike readiness. On 11 September orders were issued to Ormonde from the Secretary of State that officers were no longer obliged to 'keep their field equipage'. Unfortunately, the relaxation in the level of military readiness was accompanied by a marked deterioration in the care and attention paid by army commanders to medical matters. The sick and wounded were neglected and so badly provided for that the surgeons, left without adequate hospital support, were forced to petition the Queen. They requested her to use her influence with the Duke of Ormonde and persuade him to supply them with chests of medicines as, following the earlier seasonal reduction in troops, the monetary allowance for the provision of medicines had been reduced to a weekly allocation of only 10 styvers per company per week. Meanwhile, a general lowering of troops' morale was reflected in a steady daily rise in the numbers of soldiers reporting sick, especially those with venereal infections.[139]

Eventually, on 25 September 1712, the Secretary at War commented that he had considered a draft establishment for a hospital in Dunkirk that Ormonde had forwarded through the chain of command. He raised no objections to the proposal, providing the associated costs could be defrayed out of existing army funds and the number of medical staff employed therein was reflected in a similar reduction in the numbers of doctors employed elsewhere in Flanders.[140] There is, however, no evidence to suggest that any further action was taken to bring the proposal to fruition. Both John Hudson and Dr Coatsworth, who had replaced Isaac Teale as Apothecary General after the latter's recent death, were understandably disgruntled by the low priorities afforded medical matters by both the army commanders and the government and submitted a petition to the Duke of Ormonde, requesting reimbursement of their massive unpaid dues for the previous year. These included over 46,569 guilders for the salaries of medical officers who had served in the base and field hospitals, an outstanding sum of 31,520 guilders (over £3,000) jointly owed to Hudson and the estate of the dead Isaac Teale for services rendered during 1711 and 66,118 guilders outstanding for supplies provided in 1712. The petitioners also claimed that, if these amounts were not forthcoming, they faced utter ruin.[141]

The monetary burden carried by many regimental surgeons was also significant. On 2 June 1711 Mr Harris, the regimental surgeon of the First Foot Guards, made representations to Marlborough for reimbursement of the monies he had expended 'after the battles of Ramillies, Oudenarde and Malplaquet and other occasions when he was ordered to take care of a great number of wounded French prisoners'.

Similarly Mr De Brie, the surgeon of Lord North and Grey's Regiment, submitted a bill for the time that he had remained in Courtrai all through the winter of 1706/7 caring for the casualties of his regiment who had been left there. In the same town, an apothecary, Joseph de Mailly, submitted bills totalling 781 guilders for supplying medicines and necessaries to the sick and wounded and, in Lens, the matron of the hospital where several allied soldiers had been treated also sought to recoup her losses. In all of these cases Hudson was ordered to reimburse them for their services, charging the various amounts to his hospital accounts although, as has been shown, his outstanding dues from previous years remained unpaid.[142]

That the medical organization in Flanders should have fallen into such a sorry state so soon after the removal of the Duke of Marlborough is an indication of the influence and strict controls that he exerted throughout his tenure of office. Although heavily tempered by strict curbs on expenditure, his attitude towards hospitals and to soldiers' welfare was always positive. Scouller's claim, quoted at the beginning of this chapter, that Marlborough's medical rescources were 'remarkable for mismanagement, brutality, inhumanity and, possibly, corruption' is not merely an oversimplification but, clearly, a gross misrepresentation of the facts.[143]

The War of the Spanish Succession was not, however, only fought in Flanders. The next chapter will examine the medical provisions made for troops serving under the Earl of Peterborough, the Earl of Galway and others in Spain and Portugal where the attitudes of commanders toward the care and welfare of their men can be analysed in direct contrast with contemporary events in Flanders.

Notes

1. R.E. Scouller, *The Armies of Queen Anne* (Oxford: Clarendon Press, 1966), p. 93.
2. Ibid., p. 235.
3. BL Add. Mss, 61335, fol. 172.
4. BL Add. Mss, 61369, fol. 115.
5. BL Add. Mss, 61317, fol. 193; 61335, fol. 172.
6. BL Add. Mss, 61319, fol. 115.
7. BL Add. Mss, 61317, fol. 116; Peterkin and Johnston, pp. 1–25.
8. BL Add. Mss, 61318, fols 233–34.
9. BL Add. Mss, 61319, fol. 115.
10. BL Add. Mss, 61394, fol. 105.
11. BL Add. Mss, 61372, fol. 199; 61369, fol. 101.
12. BL Add. Mss, 61369, fol. 103.
13. J.A. Lynn, *Giant of the Grand Siècle* (Cambridge, 1997), pp. 430–39.
14. BL Add. Mss, 61335, fols. 175–6.
15. A. Peterkin and W. Johnston, p. 25.
16. BL Add. Mss, 61335, fol. 170
17. BL Add. Mss, 61369, fol. 50.
18. General R. Kane, *A System of Camp Discipline* (London, 1757), pp. 7–40.
19. Bod. L Vet. A4. fol 1286, *Rules and Articles for the Better Government of Her Majesties Land-Forces, 1702*, pp. 15–33.

20 TNA, WO 4/3, fol. 11.
21 TNA, WO 26/11, fols 214–15.
22 BL Add. Mss, 61370, fol. 158.
23 TNA, WO 4/8, fol. 63.
24 Ibid., fol. 65.
25 BL Add. Mss, 61370, fol. 1.
26 TNA, WO 4/2 to 4/10, *passim.*
27 TNA, WO 4/12, fol. 326.
28 *Cal. Treas. Books, 1709* (1949), p. 257.
29 Ibid.
30 TNA, WO 4/11, fol. 9.
31 BL Add. Mss, 61369, fol. 116.
32 A. Peterkin and W. Johnston, p. 18.
33 BL Add. Mss, 61370, fol. 139.
34 TNA, WO 4/2, fol. 28.
35 BL Add. Mss, 61395, fols 21 and 178.
36 Ibid., fol. 187.
37 Ibid.
38 Ibid., fol. 230.
39 Ibid.
40 Ibid., fol. 220.
41 BL Add. Mss, 61395, fol. 254.
42 Ibid.
43 Ibid., fol. 67.
44 BL Add. Mss, 61370, fol. 367.
45 Ibid., fol. 425.
46 Ibid., fols 425 and Add. Mss, 61408.
47 BL Add. Mss, 61396, fol. 124.
48 BL Add. Mss, 61408 and 61370, fol. 119.
49 Sir G. Murray, *The Letters and Dispatches of John Churchill, Duke of Marlborough, 1702–1712* (4 vols, London, 1845), vol. 1, p. 321.
50 BL Add. Mss, 61408.
51 BL Add. Mss, 61370, fol. 425.
52 BL Add. Mss, 61396, fol. 195.
53 Ibid., fol. 201.
54 Ibid., fol. 223.
55 Ibid., fol. 206.
56 Ibid., fols 194–5.
57 Ibid., fols 211, 236–7.
58 Ibid.
59 TNA, WO 4/5, fols 185–6.
60 TNA, ADM 99/5, n. fol.
61 Ibid.
62 Ibid.
63 Ibid.
64 TNA, WO 4/3, fol. 186.
65 Ibid.

66 Ibid., fols 190–91.
67 TNA, WO 4/13, fol. 71.
68 Ibid., fol. 195
69 TNA, WO 4/4, fol. 32.
70 TNA, WO 4/6, fol. 8.
71 TNA, WO 4/7, fol. 213.
72 TNA, WO 4/4, fols 38 and 39.
73 *Cal. Treas. Books, 1706* (3 vols, 1950), vol. 3, pp. 225 and 613.
74 BL Add. Mss, 61318, fol. 275 and 63196, fol. 301.
75 Ibid., fol. 277.
76 BL Add. Mss, 61370, fol. 408.
77 TNA, WO 4/3, fol. 170.
78 BL Add. Mss, 61317, fol. 196.
79 BL Add. Mss, 61318, fol. 279.
80 Ibid., fol. 273; *Cal. Treas. Books, 1705–1706* (3 vols, 1952), vol. 2, p. 66.
81 Ibid., *passim*.
82 BL Add. Mss, 61397, fol. 125.
83 BL Add. Mss, 61395, fol. 243.
84 BL Add. Mss, 61397, fol. 155.
85 F. Taylor, *The Wars of Marlborough, 1702–1709* (Oxford, 1921), p. 298.
86 Ibid., pp. 254 and 298.
87 Ibid., fol. 255.
88 Ibid., fol. 285.
89 BL Add. Mss, 61318, fol. 248.
90 Ibid., fol. 249.
91 Ibid., fol. 152.
92 Ibid., fol. 256.
93 Ibid., fol. 246.
94 Ibid., and fol. 255.
95 *Cal. Treas. Books, 1705–1706* (3 vols, 1952), vol. 2, p. 66.
96 TNA, WO 4/4, fol. 189.
97 BL Add. Mss, 61371, fols 131–2.
98 TNA, WO 5/11 n. fol.
99 T. Lediard, *The Life of John, Duke of Marlborough* (3 vols, London, 1736), II, p. 33.
100 G. Guyot, *L'ancienne abbaye de La Ramée* (Brussels, 1978), *passim*.
101 BL Add. Mss, 61318, fol. 257.
102 Lediard, II, p. 57.
103 BL Add. Mss, 61206, fol. 123.
104 BL Add. Mss, 61371, fol. 495.
105 BL Add. Mss, 61305, fols. 121–2.
106 BL Add. Mss, 61371, fol. 495.
107 BL Add. Mss, 61397, fol. 339 and 61398, fol. 82.
108 BL Add. Mss, 61371, fol. 495.
109 BL Add. Mss, 61379, fol. 170r.
110 Ibid.
111 TNA, WO, 4/5, fol. 176.

Hospital Provision during Marlborough's Campaigns

[112] BL Add. Mss, 61371, fols 473–97.
[113] Ibid.
[114] BL Add. Mss, 61272, fol. 232.
[115] BL Add. Mss, 61399, fol. 428.
[116] Ibid.
[117] BL Add. Mss, 61312.
[118] BL Add. Mss, 61400, fol. 189.
[119] BL Add. Mss, 61399, fol. 491.
[120] Ibid., fols 418–19.
[121] BL Add. Mss, 61272, fol. 200.
[122] Ibid.
[123] TNA, WO 4/7, fol. 270
[124] BL Add. Mss, 61318, fol. 243.
[125] TNA, WO 4/8, fols 333 and 337.
[126] TNA, WO 4/10, fol. 2.
[127] Ibid., fol. 208.
[128] BL Add. Mss, 61372, fols 135–7.
[129] Ibid., fol. 132.
[130] BL Add. Mss, 35455, fol. 41.
[131] TNA, WO 4/8, fol. 353.
[132] BL Add. Mss, 61401, fol. 1660.
[133] Ibid., fol. 16.
[134] TNA, WO 4/10, fols 265–6.
[135] BL Add. Mss, 61318, fol. 297.
[136] Wellcome Library for the History of Medicine, RAMC 1299, *passim*.
[137] BL Add. Mss, 61402, fols 206–7.
[138] R. Kane, *Campaigns of King William and Queen Anne from 1689–1712* (London, 1745), p. 102.
[139] Wellcome Library, RAMC 582.
[140] TNA, WO 4/13, fols 101–2.
[141] Wellcome Library, RAMC 583.
[142] BL Add. Mss, 61402, fols 79, 85 and 113.
[143] Scouller, p. 235.

Chapter 7

The Army's Hospitals in Spain and Portugal

At the outbreak of war in 1702, when the British government decided to support the Austrian claim to the throne of Spain, a joint army and naval force was dispatched on a mission to capture Cadiz. As the principal naval arsenal of Spain and the main port for trade with South America, the city was a choice target where the capture of the fortress and harbour would have dealt a serious blow to the economy of Bourbon Spain. The naval elements of the expedition, some fifty ships, were commanded by Admiral Sir George Rooke, while the land force of 10,000 English and 4,000 Dutch soldiers, was led by the Duke of Ormonde.

In the event, the expedition was conducted in such a half-hearted manner that after only a month on shore, and with nothing to show for his men's exertions, Ormonde re-embarked his troops intending to return to England. On 17 September news reached the fleet that a combined French and Spanish treasure fleet had entered Vigo harbour. In response, the British fleet diverted to attack them and, in a combined land and sea attack, the port and enemy fleet were captured along with £1,000,000 in booty. Ormonde wanted to over-winter in Vigo but Rooke was unwilling to detach ships in sufficient numbers to act as the supply vessels that would be necessary to maintain the troops in provisions. As a result, the soldiers, including the sick and wounded, were re-embarked and the fleet returned to England.[1]

Apart from the surgeons attached, as normal, to individual ships and regiments, very limited medical facilities had accompanied the expedition in the belief that neutral Portuguese hospitals would be willing to open their doors to British casualties. Ostensibly, this was a reasonable assumption, given that a similar approach was adopted by Marlborough in Flanders. The difference was, however, that the forces in the Low Countries were accompanied by a British hospital, the staff of which had seen recent service under William III. Equally, despite their widely publicized differences, there was a much closer liaison and understanding between the British and Dutch governments than was the case in Portugal, where inadequate preparation and a distrustful negotiating atmosphere between allied politicians made the task of developing good working relationships much more difficult. A complicated chain of correspondence was insisted upon whereby Martin Llewellyn, the army's Commissary General of the Provisions, was instructed to apply initially to his Commander in Chief for instructions:

particularly in reference to the Hospitals and the care which is to be taken by the Portuguese of the sick and maimed soldiers of our Army ... In cases of dispute you are to refer to our Chief minister at the Court of Portugal.[2]

Discussions would then continue at a diplomatic level but, as the Portuguese Court was renowned for the Byzantine nature of its communication and decision-making, any such application procedure would involve a long, drawn-out process.

As regards the return of Rooke's and Ormonde's casualties to England, although the Secretary of State, the Earl of Nottingham, gave the Commissioners for Sick and Wounded Seamen advance warning on 16 October 1702 of the precipitate return of the fleet, the initial burden of caring for the casualties fell, as usual, upon the ports of disembarkation. In addition to caring for sick and wounded seamen, the Commissioners were also responsible for the care and supervision of prisoners of war. Always reluctant to accept responsibility for wounded soldiers, they claimed, correctly, that army personnel were not included in their terms of reference and obstructed any attempt to involve them in such matters. At times they seem to have paid more attention to the prisoners than to the care of their own forces. For example, in contrast to the shortage of funds made available to local inhabitants for the care of casualties, the Committee Treasurer, Mr Povey, escorted on each journey by a corporal and six soldiers of the Horse Grenadier Guards, made almost weekly trips from London to ports such as Harwich, Portsmouth and Plymouth, carrying funds destined to pay for the housing and sustenance of prisoners of war.[3]

As the Commissioners' primary role was to care for naval personnel, it was necessary for the Secretary of State to submit a request to the Lords of the Admiralty before they would take care of any sick and wounded soldiers who might be landed. It was also necessary for him to specify that this work was to be conducted in the same manner as they would treat sick and wounded seamen and it was made perfectly clear that separate accounts were to be maintained for each of the two services so that, later, bills could be directed to the correct source of funding.[4] This tenuous relationship permeated correspondence between the Secretary at War and the Committee. For example when, in 1705, they were asked by Henry St John to assist in providing 'necessaries' to sick and wounded men in Gibraltar, the Commissioners 'observed that there being no seamen now at that place, the furnishing of those things does not relate to the business of their office'. The 'necessaries' in question related to simple foodstuffs, such as rice, currants, raisins, oil and wine, items that were regularly supplied to the hospitals in Flanders, as noted in the previous chapter. In this instance, the request related to the care of sick and wounded soldiers left in Gibraltar after their regiments had departed on posting elsewhere. Initially, the Committee exhibited their usual reluctance to become involved but, eventually, St John issued a direct order 'that care is to be taken by you for the supply of such necessaries of that kind as the sick and wounded men of the land forces in that garrison shall stand in need of'.[5] He also instructed the Commissioner of Transportation to convey the goods directly to the Governor of Gibraltar 'in regard there is no particular person to whom the care of the sick and wounded land soldiers does properly appertain'. This last statement reached to the heart of a problem that will be addressed in greater depth later in this chapter.

Meanwhile, on 16 May 1703, a treaty had been signed in Lisbon whereby Portugal agreed to join the allies in offensive operations against the armies of Bourbon Spain and France. Under the terms of this agreement the opportunity arose to launch joint naval and military expeditions against Barcelona, Cadiz and Minorca during 1704 using a combined English, Dutch and Portuguese force. Medical preparations started during the autumn when the Apothecary General, Isaac Teale, was ordered to prepare eight 'double chests of internal and external medicines' for a regiment of Horse, another of Dragoons, and six Foot regiments for the use of the regimental surgeons of these units.[6] These were subsequently inspected by Dr Morley and Dr Adams, two of the Commissioners for Sick and Wounded Seamen, as regards quality and value for money prior to dispatch. Then, on 1 September, the Secretary at War wrote to the Commissioner of Transportation instructing him to arrange for various chests of medicines and equipment destined for Portugal to be loaded onto transport ships at Spithead.[7] In due course William Blathwayt, who held the appointment of Secretary at War at that time, sent an invoice of these medicines to the Duke of Schomberg, the commander of the British contingent, for his approval and signature, although by then, 2 November, the chests were already in passage to Portugal.[8]

As time passed it became obvious that the Portuguese army was poorly equipped, their magazines were empty and their fortresses in ruins. Local transport was non-existent.[9] The allied commanders quarrelled and went their own ways and, subsequently, Schomberg was removed from command and replaced by the gout-ridden Earl of Galway. Not surprisingly, the ensuing campaign was a shambles. The capture of Gibraltar by a naval and marine force in July 1704, initially regarded as a secondary option if all of the others proved impracticable, was the single major achievement of British arms in either Spain or Portugal that year.

On 10 July, a royal warrant authorized rates of pay for 'two surgeons at 10s per day plus four mates at 5s per day for the service of the hospital in Portugal'. Three weeks later, on 31 July 1704, approval was given for an advance of three months' pay to be paid to Richard Pearce, master surgeon, and four surgeons' mates 'to enable them to prepare for their voyage'.[10] Eventually Pearce, the four hospital mates, and six additional surgeons travelled to Lisbon together with sufficient drugs and equipment to establish a general hospital.[11]

The following March the Apothecary General was paid £654 5s 4d for a supply of drugs, medicines and surgeon's instruments dispatched by him to Portugal, representing the hospital's annual consignment for 1705.[12] It had been intended that the full complement of hospital staff would travel on the first available convoy but, by 8 January, some of the appointments remained unfilled. St John attempted to inject a degree of urgency into the matter by writing to the Secretary of State inferring that the Surgeon General, who was responsible for selecting medical personnel 'such as are able and fit for the service', had been dilatory in his duties.

In truth, Whitehall had omitted to publish an approved hospital establishment and it was, therefore, not surprising that the formation of the hospital was tardy!

With the arrival of spring it was decided to launch two distinct expeditions against the Iberian Peninsula. One, commanded by the Earl of Peterborough, numbering 6,500 men, was sent to Catalonia in early May with the capture of Barcelona as its objective. Dr Friend and Cornelius Dummer accompanied the commander's retinue as Physician General and Surgeon General respectively.[13] The second force, some 3,000 British troops, arrived in Lisbon early in May 1705 but the Earl of Galway, who had spent the winter months in England, did not land until 10 August. Peterborough's force was successful in taking the city of Barcelona on 9 October but further operations were halted due to a lack of money and supplies.[14] It is difficult to determine whether each or either of the two expeditions was accompanied by a hospital. It is, however, clear that a virulent illness, probably dysentery, broke out among Peterborough's troops and was soon so widespread that the only course of action was to disperse and relegate the troops to garrison duties among the Catalonian fortresses during the ensuing winter. Overall responsibility for supervising the standard of care provided to sick and wounded soldiers had, once again, been delegated to the Commissary for Provisions, Charles Medlicot, rather than a medical man.[15] On this occasion, in the event of difficulties arising between the British and Portuguese civic or hospital authorities, Medlicot's powers of action were strictly limited to referring the matter to the British Representative in Lisbon.

In the autumn of 1705, having accepted that it had been remiss in failing to provide adequate hospital facilities for either the Spanish or Portuguese expeditions, Whitehall responded at its usual slow pace. Wide-ranging discussions were held in London regarding the financial implications. Initially, Parliament granted £244 'for the hospitals in [both] Spain and Portugal' for the year 1705. Exactly what this sum was intended to pay for is unclear as the drugs, instruments and staff had already been committed and paid for. Later, on 7 December 1705, a further £244 was added retrospectively for the employment of 'two surgeons and four mates for the hospital in Portugal' between 25 August 1704 and 25 December 1705.[16]

In due course, a letter from Brigadier Stanhope, the British ambassador to Archduke Charles, the Austrian pretender to the throne of Spain, arrived on the desk of the Secretary of State asking specifically for a properly staffed hospital to be sent to Spain. This missive seems to have spurred the government into greater action as, in response, the Council of State decided to allocate the more realistic sum of £250,000 to pay for Parliament's military commitment in Spain in the coming year.[17] It was further agreed that £6,000 of this money would be earmarked for the provision of a hospital in Catalonia. Seven days later St John wrote to James Brydges, the Paymaster General, authorizing him to issue sufficient funds from this £6,000 to cover the cost of providing a physician general, a surgeon general, a purveyor, two physicians, two surgeons, four surgeons' mates and two apothecaries 'to attend the hospital in Catalonia'.[18] His note also included a request for Brydges to advance £800 to the purveyor as soon as possible so that he could purchase sufficient mattresses, blankets, shirts and caps, as well as 'other necessaries and utensils for the kitchen, besides such sort of provisions as are useful in an hospital and are not to be had in those parts', in England before his departure.

St John justified his staff list and the associated expenditure to the Secretary of State, Sir Charles Hedges, by commenting that the sums quoted were the minimum 'as the nature of the service will require and in proportion to the number of officers employed in the hospital in Flanders'.[19] As a compensatory proviso, to offset this expense, 5d was to be deducted from every non-commissioned officer and soldier admitted to the hospital for every day that they remained as in-patients as a contribution towards the cost of their treatment, but St John also hinted at recruiting difficulties in raising sufficient numbers of medical staff when he claimed that, although the rates of pay were set at the normal level for the job, they were 'as low as it will be possible to procure any persons valuable to go so far for'.[20]

Military service was unpopular among physicians and surgeons as private professional practice in England was more lucrative than a fixed army salary with little opportunity to acquire additional income. Equally, service in Flanders, under the command of Marlborough, might have been regarded as a potential stepping-stone to higher things by garnering reflected glory, especially if the candidate was noticed by the Commander in Chief. A posting to either Spain or Portugal, where the Commanders in Chief did not attract the same social or professional status, was seen as a very poor alternative, especially in view of the greater distance from England. Strangely, there was no mention of a hospital in Portugal in any of the government's discussions but, on 1 February 1706, St John wrote again to Paymaster General Brydges, this time to confirm the final list of personnel who would make up the staff list of the hospital destined for Spain (see Table 7.1).

Table 7.1 Staff list for the hospital in Catalonia, December, 1705

Mr Charles Watkins, as Director and Purveyor at 15s per day
Two clerks at 5s each per day
Dr Friend and Dr LeCaan, physicians, at 15s each per day
Cornelius Dummer and William Neilson, master surgeons, at 10s each per day
Thomas Bailey, Pelham Johnson, Thomas Phillips and Robert Nelson, surgeons' mates at 5s each per day
Rowland Saise and William Collet, apothecaries, at 5s each per day

Source: TNA, WO 4/4, fol. 68.

Included with the document was a statement that 'no surgeon or surgeon's mate belonging to any of the regiments shall be at the same time a surgeon or surgeon's mate of the said hospital'.[21] On the same day orders were issued for the nominated personnel to travel to Portsmouth, where a convoy was preparing to set sail for

Catalonia. Isaac Teale was also requested to load the previously ordered medical supplies onto the same ships.[22]

Meanwhile, Peterborough had successfully secured Barcelona, where, among a vast hoard of military supplies, 'three large [enemy] hospitals of sick and wounded, being it is thought, about 5,000' were also captured.[23] The former French commander, Marshall Compte de Tessé, subsequently wrote to Peterborough requesting that he ensure the safety and proper treatment of the French sick and wounded. A guard was posted but not, unfortunately, before local micquelets (guerrillas) had broken into the hospital and murdered some of the patients. Matters improved somewhat once the city had been fully secured and a British army hospital established within its walls.[24]

In January 1706 Peterborough went on to capture Valencia, thereby clearing his road to Madrid from the east. Galway, advancing from Portugal, achieved his main objective when he captured Madrid four months later. This major achievement should have placed the allied cause in the ascendant but, instead, Galway discovered that the sympathies of the local population were almost entirely with the Bourbons. His lines of communication rearwards to Lisbon were cut, his force was over-exposed to danger from a larger French army and his three appeals for assistance from Peterborough in Valencia went unanswered. Eventually, in August, after a personal appeal by Archduke Charles, Peterborough responded and, with Charles alongside him, he marched into Madrid with just 400 dragoons. Just four days later Peterborough returned to Valencia, abandoned his command, boarded a ship and travelled to Genoa for a private visit to the Duke of Savoy. Recalled to England in February 1707, he was summoned to appear before Parliament and asked to explain his actions. When he was subsequently relieved of his command, the associated disgrace destroyed his social as well as his professional life and he spent the rest of his days in obscurity.

Reluctantly, Galway assumed overall command of the troops in Spain as well as those based in Portugal, a position that he held until February 1708. Meanwhile, the two armies continued to be regarded as separate entities by London. Although the capture of Madrid had fulfilled the allies' main war objective, widespread revolt, desertions and the outbreak of disease, especially typhus, among the troops combined to reduce significantly the strength of the allied forces. As a result, it was decided to abandon the capital and move the headquarters across Spain to the port of Valencia where the army could receive supplies and the troops could move into winter quarters. It is assumed that the general hospital also moved to Valencia at that time. On 8 January 1707 a roll call of British soldiers was taken. The results, reproduced in Table 7.2 indicate that, as a result of sickness and other factors, such as absence, deaths, desertions and chronic undermanning, his effective force had been reduced by more than one-fifth of its supposed establishment.

Table 7.2 Account of the effective men, including corporals, in each regiment of foot in Portugal, January 1707

Regiment	Establishment	Effective	Absent	Sick
Lord Portmore's	698	593	62	43
Lt General Stewart's	698	647	26	25
Brigadier Blood's	698	495	66	137
Brigadier Brudenell's	698	499	134	65
Col Wade's	698	538	111	49
Totals	3,490	2,772	399	319

Source: TNA, SP 41/3, fol. 69/1.

It is probable that, as in Flanders, the hospitals in Spain and Portugal closed during the winter months. Certainly many senior officers returned to England at that time. On 1 February 1707 the hospital officers were called forward for the coming season's campaign and ordered to join a convoy preparing to sail from Portsmouth. That same day Dr Thomas Lawrence, the Physician General, was requested to 'hasten away the physicians for the hospital to Portsmouth' after applying to James Brydges, the Paymaster General, for an advance of 84 days' pay to be given to those travelling. The Surgeon General received a similar missive ordering the departures of two surgeons and four mates.[25]

Troop reinforcements had already been dispatched from England to Lisbon in late 1706 but, with Galway in Valencia, the draft was subsequently rerouted to that port. Among the transport ships was the *Charles*, a vessel of some 25,914 tons commanded by Master Henry Brand which had been fitted out to carry five members of the hospital staff, Commissary Douglas and four others, as well as the hospital's surgeons' chests.[26] Unfortunately, during the extended voyage, undertaken at the height of the winter gales, 50 per cent of the troops in the transports succumbed to a combination of typhus and exposure.

On 25 April 1707 Galway fought a disastrous action at Almanza against a French army under the command of the Duke of Berwick during which the British and their allies lost about 4,000 men killed or wounded. Some 3,000 were taken prisoner. In the aftermath of the battle Galway retired to Barcelona, where total confusion reigned. It appears that no accurate statistics of overall losses were recorded, although a list of English officers who were either killed or taken prisoner does survive. The casualties included a major general, a brigadier, seven colonels and twelve lieutenant colonels, as well as the regimental surgeon and mate of Southwell's Regiment. The list is summarized in Table 7.3.[27]

Table 7.3 English officers killed or taken prisoner at the battle of Almanza, 25 April 1707

	Killed	Prisoners
Horse	18	9
Dragoons	18	51
Foot	77	261
Marines	2	0
Totals	115	321

Source: BL Add. Mss, 22,264, fol. 42.

Poor record keeping was endemic throughout Galway's army. In the words of one contemporary writer, 'a great number of soldiers were sick in hospitals in Spain and Portugal of which no particular [number] can be given, as well as that diverse soldiers have been discharged and sent home just before the battle of Almanza'.[28] That such a state of affairs was condoned at the highest level is evident in a letter directed to Galway as early as 23 February 1707 by the Secretary of State which shows how a false sense of security and poor awareness of the true nature of the situation permeated their deliberations:

> Her Majesty observes that the methods of discipline there make it impossible to know the number of those troops with the same smartness as is practised in other parts and, considering with what cheerfulness and success they marched through Spain to Madrid, and the losses they sustained, and being very well assured that the King of Portugal has lately raised and is still raising a considerable number of forces, Her Majesty has not thought it advisable to make too nice an enquiry into the state of those troops especially since the enemy is making continual application to break an alliance of so great importance to the common cause.[29]

Ten months later the Secretary at War, Henry St John, was informed by the Secretary of State, Robert Harley, that the House of Commons required clarification of certain specific points relating to the army in Spain and Portugal. The two most important of these were, first, to establish the actual number of Portuguese troops provided on an annual basis since the treaty with that country had been signed in 1703 and, second, the number of soldiers present at the battle of Almanza together with those serving elsewhere in Spain at that time. In his reply, sent on 24 December, St John was forced to admit that he could not immediately provide a comprehensive reply. He had never been told the condition or strength of the troops provided by Portugal, either by Ministers of the Crown or by the General Officers serving abroad. Having been asked to find out, he made wide-ranging enquiries seeking accurate information but the replies that he received were all unsatisfactory while the accounts attached to these answers were always muddled and difficult to interpret. Despite large amounts of clothing, arms and equipment having been sent from England, many were unaccounted for and, in response to Parliament's demand for a statement of the numbers of regiments and troops in English pay at the time of the battle of Almanza, St John could only reply that

> the best information as can be had from the General Officers now here [in England] who were at the battle of Almanza shall be got for the satisfaction of the House, there being no other way of coming at the knowledge of what numbers these regiments in English pay consisted of at that time.[30]

The Secretary at War's correspondence with senior officers who had been present in Spain at the time of Almanza continued for many months. Various supposed lists detailing the numbers of troops present in Spain during 1707 were sent to the Secretary of War but, as late as January 1711, St John's successor, George Granville, eventually admitted that 'under our present state of uncertainty as to the condition of the army in Spain, I do not see how it is possible to make an exact estimate of the charge of the war in that country'.[31] In a final resigned acceptance of this situation, instructions were issued on 13 February 1711, ordering commanders to submit exact lists of troops present in their forces at both the beginning and end of every future campaign.[32]

As the information regarding the numbers of troops present emerged, it became clear that the number of British soldiers captured by the French at Almanza was so large that a paymaster dedicated solely to administer their affairs was required. John Arnott was appointed to this position and, between January 1708 and February 1710, he was granted the freedom to travel around the area between Paris and Valenciennes, where the majority of the prisoners were held, to distribute their subsistence money. He was provided with a French clerk, who was paid £196 for his services, while the hire of horses to facilitate these journeys cost £164.[33]

Several other officers, some prisoners of war themselves, were employed on similar duties. In due course, on 14 November 1709, one of these, Lieutenant John Adams, submitted a petition seeking reimbursement of his expenses. Having been captured at the battle of Almanza, he was taken to Bayonne in France where Major General Shrimpton, the senior local British officer, ordered him to 'subsist and take care of the prisoners as they came from Spain'. In the course of these duties he not only arranged for the prisoners to be fed but also attended the hospitals every day as an interpreter between the sick and their physicians. This, he claimed, had been 'to the great prejudice of his health and that he had been discharged of the said trust and had paid his account but has not yet been reimbursed'.[34] That same year, some two years after the battle of Almanza, the Paymaster General eventually allocated the sum of £5,875 for subsisting prisoners of war in France and Spain.[35]

Captain Thomas Hyde was another officer who had been employed in caring for the needs of British prisoners of war.[36] Following his return to England he petitioned for appointment as Sub-Major at the Royal Hospital at Chelsea, claiming that he was taken prisoner by the Duke of Berwick's army during the siege of Elcha and subsequently made responsible for the care of 400 English prisoners.

Every week for some thirteen weeks he had travelled a distance of 20 leagues 'from Monla Castle to Moncha', accompanied by guides that he hired at his own expense, to enable him to fetch money for the men's subsistence and thus prevent them from enlisting into the enemy's service. On one of these journeys he was robbed by local Spanish brigands of over 300 pistolles, a week's subsistence allocation, a sum that he had subsequently made good out of his own money. For four months he had survived on a diet of bread and water.

It is not known if Hyde's petition was successful but reimbursement of monies expended by individual officers and others on government service was seldom recovered speedily. For example, Paymaster Arnott had to wait until 1724 before he received a final payment of £850 12s 1d relating to monies owed to him for duties that he had carried out fifteen years earlier.[37] The treatment received by other officers was not much better. Earlier, in July 1706, Galway had written to St John regarding the plight of Captain Hugh White, who had been badly wounded in March 1705. The captain had already petitioned the government for reimbursement of the additional expense that he had been put to during the previous fifteen months as a result of a fractured leg that was, even then, not yet healed. White required a further surgical operation, which would attract even greater expense. In this case St John recommended that White should receive £60, the same amount as that paid to Marlborough's officers wounded at Blenheim.[38]

Meanwhile, in March 1707, Major General John Richards had been appointed Governor of the fortress of Alicante, the last stronghold in Valencia still held by the allies. It became obvious that, sooner or later, the French would lay siege to the town and, on 3 April, Richards reported to Galway that, in answer to an instruction received earlier regarding the evacuation of his sick and wounded, 'everything shall be done in relation to the sick and to the hospital in the manner you have ordered'.[39] Four days later, Richards told Galway that he had

> taken all the pains imaginable to get the remains of the sick people from Kirona but for want of carriage and the disobedience of the country people there still remain 30 or 40. I have hyred a ship, for boat there is none, and the Dutch have done the same, who at one will carry away all that we have together with the hospital to Denia at the rate of a dollar a head, the ship finding them with wood and water which is the cheapest I could get it done.[40]

Even so, all did not go well as, on 19 April, Richards instructed the Commissary at Kirona to continue providing medicines and food to the sick who remained there due to the non-availability of ships to evacuate them.[41]

On the same day Richards also informed Galway that he had received a demand for payment from the Duke of Berwick in respect of British troops captured by the French. He requested clarification of the current policy regarding the exchange of prisoners of war, 'it being a great expense and lots of time to bring them back here'. He enclosed the Duke of Berwick's letter 'in which he pretends we must pay for the bread they give our prisoners' with a request for confirmation that the French were making reciprocal payments in regard to their troops.[42] As has been previously discussed in Chapter 6 above, this was indeed common practice in Flanders and, in reply, he was assured that the French demand was not unusual but had in fact been the norm for some time past.[43] Even so, only one month later, Galway himself was to complain that prisoners were being taken to Flanders for exchange and thereby lost to his command. Had they been exchanged locally, he claimed that he 'could have raised about 12 good battalions'.[44] Meanwhile, Richards and 53 of his men were killed when a mine was exploded beneath the walls of Alicante and, following the subsequent surrender of the fortress, the remnants of the garrison were transferred to Minorca.

The situation continued to deteriorate when, on 12 November 1707, Lieutenant General Charles Wills, commanding the British troops serving with the Portuguese army in Lerida, wrote to Galway informing him the he had been forced to surrender the castle and garrison to the French after a four-month siege. He informed his Lordship that although he, Wills, had been obliged to capitulate, he was hopeful that the terms of surrender would allow him to rejoin Galway's forces with the survivors of his six battalions but, regretably, the debilitating effects of a prolonged siege and poor nutrition had taken their toll. The poor health and condition of the garrison forced Wills to 'leave a great many sick and wounded officers and soldiers behind me until they are in a condition to march to the camp or quarters of your Lordship'.[45] Fortunately, the articles of capitulation signed the previous day included an agreement that all of the flour, wine, medicines and other necessary provisions held in the store were to be given to the hospital staff for the benefit of the sick and wounded, although a proviso was set whereby the new French Governor was to arrange distribution of these items.[46]

It was obvious that the forces in both Spain and Portugal were in disarray. Questions were even asked in Whitehall about why the army in Spain, with twenty regiments, had only six general officers compared with the nine serving in Portugal where there were only sixteen regiments. Urgent demands were made for the situation to be rectified.[47] Despite their losses a sizeable body of British troops remained in Spain needing properly organized medical support. Although physicians, surgeons, drugs and equipment were dispatched from London in quantities that equalled those sent to Flanders, when these arrived at their destination, the army's administration had, for several years, failed in many respects to ensure that the troops gained maximum benefit from them.[48] In January 1708, Dr Amyott, Physician to the Commander in Chief of the Forces in Spain, had received the meagre sum of £300 for hospital medicines but, shortly afterwards, Dr LeCaan, who had been serving in Spain since 1705, was appointed Physician General in Spain. From this time it is possible to discern an improvement in both the reporting of medical affairs and general attitudes towards soldiers' care and welfare.[49] As noted in the previous chapter, LeCaan had previously gained considerable experience on active service in Ireland and Flanders and, in his new position, he began to exercise his authority in a letter to the Secretary at War in which he graphically described the sorry state that he had found during an initial inspection of the hospital. 'Patients were left naked to the cruelties of the weather', the smell was nauseous and, for want of adequate medicines and supplies, the patients 'could get no relief and the wounded cannot be dressed, and for want of sheets, blankets and other things (which cannot be purchased for money in that country) the poor men cannot be kept clean or warm'.[50] He then proceeded to describe how, as a direct consequence of these shortages, patients contracted highly contagious diseases that 'the officers and servants of the hospitals were not able to attend ... without the greatest and most constant danger of their lives' thereby rendering 'the conditions of the patients irrecoverable'.

Naturally, members of the hospital staff were not immune to disease and LeCaan emphasized that several surgeons and apothecaries had already died as a result of infection. He pressed for the supply of 600 single sheets, 400 double sheets, 500 beds and bolsters, 1,000 shirts, 600 single and 400 double blankets plus oatmeal, flour and medicines, identifying hospitals at Gibraltar, Alicante, Denia and Catalonia as the units whose needs were greatest.[51] Eventually, six months later, the effects that LeCaan's words had on Whitehall became evident when, on 26 June 1708, his demands were met and an order issued for £6,000 to be allocated out of the profits of the East India Company.[52]

By February 1708, advancing age and increasing debilitation had forced Galway to plead with London to be replaced in Spain. His request was partially accepted and Count Guido von Staremburg, an Austrian field marshall, was appointed to the overall command of allied troops in Spain. Galway, however, was to remain as Commander in Chief in Portugal and, on 9 February, he returned to Lisbon where, despite his continual requests for retirement, he was to remain for two further years as Commander in Chief. In Spain, Major General Stanhope, the English ambassador to Archduke Charles, was given the rank of Lieutenant General and placed in command of the English contingent, while also retaining his diplomatic post.

Little change had been made in the reception arrangements for casualties who survived long enough to be repatriated and, on arrival back in England, the problems of these men were far from resolved. As mentioned in Chapter 6 above, the coastal towns of the south and east had little option but to shoulder the acute financial burden imposed upon them by the continuous arrival of military casualties from overseas. Despite the problems noted earlier regarding the attitude of the Commissioners for Sick and Wounded Seamen when asked to provide care for soldiers evacuated by Admiral Rooke's fleet in 1702, no alternative official body was nominated to be routinely responsible for evacuated soldiers until, in 1709, after a shipload of men invalided from Portugal had been turned adrift in the streets of Penrhyn, penniless and reduced to begging for charity, the task was peremptorily thrust upon the Commissioners of Transport.[53] Unfortunately, this arrangement did little to ease the confusion or various conflicts of interest.

In July 1709, despite the continued absence of any monetary provision for casualties landed at Harwich from Flanders, just such an allowance was approved in respect of disabled soldiers brought from Portugal to Falmouth. From December 1706 onwards, a house had been hired in the Cornish port 'for use in taking care of land soldiers disabled in service abroad' at a cost of £30 per year.[54] Now, the newly introduced allowance, set at 6s 8d for treatment, was augmented by a further 1s per night for lodging until the patient was cured and another £1 for conduct money, calculated at a penny per mile, to cover transportation costs. To further standardize procedures, the duty of care for sick and infirm soldiers landed in Falmouth was delegated to a nominated local surgeon, Thomas Code, who received a retainer of £25 a year for services in such matters in addition to his agreeing to act as the local agent of the Commissioners for Sick and Wounded Seamen.[55]

Code was obviously kept busy as, on 19 July 1709, the Queen's Remembrancer at Exeter wrote to Secretary at War, Walpole, requesting that the large sum of £306 6s 4d be issued to Code for 'quarters and cure of sick and wounded soldiers put on shore at Falmouth between 1 September 1706 and 30 September 1708'.[56] On 1 July 1709, the Commissioners for Sick and Wounded Seamen attempted, with limited success, to extend this move towards standardization by indicating to the Lord Treasurer that the system and level of remuneration should be standardized throughout all ports and harbours, both large and small.[57] However, it was not only casualties returning to England from overseas who required care and attention. Recruits and reinforcements awaiting departure for foreign parts frequently fell sick due to delays caused by bad weather and other factors. Convoys making ready to sail overseas were frequently forced to remain in harbour for long periods while awaiting a favourable wind. Crammed into constricted spaces on board transport ships, the embarked soldiers quickly fell victim to a variety of communicable diseases. Such was the case in 1708 when General Earl wrote to the Secretary at War requesting that, having been forced to send a large number of men from an outward-bound convoy into the naval hospitals at Dover and Portsmouth, the necessary authority be granted for their continued care under naval auspices.[58] This was done. Later, when the men had recovered sufficiently, they were sent to the Isle of Wight to await onward transport to their units. As previously noted, this was a measure frequently adopted in an attempt to reduce the high rate of desertion prevalent among troops bound for unpopular duty on the Iberian Peninsula.[59]

The confusion and difficulties that existed regarding the financial arrangements for the care of repatriated sick and wounded mirrored the general state of the army's administrative affairs as it attempted to fight a war on several fronts. By August 1709, permanently frustrated in his relationships with his country's allies, Galway expressed his utter desperation in a letter to the Secretary of State in which he complained bitterly of the chicanery of both the court and the King of Portugal:

> When I represented to them the miserable state of their cavalry, their horses perishing for want of barley, their soldiers without pay or bread, the easiness with which the Marquis de Bay can overrun their country, they are as insensible and give as little attention as if I was talking to them of the Czar's affairs, so I see no manner of way to waken them from their lethargy, besides the court is in the utmost confusion. The Marquis d'Alegrette, who has hitherto chiefly governed, is dying. The [Portuguese] King's health is very suspicious ... The Queen has no manner of authority and nobody appears in the government of affairs, neither do I know any among them capable of it to whom I could address, so your Lordship's sees what can be expected from hence.[60]

Communication difficulties between the commanders on the ground and Whitehall were a continuing major problem and came to characterize the Spanish and Portuguese campaigns. While natural delays occurred in the conveyance of dispatches by sea between London and the Iberian Peninsula, many additional factors existed. The commanders in the field seem to have developed a particular reluctance to communicate with Whitehall. Inevitably, this unfortunate tendency frequently initiated or exacerbated pre-existing problems. A clear example can be noted in the way that personalities were nominated to fill vacant appointments. On 9 May 1709 the Earl of Galway complained to the Earl of Sunderland that, although he had been granted authority to fill vacant positions locally when necessary, the Queen continued to nominate her own appointments for the same vacancies.[61] Perhaps the case of Dr William Neilson, who was appointed by Whitehall to the supposedly vacant post of Director of the Hospital in Portugal in March 1709, was the most prominent example of this situation.[62] Neilson had seen a considerable amount of former service as Physician to the Hospital in Spain under Peterborough but, before he could assume his new post, Galway, 'not knowing that your Petitioner was then serving in Spain', appointed another by the name of Oates to the same position. When Neilson arrived in Lisbon to assume his duties he found himself out of a job and was obliged to return home at his own expense, taking his clerks with him, having sold all his equipment in order to pay for the journey.

On receipt of Neilson's subsequent plea for redress, the Queen referred his plight to the Secretary at War for investigation. In due course Colonel Bladon, the Earl of Galway's military secretary, advised Neilson that he was convinced, for whatever reason, that his service was unacceptable to the Earl and advised him to accept a douceur of ten shillings a day (half pay) as a retainer. Meanwhile, he was further advised to remain in England until, at some point in the future, Galway decided how to employ him. As Neilson was technically under Galway's command, the doctor accepted these terms believing that he had no option but to comply.

By this time, the Earl of Galway had suffered further physical decline. At the age of 62, overworked and suffering from the loss of an eye, gout and rheumatism, he had been pleading for several months to be relieved so that he could retire. On 20 January 1710, tired and worn out, he wrote in his own hand to the Secretary of State complaining that he was very ill and could no longer carry on.[63] He asked to be allowed to return and spend the remainder of his life in retirement on his estates. Two months later, in the absence of a reply, he wrote again. A prolonged attack of gout, added to his other infirmities, had left him afraid that he would never ride a horse again and he indicated that, as his memory was impaired, he felt unable to act as the Queen's ambassador. As a result of his illness he could no longer sign his own name.[64] Shortly afterwards, in October 1710, Galway was finally relieved and replaced as Commander in Chief in Portugal by someone even less well motivated, David Colyer, the Earl of Portmore.

In due course Neilson applied to the new commander who, in turn, promised the doctor that he could assume his appointed post. Somewhat relieved, Neilson embarked once again for Portugal on board the same ship as Portmore and his entourage but, 'to your petitioners great surprise', when he landed once more at Lisbon, he found a certain Mr Charles Shadwell, 'a person in no way qualified for that post', acting as Director of the Hospital in accordance with a commission from the Earl of Galway. Such was the state of confusion over the powers of commanders to make appointments that, when Neilson turned to Portmore for redress, the Earl replied 'that it was no act of his' and, if Neilson could determine the Queen's wishes in the matter, he would be only too happy to restore the doctor to his rightful post. As matters stood, Neilson was not in a position to return home and obtain the support of the Queen as his financial circumstances were such that his 'creditors, from whom he had had to borrow money in expectation of receiving his pay, would put him into gaol upon his return to England'.[65] In the event Neilson was forced to send Andrew Tate, one of his clerks, back to England to solicit friends in order to obtain the Queen's commission.

Seven months after Neilson's initial appointment date, Walpole informed Henry Boyle, one of the Principal Secretaries of State, that the situation was much more complex than had initially been thought. In a piece of typical Whitehall subtlety, Walpole attempted to rationalize matters by admitting that 'for some years past', despite the obvious presence of such a unit, the establishment for a hospital in Portugal had not been officially authorized. As a result, the Queen's appointment of Neilson to the post of Director had, in legal terms, created a new office and, it was noted diplomatically, did not in any way interfere with the powers given by Her Majesty to her Generals abroad to dispose of vacant commissions. The absence of an official hospital establishment goes a long way towards explaining the confused state of affairs in everything relating to the hospital facilities in Portugal.

However, as Neilson had already been superseded in his former post as Physician to the Hospital in Spain by Dr LeCaan, he now stood in danger of losing both his new post and his livelihood to Lord Galway's nominee.[66] The entire matter hinged upon a single point – was the commission granted by the Earl of Galway sufficient to supersede that granted by the Queen? This was particularly relevant in light of the fact that, at the time that the Earl gave a commission to Shadwell, he had not only known that the Queen had already granted one for the same office to Neilson but had also acknowledged the situation by bringing pressure to bear upon the doctor to force his acceptance of a 'pension' in lieu of pay for the duration of the time that he, Galway, remained in command in Portugal.[67]

The full reasons for Galway's reluctance to agree to the doctor's appointment will probably never be known. In due course Shadwell submitted a counter-petition in which he claimed that several general officers supported his cause and that he had 'put the hospital into much better method than previously'. Even the Earl of Portmore commented that 'Dr Neilson, who professes physic, may not be a fit person for that employment' but, for the good of the service, since the Queen had declared that Neilson's commission was to stand, Shadwell had no alternative but to quit his office. In the event, to ease his burden, Shadwell was authorized to receive the ten shillings per day formerly paid to Neilson until other employment could be found for him in Portugal.[68] The affair continued to grumble on until eventually, in February 1712, the Queen resolved the situation when, following the death of Dr Dunoon, the Physician General in Portugal, she suggested that Neilson be appointed in his place and the post of Director of the Hospital be given to Shadwell. Subsequently, in a letter dated 9 May 1712, Lord Lansdowne expressed his thanks to Portmore for informing him that, finally, the Neilson versus Shadwell affair had ended in accordance with the Queen's wishes.[69]

Problems associated with the control and direction of officers' movements and appointments were more extensive than the occasional individual dispute might imply. Normally a reasonably complex process, the filling of officers' vacancies and appointments was made more complex by the need to provide appropriate people, many on a temporary basis, to fill vacancies caused by the huge losses sustained at the battle of Almanza. This entailed sending a significant number of junior officers, lieutenants and captains, from England and Flanders, to fill vacancies left by those recuperating from wounds or held as prisoners in France. In some cases this resulted in individuals holding, on paper, two appointments at the same time. The case of Joseph Ankott, a master surgeon, who was sent to serve with the army in Spain, was typical. Ankott had been serving as the regimental surgeon of Colonel Hill's Regiment in Flanders when he was posted to Spain. He officially retained this appointment in addition to his new role which was, presumably, to act as surgeon to Southwell's Regiment whose normal doctor had been captured at Alamanza. In such cases, many even retained an entitlement to two salaries as when, in due course, Ankott's wife Jane petitioned for financial support, she was granted her husband's pay as the surgeon of a regiment in Flanders while, presumably, he continued to draw a salary for his work in Spain.[70] The sum that Mrs Ankott received was paid to her out of a fund of £12,000 set aside by the government for the pay of the seconded officers and, presumably, to provide the money needed to pay second salaries to those so entitled. Later, when officers held by the French were exchanged or released from imprisonment and returned to duty, those who had been seconded to fill their vacant posts either went back to their original regiments or were retired on half pay.

Meanwhile, in the early spring of 1710, von Staremburg who, as previosuly noted, had relieved Galway in command of the forces in Spain two years earlier, decided to mount an offensive campaign during which his troops successfully took Saragossa and Castile and recaptured Madrid. By then, however, the sympathies of the Spanish people were almost entirely pro-French. Short of supplies and plagued by continual desertions from his army, Staremburg took the fateful decision to divide his force into its constituent national components. The bulk of the English troops in Spain had taken up quarters for the winter in Brihuega, where they were surprised, trapped and besieged by a superior French army. On 9 December 1710, after a fierce resistance, they were overwhelmed and the castle surrendered. General Stanhope, with almost 2,000 of his soldiers, was captured. He spent the next two years as a prisoner of the French.⁷¹ The following day, in an attempt to relieve Brihuega, Staremburg's forces also suffered heavy casualties at Villa Viciosa, and retreated.

The combined effects of these setbacks left the whole of Spain, effectively, in enemy hands. In May, with Stanhope in captivity, command of the English troops in Spain was handed to the Duke of Argyle. The confusion that permeated everything concerned with the administration of the army in the Iberian Peninsula also disrupted the efficient distribution of drugs and equipment. In the spring of 1711, a cargo of medicines valued at £1,632 6s 10d, supplied by apothecary William Lilly, was dispatched on board the transport ship *William* for the use of the hospitals in Spain.⁷² When, in due course, a bill for this cargo was presented to the Paymaster General, the latter's immediate response was to claim that 'the deficiencies of the current year were so great' there was not enough money available to pay for them.⁷³ This was yet another example of poor or faulty communication. The Duke of Argyle had circumvented the normal channels by submitting the annual Spanish order for drugs directly to Lilly. Reaction was not long in coming from an irate Apothecary General and, on 12 March, the Secretary at War responded by writing to the Duke enclosing a letter from an annoyed Isaac Teale complaining that he, Teale, by virtue of his commission, held the sole right to supply medicines to the forces and reminded all concerned of the Act of Parliament that required medicines and goods to be inspected by appropriate authorities at Apothecaries' Hall prior to dispatch.⁷⁴ Teale also alleged that, in obtaining the order, Lilly had 'made use of his [Teale's] name without good reason'.⁷⁵ Argyle was then asked to state what objections he had, if any, to medicines being provided through the normal channels. Protracted arguments ensued that centred on whether the goods should be paid for and, if so, by whom. More than a year passed before a way around the impasse was found and it was decided that Lilly had supplied the drugs in question before the quoted Act of Parliament had been passed. Lilly was eventually reimbursed with the full value of the cargo.⁷⁶

Lilly's trials were serious enough, but they paled into insignificance alongside those of another apothecary, Mr Richard Lawrence. On 10 March the Secretary of State informed Dr Dunoon, Physician General to the army in Portugal (who was at that time in London, having spent the winter months in England) that his recent order for medicines for the hospital and regiments in Portugal had been prepared by the apothecary, Richard Lawrence, and was awaiting inspection by Dunoon himself, accompanied by Dr Thomas Lawrence, the Physician General to the Army, prior to their dispatch.⁷⁷ On 20 March 1711 Dunoon certified that this had been done but, subsequently, a further order was issued that required a second inspection, this time by the Physician General accompanied by Alexander Inglish, Surgeon General of the army. This was in accordance with existing regulations that stipulated a surgeon's assessment was required in addition to that of a physician. This was done on 20 March and, six days later, Richard Lawrence confirmed that he had personally supervised the loading of the goods packed into seven crates aboard the *Union* transport. Of these, six were destined for the hospital while the seventh contained 40 regimental chests that had been loaded in accordance with an order issued some ten days earlier by the Commissary of the Train. All were marked for delivery to Dr Dunoon on arrival in Lisbon. In due course, on 27 April, a Royal Warrant was issued for Lawrence to be paid £1,314 10s 1d for the items that he had dispatched, but the matter did not end there.

The nefarious means by which many office holders conducted their business is brought into stark relief by subsequent events. Sometime after the drugs, medicines and instruments had arrived in Portugal, Dr Neilson wrote to Lawrence saying that he, Neilson, had first claim upon any reimbursement of outstanding dues and was apprehensive that Lawrence's claim would hinder or delay any outstanding payments due to him. He went on to inform Lawrence that a clerk was on his way to England carrying documents stating that, unless Lawrence consented to having his payment warrant altered in favour of 'the Army Contingency Fund for Portugal', Neilson would deliver certificates to both the Lord Treasurer and to Lord Portmore claiming that part of the goods sent by Lawrence were 'not good'.[78] Perhaps Neilson's willingness to engage in this form of thinly veiled and underhand threat displays a character trait of which Galway had been aware when he had earlier refused his services! Shortly afterwards Portmore, no doubt at Neilson's behest, adopted an even more aggressive attitude. He sent his personal secretary to call upon Lawrence and inform him that unless he, Lawrence, agreed to these proposals, payment of his dues would be stopped completely. Lawrence appealed to the Secretary at War and, in reply, was reassured that none of this was acceptable and that it was impossible for him to comply with Lord Portmore's demands.

On 12 November 1712 the Paymaster General requested the Secretary at War to provide him with a list of everyone who had submitted demands for reimbursement of monies expended in supporting the hospital in Spain together with an 'account of the state and condition of the hospital' and its means of funding.[79] Two months later, on 20 January 1713, a report from Lawrence listing the drugs and materials that he had supplied was referred to Lord Portmore for his comments. In his reply, the Earl rejected any personal responsibility for the initial order, claiming that he would never have sanctioned such large quantities, and refusing to sanction the notion that he had ever given directions for sending such a large quantity as was listed in Lawrence's inventory. As regards their quality, Portmore referred to a certificate, purportedly signed at the time by the director, physician, master surgeon and master apothecary of the British hospital in Portugal, in which it was reported that, when the drugs arrived in Lisbon, the greater part were found to be bad and unfit for service. As a result, the warrant obtained by Lawrence for £1,214 10s 1d for the said drugs was withheld until, upon further examination, it could be established how much was salvaged and actually used in the service.[80]

Eventually, some five months later, on 13 May, the Comptroller of Army Accounts confirmed that the original acceptance certificate was to stand. The Paymaster General, Brydges, added his comment that as the William Lilly, whose case was described earlier, had supplied an even greater quantity of drugs to the hospital in Spain at the same time, for which he had been paid, it would only be fair if Lawrence should now receive his money. Eventually, on 13 June 1713, as a result of yet another appeal, to which he appended copies of all the documents that supported his petition, 'delayed as a result of Lord Portmore's inconvenience', Lawrence finally received his warrant for payment of the outstanding £1,314 10s 1d in full.[81]

Apothecaries were not the only victims of parsimony. Most military surgeons who served in Spain and Portugal faced similar difficulties in gaining adequate remuneration for their work. James Maxwell had to wait until February 1710 before he received reimbursement of £31 5s 0d in respect of medical supplies that he had provided to soldiers at the battle of Brihuega some four years earlier.[82] Peter Rouviere, who had been sent by the Earl of Galway to take care of British soldiers captured by the French at the battle of Almanza (25 April 1707), had to wait even longer. He had continued in this duty for some five months, incurring considerable personal expense. Later, at Brihuega, he had himself been taken prisoner and had lost all his baggage. In 1713, with peace in Spain concluded, he was destitute and requested the half-pay pension that was due to him as a result of his length of service. His petition, supported by references provided by several high-ranking officers, was eventually granted at the rate of 5s per day back-dated to 24 December 1712.[83]

The cost of living throughout the Iberian Peninsula had risen dramatically while the war continued. In March 1711, shortly after his arrival, Portmore discovered that he had inherited a system whereby Galway, in order to save his troops from starvation, had paid his dragoons at a rate higher than their normal pay entitlement.[84] In requesting more money, Portmore also asked for an extra physician, an assistant apothecary and a clerk to be added to the establishment of his flying hospital. No other mention has yet been found to indicate that the army's hospital in Spain possessed, or indeed practised, a capability to form a mobile sub-unit similar to that employed in Flanders. Having originally been designed to accommodate 400–500 patients, the hospital in Spain would certainly have resembled the size of its counterpart and it would not have been impossible for such a use to have been implemented. Although there was no mention of any such facility in the official published establishment, in all probability the Earl's request mirrors a local, unsanctioned arrangement about which London had not been informed.

This is yet another example of poor documentation and begs the question 'why was the medical administration in Spain and Portugal so lax?' In Flanders, strict control was exerted over the structure and performance of medical units. The work of the hospital director, especially his expenditure, was carefully monitored by regular checks undertaken by senior officers. It has to be said, however, that similar moves were attempted at various times in Spain and Portugal but these did not involve inquisitive senior officers and, as a result, met with only limited success. On 11 September 1711, in the absence of any other responsible authority, the Commissioners for Sick and Wounded Seamen were asked to provide an account of their agents abroad, especially those employed to care for seamen in Spain and Portugal.[85] The same day a memorandum required them to send envoys to Spain and Portugal to inspect the entire system of hospital provision and accounting as well as to inspect and report upon the methods whereby checks, controls, inspections and surveys were conducted, and by whom.[86] Additionally, they were to carry with them copies of the accounts held in London for comparison with documents held locally. Sadly, no report of the Commissioners' findings has yet been found, nor does there appear to be any indication of the effect, if any, that their visit had on subsequent hospital administration policy. The only positive additional measure known to have been taken at that time was an agreement whereby the sum of £2,045 18s 8d was set aside to boost the fund for the relief of widows of officers killed in Spain and Portugal previously discussed in Chapter 6 above.[87]

A decision by the British government to withdraw from any involvement in further military action brought an end to the fighting in Spain and Portugal. On 16 September 1712 orders were given for the disbandment of several regiments where they stood. This action left large numbers of soldiers homeless and destitute. Officers were ordered to return home immediately while the majority of the troops were withdrawn to Gibraltar and Minorca.[88] Many sick and wounded soldiers unfit to travel were left behind until Thomas Peace, a local agent for the Commission for Sick and Wounded Seamen in Lisbon, brought their plight to the attention of Major General James Pearce. In May 1712, Pearce had been sent to take over command in Portugal from Portmore and to wind up affairs after the latter's departure. In his letter, Peace complained to Pearce that no instructions had been issued on how he was to pay the officers and troopers who had been reduced to half pay by the disbandments and were now in need of care and attention. Naturally, in line with contemporary practice, the army's hospital in Lisbon had closed when the regiments departed and yet there remained 300 sick men who required ongoing hospital care. Pearce had no option but to agree that these men should be admitted to Portuguese hospitals but he held no funds from which to pay hospital bills or any other contingencies. Prior to his departure for England, Neilson, the former director, had entered into an agreement whereby the naval hospital in Lisbon would accept soldiers but, on enquiry, Peace came face to face with yet another inter-service problem. He discovered that the admission of soldiers to the naval hospital would attract charges of 1s 3d per man per day over and above a separate entrance fee that was being demanded by the resident naval surgeon. As a result his only option was to seek permission and find sufficient funds to enable him to hire carts so that he could transport the sick to Lisbon for embarkation and repatriation to England. He also requested that he be permitted to take on a small personal staff, a secretary and a physician, who could supervise the care of army patients when they were admitted to 'the Misericords', the Portuguese name for local poor hospitals.[89]

Financial authority was granted and the subsequent extent to which local hospital facilities were used can be assessed from a letter, dated 5 November 1713, sent from the Treasury to the Secretary at War, requesting him to prepare a warrant for the payment of £3,010 6s 9d to General Pearce. This huge sum reflects the amount that he had expended in providing care for sick soldiers in Portuguese poor hospitals between 21 September 1712 and 10 January 1713. Eight days later the necessary funds were raised by the release of government stock held in the South Sea Company.[90]

Itemized bills provided in support of Pearce's claim indicate that the 'misericordia' or 'house of pity' at Estremos was used as the main collecting centre for the sick and wounded brought in from other disparate locations including those at Vlla Vicosa and Redondo, both located about twenty miles from Estremos, and that of Beja, some sixty miles further south.[91] The invoices submitted for payment by these hospitals included charges for supplying the patients with meat, wine, bedding, fuel, water and oil at a standard rate of 9d a day per man. This element of the overall bill was divided for payment between the regiments to whom the patients belonged, calculated at 5d per day for each man, and charged as subsistence. The Major General paid the remaining 4d on behalf of the government. There were also charges listed for other elements, described vaguely as 'additional items' and 'senior officers', as well as the provision of mules, although transportation costs to convey patients from various outlying hospitals was invoiced separately.

Although the war in Spain had eventually spluttered to a desultory end in 1712, it took until June 1713, long after the forces in both Spain and Portugal had been disbanded, before any form of centralized statement of pay due to the army's hospital staff was completed. The final account, which was by no means comprehensive, and provides only a partial glimpse of the final hospital establishment, is shown in Table 7.4.

Table 7.4 Final payment to medical staff on disbandment of the hospital in Spain, for services provided between 25 December 1709 and 23 December 1710

Vincent Chabane, Director of the hospital in Spain: £456 5s
James Penman, Master Surgeon of the hospital in Spain: £182 10s
Dr Alexander Innes, Chaplain to the hospital in Spain: £21 13s 4d.
Rowland Size, Apothecary at the hospital in Spain: £91 5s
Richard Quinn, Surgeons' Mate at the hospital in Spain: £91 5s
John Cole, Surgeons' Mate at the hospital in Spain: £91 5s
John Hawkins, Surgeons' Mate at the hospital in Spain: £91 5s

Source: *Cal. Treas. Books, 1713* (2 vols, 1955), pp. 260–61.

In addition to the above, Charles Shadwell, by then restored to his post as the Director of the British Hospital in Portugal, received £91 10s for his services between 23 December 1711 and 22 June 1712.[92] On the other hand, surgeons' mates William Elphinstone, Robert Napier, Robert Maitland and John Mylne, who had been granted advances of three months' pay in April 1710 to enable them to travel to Spain, are not mentioned in this financial summary.[93]

As has been shown earlier in this work, the hands-on daily care of patients was normally the function and responsibility of nurses employed specifically for that purpose. While nurses and ancillary staff were certainly employed in Spain and Portugal, who they were or where they came from remains an enigma, although much can be inferred. For example, it can be shown that wives certainly accompanied the troops as, in July 1704, five women applied to go to Portugal to join their husbands who were serving there in General Stewart's Regiment. Following correspondence with the regiment's commanding officer in which enquiries were made into the practicalities of agreeing to such a request, St John was informed that the regiment would welcome 'necessary women'. The appropriate passes were subsequently issued.

In April the following year St John wrote to the Commissioner of Transportation offering guidance regarding the allocation of shipping to the regiments then ordered to Jamaica and there is no reason to suggest that the advice offered varied to any great extent from that relating to Spain or Portugal.[94] His letter included a directive that a regiment was to be calculated as numbering 834 men, including commissioned officers and their servants but, in addition to that number, provision was also to be made for 48 'necessary women' per regiment. This represented an allocation of four women per company. Later the same day these calculations were amended by a second letter that reduced the figure to three women per company – 36 women per regiment.[95] It can therefore be deduced that considerable numbers of women were available with the army to provide female nurses in the hospitals on the Iberian Peninsula.

Regrettably, the surviving information relating to the day-to-day work of the army hospitals is almost entirely limited to warrants authorizing payments of salary, bills for the supply of drugs and equipment, and the desperate pleas of medical staff seeking reimbursement of funds expended on hospital business. This is not surprising given the general lackadaisical approach to control, administration and commitment that is evident in the attitude of the commanders despite the good intentions of Whitehall. Where then does the root of the problem lie? Throughout most of the years that the campaign in Flanders and Germany was fought, a competent commander, assisted by an equally brilliant quartermaster general, exerted genuine and continuing personal interest in the lives and the welfare of their troops. In Spain and Portugal, where a series of self-interested and incompetent leaders held command, little thought was given to these matters and the medical service provided to soldiers suffered as a result.

Notes

1. Hon. A. Parnell, *The War of The Succession in Spain* (London: George Bell, 1905), pp. 21–50.
2. TNA, WO 26/11, fols 67–71.
3. TNA, WO 4/2, 4/3 and 4/4, *passim*.

4   *Cal. S.P. Dom., 1702*, p. 270.
5   TNA, WO 4/4, fols 16–8.
6   Ibid., fol. 71.
7   TNA, WO 4/2, fol. 28.
8   Ibid., fol. 84.
9   Fortescue, vol. 1, p. 447.
10 Ibid., pp. 120, 300 and 321.
11 *Cal. Treas. Books, January 1704–March 1705*, p. 229.
12 Ibid., p. 544.
13 TNA, WO 4/4, fol. 246.
14 *Cal. Treas. Books, January 1704–March 1705*, p. 463.
15 TNA, 26/12, n. fol.
16 BL Add. Mss 22,264, fol. 10; *Cal. Treas. Books, January 1704–March 1705*, p. 430 and *1705–1706* (3 vols, 1952), vol. 2, p. 243.
17 Ibid., fols 67–8.
18 TNA, WO 4/4, fols 62–3 and WO 4/7, fols 79 and 226.
19 Ibid.
20 Ibid.
21 TNA, WO 4/4, fol. 68.
22 Ibid., fol. 141.
23 HMC, *Cholmondeley Mss*, Appendix, p. 348.
24 Ibid.
25 TNA, WO 4/4, fols 141–42.
26 BL Stowe, 471, fol. 57.
27 BL Add. Mss, 22,264, fol. 42.
28 Ibid., fol. 16.
29 Ibid., fol. 18.
30 TNA, WO 4/7, fols 81–2.
31 TNA, WO 4/10, fol. 94.
32 Ibid., fol. 185.
33 BL Add. Mss, 22,616, fol. 176.
34 *Cal. Treas. Books, 1709* (1949), p. 424.
35 Ibid., p. 211.
36 TNA, SP 34/33, fols 199–200.
37 BL Add. Mss, 22,616, fol. 177.
38 TNA, WO 4/5, fol. 9.
39 BL Stowe, 474, n. fol. entry for 3 April 1707.
40 Ibid., entry for 8 April 1707.
41 Ibid., entry for 16 April 1707.
42 BL Add. Mss, 61504, fol. 40.
43 Ibid., fol. 43.
44 BL Add. Mss, 61504, fols 44–5.
45 BL Add. Mss, 61504, fol. 79.
46 Ibid., fol. 73.
47 TNA, WO 4/10, fol. 39.
48 BL Add. Mss, 22,264, fol. 36.
49 *Cal. Treas. Books, 1707–8* (1950), p. 74.

50 Ibid., pp. 176–7.
51 Ibid.
52 Ibid., p. 288.
53 *Cal. S.P. Dom., 1711*, p. 21; Fortescue, vol. 1, p. 562.
54 TNA, WO 4/4, fol. 7.
55 *Cal. Treas. Books, 1707–8*, pp. 257 and 566.
56 *Cal. Treas. Books, 1709*, p. 259.
57 Ibid.
58 TNA, WO 4/7, fol. 304.
59 Ibid, fol. 327.
60 BL Add. Mss, 61506, fol. 61.
61 Ibid., fol. 27.
62 TNA, SP 34/28, fol. 8; WO 4/8, fol. 148.
63 BL Add. Mss, 61506, fol. 124.
64 Ibid., fols 183–6 and 194.
65 Ibid., fol. 8v.
66 Ibid., fol. 9v.
67 Ibid., fol. 9v.
68 TNA, SP 34/15, fols 97–8.
69 TNA, WO 4/13, fol. 125.
70 TNA, WO 4/8, fol. 147.
71 Parnell, pp. 289–92.
72 TNA, SP 34/28, fol. 54.
73 *Cal. Treas. Books, 1711* (2 vols, 1950), vol. 2, p. 463.
74 TNA, WO 4/12, fol. 233.
75 TNA, WO 4/10, fol. 274.
76 *Cal. Treas. Books, 1712* (2 vols, 1954), vol. 1, p. 43 and WO 4/12, fol. 233.
77 TNA, WO 4/10, fol. 269.
78 BL Add. Mss, 22,616, fols 165–68.
79 *Cal. Treas. Books, 1712*, vol. 1, p. 509.
80 Ibid., p. 86.
81 BL Add. Mss, 22,616, fols 165–168.
82 *Cal. Treas. Books,1713* (2 vols, 1955), vol. 1, p. 186.
83 Ibid., p. 299.
84 TNA, WO 4/10, fols 313–5.
85 *Cal. Treas. Books, 1711* (2 vols, 1961), vol. 2, p. 443.
86 Ibid., pp. 95 and 443.
87 Ibid., p. 96.
88 TNA, WO 4/13, fol. 99.
89 TNA, SP 41/4, fol. 120.
90 *Cal. Treas. Books, 1713,* II, p. 430.
91 Ibid., pp. 420–21.
92 Ibid.
93 TNA, WO 4/9, fol. 428.
94 TNA, WO 4/3, fol. 226.
95 Ibid., fol. 227.

Chapter 8

Evaluation

At the beginning of the period under discussion the British Standing Army was a fledgling organization attempting to find its feet after the wholesale demolition of its predecessor, the New Model Army of the Commonwealth, following the Restoration of the Monarchy. The destruction of the hospital facilities that had been established by Parliament during the preceding twenty years left a vacuum that was not immediately filled. Little consideration was given to providing a medical service in support of the pitifully small body of soldiers authorized by a government who, in view of the recent past, were understandably fearful of a large standing army. Parliament saw no reason to add to its financial burden by providing medical facilities for an organization whose perceived role was limited to the protection of the King and his royal palaces, especially when the existing services of the London Poor Hospitals, working in conjunction with unit and garrison surgeons, appeared to provide adequate cover for the soldiers' needs.

The acquisition of Tangier dictated the dispatch of a sizeable British garrison, recruited mainly from former Parliamentary soldiers then serving in Dunkirk, to defend the new colony against marauding local tribesmen. Of necessity, this entailed the provision of medical facilities, however basic, for the sick and wounded casualties that would and did inevitably ensue. The government's lack of enthusiasm for the task mirrored the disastrous earlier response by the Commonwealth government to the provision of medical facilities during Cromwell's 'Western Design' expedition to the West Indies in 1655, and for the campaign in Flanders during 1657.[1]

Despite its unsuitability, the building requisitioned for use as the garrison's hospital at the start of the colony's existence continued in use as such throughout the time that Tangier remained in British hands. This was despite the urgings of local governors and moves by engineers to promote the construction of a purpose-built facility. As discussed above in Chapter 1, even though their efforts met with little success, the plans submitted in support of their arguments survive to provide evidence of the changes taking place in contemporary thinking regarding the design and construction of hospitals, concepts that may be seen today in the design and structure of such important landmark buildings as the Royal Hospital, Chelsea and the Hôtel des Invalides in Paris.

The proposal for the construction of a lazarette was equally important. Whereas England's position as an island may have promoted a false belief that the sea provided a barrier against infection from overseas, the formulation and submission of a design for a designated isolation facility enabled the colony's engineer and indirectly the Tangier Board members to broaden their experience of such structures through comparison with those existing in other Mediterranean countries. It also introduced the doctors to the relatively unfamiliar concept of preventive medicine. Although this first period of England's involvement in Africa was conducted at a time when the army's medical services and hospital facilities had reached the nadir of their fortunes, the physicians and surgeons of the garrison certainly acquired experience in active disease prevention that were to serve to the army's benefit in later years. As a result the garrison's physician, Dr Thomas Lawrence, who in later life served as Physician General in the armies of William III and Marlborough, was well equipped to become these latter commanders' senior medical adviser. Despite a widespread lack of motivation among senior officers of the garrison towards improving their poorly funded and ill-supported hospital facilities, the occupation of Tangier stimulated a broader understanding of the effects of diseases in hot climates among an army engaged in a long-term struggle against an indigenous people. It is questionable whether this knowledge was utilized to the best effect in the garrisons subsequently established elsewhere.

Back in England, although the Savoy Hospital was reopened during the second and third Dutch Wars, this arrangement did not survive the end of these wars and the hospital was closed again each time peace was declared. The only remaining effective acute hospital care available to sick soldiers was provided by small regimental hospitals and the continued traditional use of the Poor Hospitals of London, St Bartholomew's and St Thomas'. The use of British soldiers as mercenary troops in the service of France during the 1670s did, at least, achieve the benefit of widening their officers' understanding of continental methods. Regimental surgeons also gained a broader experience of providing care to troops in battle, while there was an increasing awareness of the actions taken in France to alleviate the lot of discharged veterans such as Louis XIV's establishment of the Hôtel des Invalides.

At this time a general thirst for scientific experimentation (typified by the formation of such learned bodies as the Royal Society) and the spread of alternative ideas and increased knowledge exerted a significant influence on military medical thought during the remainder of Charles II's reign and that of his brother, James II. The desire of Charles not to be outdone by his French cousin led directly to the foundation of the two royal veterans' institutions at Kilmainham and Chelsea while his brother James, with his close interest in the army as a pillar of his personal power-base, introduced several improvements in the field of soldiers' welfare, including enhanced benefits payable to soldiers or their dependants following death, injury or discharge from the service. An increasing awareness of the benefits to be gained from conserving manpower by paying attention to the health and well-being of the soldiers, rather than increasing wastage through neglect, is evident from the trouble taken to construct a hospital close by the camp established on Hounslow Heath during each year of the new monarch's reign. There, for the first time since the Restoration (apart from Portsmouth's short-lived garrison hospital), a dedicated military hospital facility, with a permanent staff of doctors, nurses and administrators, was opened specifically to cater for the needs of sick or injured troops. This was a highly significant event in the history of the army's medical services and it is interesting to speculate what would have developed out of this establishment had the so-called 'Glorious Revolution' of 1688 not occurred. As it was, soldiers at the time, and in the years that followed, were fortunate that the services of St Bartholomew's and St Thomas' hospitals were available to fall back on in times of need.

Following the accession of William III, the disastrous start to the wars in Ireland acted as a catalyst for change in the provision of military hospitals and general medical support for Britain's army. The subsequent introduction of Dutch army methods included the formation of mobile field hospitals which brought, for the first time, a capability to provide integrated and continuous close medical support to the fighting troops. The practice of maintaining mobile field hospitals was carried forward into William's later campaigns in Flanders and, in essence, remains a cornerstone of field medical support to the present day.

Contracting for hospital services was a system widely used by the Dutch and French armies. In the latter case it provided the means whereby fifty or so military hospitals were sited along the northern and eastern borders of France. It was, therefore, neither an unusual nor unique concept when it was introduced to the English army at a time when the King and Parliament were continually searching for the cheapest option, bearing in mind the country's parlous financial state. The Nine Years' War cost the country an average of five million pounds annually and the War of the Spanish Succession over eight million.[2] Entrepreneurs providing services to the government were naturally in business to make money but, coincidentally, despite the country's fiscal difficulties, the same approach was adopted by holders of the major Offices of State, such as the Paymaster General to the Forces. Parliament allocated an annual budget to these officials and seems to have turned a blind eye when any surplus found its way into the post-holders' pockets. The scandal that arose when the Earl of Ranelagh was impeached after being found guilty of misappropriating huge sums during his time as Paymaster General was an exception to the norm. The ability of his successor, James Brydges, Earl of Chandos, to accumulate vast wealth during his years in office provides a clear example of how it was generally understood that incumbents would derive personal profit from their time in office.[3] Even so, while personal interest and greed were undoubtedly ever-present factors, the typical characteristics of financial administration in the years following the Restoration have been described more charitably by Ogg as 'not dishonesty, but clumsiness and wastefulness'.[4] Much the same could be said about many other elements of contemporary public service. During the 1690s the foundation of the Bank of England and the establishment of a National Debt funded by loans from City financiers enabled the King and Parliament to wage war on almost endless credit without any serious attempt being made to balance the books.

William III was an unlucky monarch in war. His military defeats were suffered more as a result of misfortune than through any deficiency in his command ability.

His army was also unfortunate in the poor choices made when selecting contractors for providing services to the army that was sent to Ireland in 1689 and for the hospital services provided in Flanders during 1692 and 1693. While the troops suffered, individuals such as Shales, Harbord, Keggelaer and Samuel Venner milked the system for all it was worth. It was not until Patrick Lamb, an honest member of the King's personal household with experience and expertise in personnel, stores and food management, was appointed as contractor for the army's hospitals that a workable and relatively efficient system was achieved.

The example of hospital provision established during the Williamite wars was followed, more or less, and developed by the Duke of Marlborough's army. The Duke was astute in his choice of both Cadogan for his Quartermaster General and John Hudson as his hospital contractor. It was also fortunate that the army could continue to call upon Dr Thomas Lawrence, the Physician General, with his many years' experience with the army both at home and overseas, to act as medical adviser as well as a group of committed and efficient physicians and surgeons. Equally, the contribution made by nurses to the efficient functioning of the military hospitals in Flanders has previously been either ignored or dismissed as of little importance. Their significance can however be hinted at when the numbers employed in just one establishment, the Bijloke Hospital in Ghent, during the years when that facility functioned as the army's main base hospital in the six years from 1706 to 1712, are examined (see Table 8.1).

Table 8.1 Nursing staff numbers at the Bijloke Hospital, 1706–1712

Year	June	July	Aug	Sept	Oct	Nov
1706	18	24	30	50	52	60
1707	42	40	40	55	63	–
1708	67	60	42	*	*	*
1709	50	47	46	52	55	55
1710	48	55	40	†	†	†
1711	20	27	30	15	12	–
1712	22	18	33	48	50	35
Average	38	39	38	44	46	50

* : Ghent in French hands
† : Base hospital moved to Lille

Source: BL Add. Mss, 61318, *passim*.

Similar numbers of nurses were employed in the army's other hospitals during both the Nine Years' War and the campaigns of Marlborough. There can be little doubt that the lot of sick and wounded soldiers would have been much worse without the intervention of these men and women. While a quality assessment of care provided in the military hospitals of the late seventeenth and early eighteenth centuries in twenty-first-century terms would be anachronistic, and in any case would be impossible, perhaps some indication of the worth and efficiency of these establishment can be viewed in the light of patient survival. Statistics do not exist in sufficient quantities and detail to permit a full analysis of survival rates. Accurate records of admissions to the Royal Hospital, Chelsea are not available prior to 1715 but an examination of 1,703 records compiled during the medical examination of applicants for admission to that establishment from 1715 to 1732, as well as 229 records relating to The Royal Hospital Kilmainham over a similar time scale, were examined. Due to the limited nature of the entries compared with those of Chelsea, the Kilmainham records have been excluded from the following statistical analysis. The injuries sustained are listed in Table 8.2.

Table 8.2 Analysis of injuries suffered by applicants for admission to Chelsea Royal Hospital, 1715–1732

Leg wounds	566
Chest wounds	54
Abdominal wounds	93
Back wounds	64
Head wounds	615
Unspecified	28
Multiple wounds	283
Total	1,703

Source: TNA, WO 116 and WO 117.

Of the 1,703 records initially examined, 503 were chosen for more detailed analysis. The criteria used in selecting cases required each entry to list the nature of the solder's injury, his age at the time of his application for admission to the hospital, his total length of service and, in particular, attribution of his injury to a specific major battle. The date of his injury and his age at the time of injury could then be calculated. Table 8.3 is a summary of the findings and shows that, among the 503 applicants studied, the average age at injury was 30 years and at application 55 years. Each had served an average of 27 years in the army. It is suggested that it would not be unreasonable to assume that the remaining candidates for admission would demonstrate similar figures. It is also clear that the majority of soldiers in this group soldiered on for a considerable length of time, in some cases nearly forty years, after injury. The extent and nature of individual injuries is of obvious relevance to this study and, although detailed clinical observations are not available today, the brief descriptions of the injuries contained in the records manage, nevertheless, to convey the severity of many of the injuries.

Table 8.3 Age and length of service analysis of 503 soldiers applying for admission to the Royal Hospital, Chelsea, 1715–1732

Battle	No. records	Age at injury	Age at application	Length of service
The Boyne, 1690	9	29	60	30
Aughrim, 1691	21	31	61	30
Steenkirk, 1692	14	30	62	34
Neerwinden, 1693	23	28	59	31
Namur, 1695	60	28	56	30
Schellenburg, 1704	37	34	56	29
Blenheim, 1704	68	32	54	26
Ramillies, 1706	36	32	54	27
Almanza, 1707	115	33	52	26
Oudenarde, 1708	13	28	53	26
Malplaquet, 1710	76	31	53	25
Brihuega, 1710	34	30	52	24
Villa Viciosa, 1710	7	25	49	22

Source: TNA, WO 116 and WO 117.

Appendix G lists some 14 individual wound histories of applicants for admission to the Royal Hospital, Chelsea and clearly demonstrates that it is highly unlikely that such men would have survived and subsequently returned to duty, in many cases more than once, without skilled medical and nursing care. Due consideration must be given to these aspects when statements are made regarding the efficacy of the treatments given in the military hospitals of the day.

Demonstrably, the efficient functioning of the army's hospitals throughout Marlborough's wars was a direct result of efficient supervision at all levels of military administration plus the personal involvement in such matters by the commander in chief. It is unlikely that this level of success would have been achieved without the availability of skilled medical and nursing care from the time of injury onwards. It would be pleasing if the same could be also said for the medical care provided for troops serving in Spain and Portugal. There, it must be said that, after a sluggish and confused beginning, Whitehall's attitude towards the provision of health care in that theatre of operations improved as the years passed, especially after Dr LeCaan arrived as Physician in Charge of the Hospital in Spain. But the government's initial failures pale into insignificance when compared with the performance of the various commanders in chief and their staffs whose performance was, at best, mediocre. They displayed gross ignorance, blindness, incompetence and self-interest in their attitudes towards conserving manpower to the extent that, at times, they appear to have had little idea of just how many troops were under their command. Their failure to adequately concern themselves with the maintenance of health and welfare among their troops is silhouetted in stark contrast to that so clearly demonstrated by the hands-on approach of Marlborough and his officers in Flanders. The Duke's personal involvement with the needs of the sick and wounded, as well as his concern with the welfare needs of discharged soldiers who returned to England disabled and incapable of earning their living, was exemplary. As has been shown, he went to great lengths to secure vacancies for his veterans in the Royal Hospital, Chelsea, as, at times, did various officials in Whitehall.

No similar involvement or effort has been detected among those who commanded in Spain or Portugal. Galway, Peterborough, Stanhope, Portmore and Argyle appear to have been singularly inactive in their attempts to improve the lot of their sick or wounded soldiers. It is significant that the numbers of soldiers injured during the battle of Almanza in 1707 who later sought admission to Chelsea between ten and twenty or so years after the battle – long after their former commanders had any influence over their future – far outnumbered, at 115 applicants, those wounded in any other battle, including the bloodiest of the age, Malplaquet. This lends weight to the theory that the superior care provided in Flanders resulted in a reduced requirement for ongoing hospitalization compared with that available in Spain and Portugal where facilites were less well developed. To temper this statement, it has to be accepted that any final judgement regarding the quality and quantity of health-care provision in Spain and Portugal may be coloured by the fact that whereas Marlborough's wars in Flanders were well documented, and a comprehensive series of hospital archives survives, there remains very little day-to-day medical documentation for the hospitals in the Iberian Peninsula to illuminate the working lives of those employed in the army's hospitals. This is the end result of a working environment where poor management, indifferent paperwork and lack of supervision were commonplace rather than a symptom of losses and the destruction of archives during the subsequent centuries spent in storage.

The work of John Hudson as a trustworthy director of hospitals throughout Marlborough's campaigns is particularly relevant to this discussion. In comparison with the ever-changing and variably efficient personalities who performed the same function in Spain and Portugal, where office-holders seem to have constantly changed on a yearly basis thereby obviating any continuity of practice or documentation, Hudson provided continuity and reliability. He is owed a debt of gratitude for the attention to detail exhibited in his accounts that provide us with an outstanding record of information relating to the day-to-day minutiae of the hospitals' administration and function during his time in office. Much can also be said in similar vein regarding the records left by Richard Hill dating from his time as Deputy Paymaster to the Forces under William III in Flanders during the Nine Years' War.

It is to be hoped that this study has demonstrated that the success or failure of the army's medical services during the early years of the British Standing Army formed a constantly rising and falling barometer reflecting the nature and extent of governmental involvement, as well as that of senior officials and personalities, in the welfare of soldiers. Starting with a bare slate, elements of the practices and structures necessary to provide an adequate medical support service were gradually introduced as a result of experience, suffering, trial and error. Many of the lessons learned formed the basis of systems that remain pertinent to this day.

Undoubtedly, the medical services of the period reached their apogee during the campaigns of Marlborough and it is, perhaps, a significant measure of both the effectiveness and worth of the Duke's medical arrangements that when, some 30 years later, the Earl of Stair was preparing to depart for the Continent at the outset of the War of the Austrian Succession, he requested an aide to research what arrangements his great predecessor had made for casualty care during his campaigns. The response that he received quoted the medical establishment for 1710 and, in due course, this was replicated by Stair for the coming war. In this instance imitation was not only the sincerest form of flattery but also the most appropriate course of action.

Such, then, was the nature of military hospital provision during the infancy of the British Standing Army. Many of the contemporary problems, attitudes and difficulties experienced in providing hospital care for soldiers have constantly reappeared down the centuries and continue to do so to the present day. Military medical development during the period discussed in this work has been grossly under-researched and subjected to many common, misplaced assumptions for which there is no basis in fact. As has been shown, relevant information on the care given to military casualties has to be sought among diverse and sometimes obscure sources, often with little or no apparent direct association with the history of particular campaigns, battles or individual regiments. It is hoped that the arguments offered here have demonstrated the importance of a wider appreciation of the subject and will stimulate further research into a neglected field of study.

Notes

[1] See Gruber von Arni, ch. 6.
[2] G. Holmes (ed.), *Britain After the Glorious Revolution, 1689–1714* (London: Macmillan, 1969), pp. 22–3; C. Wilson, *England's Apprenticeship, 1603–1763* (London: Longman, 1965, republished 1986); Min-Hsun Li, *The Great Recoinage of 1689–9* (London: Weidenfeld and Nicolson, 1963); D. Ogg, *England in the Reigns of James II and William III* (Oxford: Clarendon Press, 1955); L.M. Waddell, 'The Administration of the English Army in Flanders and Brabant from 1689 to 1697' (unpublished PhD thesis, University of North Carolina, 1971).
[3] J.R. Robinson, *The Princely Chandos, A Memoir* (London: Sampson Lowe, 1893).
[4] D. Ogg, *England in the Reign of Charles II* (2 vols, Oxford: Clarendon Press, 1934, republished 1962), vol. 2, p. 448.

Appendix A

The Humble Report of Henry Shere to the Rt Hon. Lords of the Treasury, Touching the Hospital at Tangier, 1 March 1683

The present old hospital, as it is much too straight, so it is very incommodiously situated being built against an old Battery where the damp and cold in the winter season greatly annoy the sick people; but may serve well enough for quarters to soldiers that are in health; and may be accordingly made quarters or stables, in lieu of such quarters or stables as the King at this day pays rent for, so that his Majesty need not be a loser by withdrawing the sick people from the said hospital.

The town house, as it is called (which was a gift of the Lord Bellasis to the Corporation), hath been ever since the beginning of the last war made use of for an hospital, is a building very commodiously situate, with a large garden and a room sufficient to make an addition for enlarging the said house to a capacity of accommodating all the sick people of the garrison, when it shall be reduced to the Establishment proposed by your Lordships. Which addition I propose shall be capable of receiving and accommodating 140 sick men, to lye in single beds, which with the number of 60 more (the proportion a little more or less the present building is capable of receiving) will yield in all accommodation for 200 sick men: which I presume (unless some very extraordinary cases) may suffice. The dimension of which additional building, the quantity and kind of materials with their respective values at Tangier together with the charge of workmanship is here presented to your Lordships.

The said Henry Shere, by the leave given him by your Lordships, further humbly reports that the hospital at Tangier hath, according to his observation, never been under any proper methods of Government, either with respect to his Majesty's service and honour or the sick people; for by the old Establishment the allowances to the hospital was the certain limited sum of £500 per annum: not to be paid quarterly, or according to the exigencies of that service, but to run in arrear as the garrison did, and to be paid as that was paid. So that when so ever the garrison happened to be in great arrear, the hospital of necessity became the greatest sufferer for, notwithstanding the long arrear due to the soldiers, the men in health receive the greatest part of their pay in provision of diet and clothing whereas the sick people in the hospital, whose allowance is fresh provision, and which provision is not being to be had by ready money or upon trust to private men, and by the aforesaid rules of payment it being impossible to support the hospital but on trust; by which means the poor sick people necessarily labour under the same distress, that all necessitous people do who live upon credit; namely, to be defrauded in both quantity and quality and price, of whatsoever their occasions call for. And as this in Charity becomes my duty to lay before your Lordships, with respect to the preservation of the lives and health of the poor soldiers. So in duty to his Majesty's better service, I presume humbly to press your Lordships for the remedy; in as much as by due and proper care in this behalf, the reputation of his Majesty's service will be thereby much better preserved: and so much a saving of charge to his Majesty by as much as four men, by good and wholesome diet, and careful attendance when sick, will be recovered and preserved alive at a less charge to the King, than one man can be raised in England and made fit for his Majesty's service at Tangier.

For the avoiding all which inconveniences to his Majesty's service and the garrison, the said Henry Shere doth humbly propose that the present arrears of the hospital may be discharged and that for the future both humbly offer this following method to your Lordships' consideration: vi^{zt}.

That your Lordships may please to appoint proper Commissioners to inspect the affairs of the hospital with instructions to transmit a monthly account to your Lordships of the charge thereof: and that the said Commissioners be likewise empowered to draw on your Lordships' Bills of Exchange for the amount of the said sum, for it is impossible to reduce the charge of the hospital to any limited expense, so by any other regulation than what is here humbly offered, the said Henry Shere doth presume, with submission to your Lordships wisdom, it will be very difficult to avoid hardships upon the soldiers, fraud to his Majesty and direct damage to his service in that place.[1]

The estimate of the Charge of erecting an additional Building to the present new Hospital at Tangier – 1 March 1683. Being in Dimension 250 foot long, 22 foot broad in the clear, with upper and lower floors: being designed for the accommodation of 140 men to lie in single beds. The Calculation being made according to the proportion of the value of materials and Workmanship at Tangier.

> For 24 loads of Oak Timber for the ground floor etc. at £4 10s per load: £108
> For 79 loads of fir timber: £276 10s
> For Ordinary deal boards: 1,600: £112
> For Elm boards for stairs, 500 foot: £5
> For Pan tiles, 15,000: £75
> For Pan tile lathes, 90 dozen: £9
> For Brads, 12,000: £5
> For Nails of all sorts: £8
> For Bricks, 225,000: £393 15s
> For Carpenters', Sawyers' and Masons' workmanship: £180
> For Labourers' work, scaffolding and all kinds of contingencies: £50
> For Bedsteads, 160 at 4s each: £32
> Total: £1,299 5s[2]

Notes

[1] Staffs. RO, D 742/0/2/29.
[2] Staffs. RO, D 742/0/2/30.

Appendix B

The Present Annual Charge of the Royal Hospital of King Charles II[1]

Appointment	Annual Salary
The Master	£430
Physician	£50
Chaplain	£80
Auditor and Registrar	£110
Paymaster	£80
Aid Major	£26
Reader	£20
Surgeon	£50
Surgeon's Mate	£20
Providore	£50
Apothecary	£20
Butler	£16
Cook	£16
Under Cook	£8
Fuel and Chamber Keeper	£16
Clerk of the Chapel	£4 10s
Chapel Cleaner	£1
Messenger	£6
Scullery Man	£12
Scullery Man's Assistant	£8
Two Kitchen Helpers (each)	£5
Waterman	£16 18s
Hall Keeper	£1
Four Porters (each)	£16 18s
Thirteen Nurses (each)	£6 10s
Clock Keeper	£6
Gardener	£16
Garden Labourer	£7
Three Porters (each)	£3
Overseer of Works and Buildings	£20

Note

[1] T. Wilson, *An Account of the Foundation of the Royal Hospital* (Dublin, 1713), pp. 132–34.

Appendix C

Abstract of the By-Laws, Rules and Orders for Staff of the Royal Hospital of King Charles II near Dublin[1]

The following oath was administered to all persons upon their admission into any employment in the hospital.

> You shall to the best of your skill and understanding well and truly exercise the Office of … of the Royal Hospital of King Charles the Second for ancient and maimed officers and soldiers of the Army in Ireland and diligently and faithfully discharge the trust reposed in you according to such orders and instructions as you shall from time to time receive from the Governor and Master of the said hospital or other your superior officers. So help you God.

Instructions to the Physician

You are to observe that … the Apothecary, inspector of the Mad-house, Nurses and others who may be concerned in administering to the sick do receive and obey such orders and directions as you shall think convenient and necessary for the assistance and comfort of the sick and, upon failure or neglect, you are to inform the Master of the Hospital that proper order may be taken.

You shall attend at least twice in every week on such days and hours as shall be appointed for the purpose at which time the surgeons, apothecary, nurses and others that are under your inspection shall also attend in their places and receive directions.

Instructions to the Head Nurse

You shall duly execute your office by taking particular care that all the nurses do diligently and faithfully perform their duty.

You shall take care that none of them do employ deputies, but such who, on account of their age or infirmities, shall for so doing have leave from the Master, to whom you may recommend such persons as you shall judge to be proper for the trust.

You shall take care that the linen be duly mended and you shall observe that any of it has been abused. You shall inform the Master thereof and the name of the nurses in whose care it was.

You shall diligently take notice of all idle or loose women that frequent or lie in the hospital and charge them to absent themselves and, in case of their neglect or refusal so to do, you are to acquaint the Master therewith and shall not fail from time to time to inform him of every nurse who shall presume to suffer any person not belonging to the hospital to lie in any room under her care. As also of all other matters (so far as the same relates to your employment) that may tend to the service of the house and the keeping both of it and all therein in that clean and decent manner they ought to be.

Instructions to Nurses

You shall execute your office by taking care that all such rooms as shall be put into your care and charge be kept clean and decent order, that each bed be made every morning, and every room supplied with a proper quantity of clean water.

You shall, at the appointed times, deliver to the Chamberlain all the foul linen belonging to the soldiers who lie in your rooms in order to their being washed and, when cleaned, shall receive them from him again.

You shall diligently supply all the soldiers under your care with their established allowances but in a more particular manner shall be assistant to those who are sick, always remembering that you are, as soon as possible, to acquaint the Physician or Surgeon with the name of any person who shall complain of sickness, in order to his having as speedy relief as may be, and that such as may not properly be continued in the house may be sent to the Infirmary.

You shall duly attend for the receiving of victuals for such men as are not able to come to the Hall and shall, at noon, bring the broth to the tables there and daily receive from the Cook the breakfast and supper for the men under your charge.

You are not to suffer any stranger or person not properly belonging to the Hospital to lie in any room under your charge.

You shall not presume to employ any deputy without leave from the Master who is empowered to make such a reasonable deduction out of your salary as may encourage a proper person to undertake it.

Instructions to the Apothecary (extract)

You are to take care that the nurses attending the sick in the Infirmary do diligently attend and faithfully discharge their duty.

Instructions to the Inspector of the Mad-house

That a convenient place in the Infirmary be appointed for the reception of sick soldiers as shall have the misfortune to become lunatics.

That the mad-house be put under the direction of the Apothecary of the hospital.

You shall from time to time exhibit such remedies as the Physician shall judge proper to prescribe for the recovery of the lunatics.

You are to take care that the porter do assist the nurses in bringing victuals to the patients and in keeping them clean, that they prevent them from being disturbed by strangers whose curiosity may lead them to see the place, and that he constantly attends them when they are permitted to go abroad.

You are likewise to take care that the lodges and yards thereof be constantly kept clean and in decent working order.

Note

[1] G. Burston, *Abstract of the By-Laws, Rules and Orders of the Royal Hospital of King Charles II near Dublin* (Dublin, 1752), pp. 21–3, 59–60 and 114.

Appendix D

Admissions to St Bartholomew's Hospital by Regiment, 1689–1697[1]

Throughout the period covered by this work, regiments were identified by the name of their Colonel who acted as the proprietor of the unit. Unfortunately, as regimental Colonels changed frequently, the name of the regiment changed just as frequently. This poses many difficulties when attempting to provide continuity in identifying the units of origin for troops admitted to hospital during a period spanning eight years. For this reason, albeit anachronistic, the system of numbering regiments introduced some years later has been adopted in this study, wherever appropriate, as the simplest means of establishing continuity for the purpose of statistical analysis.

Household Troops	*Total admitted*
2nd Troop Life Guards	2
4th Troop, The Life Guards (Scots Estab.)	1
Royal Horse Guards	64
1st Regt Foot Guards	205
2nd Coldstream Regt Foot Guards	124
3rd Scots Regt Foot Guards	7
Total Household Troops	403

Horse	
1st Horse	3
2nd Horse	2
4th Horse	3
5th Horse	1
6th Horse	1

Regiment	*Total admitted*
7th Horse	2
Col. Windsor's Regt Horse (disbanded 1697–9)	2
Col. Ingoldsby's Regt Horse (disbanded 1689)	1
Earl of Salisbury's Regt Horse (disbanded 1688)	1
Col. Windsor's Regt Horse (disbanded 1697–9)	2

Dragoons	
1st Royal Dragoons	8

3rd Dragoons	2
4th Dragoons	1
Princess Anne of Denmark's Regt Dragoons	1
Total Cavalry	30

Dutch Horse

Garde te Paard (Dutch Horse Guards)	2
Bentinck's Regt Horse	2
Total Dutch Horse	4

Foot

1st Royal Regiment	30
2nd Foot	5
3rd Foot	5
4th Foot	5
6th Foot	45
7th Royal Fuziliers	8
8th Foot	7
9th Foot	4
10th Foot	2
11th Foot	2
12th Foot	2
13th Foot	5
14th Foot	6
15th Foot	8
16th Foot	5
17th Foot	8
18th Foot	4
19th Foot	7
21st Foot	1
24th Foot	2

Regiment	Total admitted
27th Foot	1
1st Marine Regt	1
2nd Marine Regt	2
Duke of Bolton's Regt Foot	13
Col. Brudenell's Regt Foot (disbanded 1698)	2
Col. Buchan's Regt Foot (disbanded 1697)	1
M. La Caillemote's Regt Foot (disbanded 1689)	2
M. du Cambon's Regt Foot (disbanded 1697)	1
Lord Castleton's Regt Foot (disbanded 1698)	1
Col. Col.lingwood's Regt Foot (disbanded 1698)	4
Sir David Col.lyer's Regt Foot (disbanded 1700)	19
Col. Coote's Regt Foot (disbanded 1694)	2
Lord Cutt's Regt Foot (disbanded 1698)	63

Appendix D

Earl of Donegal's Regt Foot (disbanded 1698)	1
Earl of Drogheda's Regt Foot (disbanded 1691)	2
Sir James Douglas's Regt Foot (disbanded 1698)	4
Col. Farrington's Regt Foot (disbanded 1698)	5
Col. Fitzpatrick's Regt Foot (disbanded 1698)	3
Prince George of Denmark's Regt Foot	12
Sir John Gibson's Regt Foot (disbanded 1698)	1
Col. Hales's Regt Foot (disbanded 1697)	3
Earl of Kingston's Regt Foot (disbanded 1698)	1
Viscount Lisburn's Regt Foot (disbanded 1697)	3
Col. Lloyd's Regt Foot (disbanded 1689)	4
Earl of Macclesfield's Regt Foot (disbanded 1698)	1
M. de la Melloniere's Regt Foot (disbanded 1697)	8
Earl of Monmouth's Regt Foot (disbanded 1699)	2
Col. Mordaunt's Regt Foot	1
Col. Russell's Foot for Barbadoes	2
Col. Saunderson's Regt Foot (disbanded 1698)	1
Col. Skelton's Regt Foot (disbanded 1697)	1
Col. Slingsby's Regt Foot (disbanded 1689)	1
Tower of London Garrison	1
Chelsea Royal Hospital	37
Unidentified	1

Dutch Foot

Garde te Voet (Dutch Blue Guards)	6
Col. MacKay's Regt Foot (Anglo-Dutch)	1
Brandenburgh's Regt Foot	4
Rijngraaf van Salm's Regt Foot	1
van Graben's Regt Foot	3
Total Dutch Foot	15

Totals

Total Household Troops	403
Total Cavalry of the Line	30
Total British Foot of the Line	366
Total Dutch Horse	4
Total Dutch Foot	15
Total Admissions	818

Note

1 LMA, H1/ST/A91/1.

Appendix E

Inventory of Drugs, Medicines and Utensils for the Surgeon's Chests of Regiments of Horse and Foot, 1689[1]

A Regiment of Horse
Plasters
Diapalm – 2 lb
De Minio – 2 lb
Melitot – 1 lb
Parcels – 1 lb
Diachyl. Cum Gum – 1 lb
De Rains cum Mercur. – ½ lb

Ointments
Basilic – 1 lb
Arcaes – 1 lb
Populi – 1 lb
Alb. Camph. – 1 lb
Diapomphol – ½ lb
Egyptiac – ¼ lb

Oils
Terebinth – 2 lb
Lini – 2 lb
Hyperiic Comp. – 1 lb
Succin – 2 lb

Waters
Epidemic – ¼ lb

Tinctures
Cinnamom – ¼ lb
Cardiac Carni. etc – ¼ lb
Myrrh and Aloes cum. Tot. – 2 lb

Spirits
Vini. Rectificat – 2 lb
C.C. – 2 oz

Electuaries [Confections]
Diascordium – 3 oz
Theriac Andromach – 2 oz
Lenctive – 2 oz

Pills
Ex. Duobus – ¼ oz
Rudii – ¼ oz
Laudanum Lond. – 1 oz
Laudanum Liq. – 3 oz

Powders
E. Chel. Cancr. Comp. – 2 oz
Rad. Jalappae – 2 oz

Folium [Dried Leaves]
Sennae Alex. – 2 oz

Smelling Salts
Pernan – 1 oz

Roots
Rhubarb – 2 oz
Hypercocuamiae – 2 oz

Conserves
Roa Rubr. – 2 lb
Mellis Rosar. – 2 lb

Salts
Absynth – 2 oz
Prunel – ½ oz
Cathart. Amar. – 1 oz
Cremor. Tart. – ½ oz
Tartar emetic – 2 oz
Vitriol alb. – 1 oz
Vitriol Roman – 1 oz
Alum ust. – 2 oz
Terebinth venet. – 2 oz
Gambog. – 1 oz
Camphor – 2 oz
Cautharid – ¼ oz
Mercurii praecip. rub – ¼ oz
Mercurii dulc. – ¼ oz
Antimom. Diaph. – ¼ oz
Lap. Infernal – 1 oz
Ingred. Amar. – 1 oz
Succ. Liquirit – 1 oz
C.C. – 1 oz

Dried Flower Extracts
Chamaem – 1 oz
Melilot – 1 oz
Croc. – ½ oz

Equipment
Sheets – 4
Skins of leather – 4
Cupping glasses – 2
Clyster pipes – 3
Bladders – 4
Tow – 4 lb
Thread – ½ lb
Tape, broad and narrow – 3 pcs
Vials, corks and gallipots – 12
Scales and weights – 1 small pr
Tin panikins – 2
Sponges – 2
Syringes – 2
Pots, bottles and glasses etc.
Two chests covered with tarpaulin
One quire of paper

A Regiment of Foot

The Regimental Chest for a Regiment of Foot differed only in some quantities from that supplied to a Regiment of Horse, i.e.

Ointments
Basilic – 2 lb instead of 1 lb
Arcaes – 2 lb instead of 1 lb

Pills
Ex. Duobus – ½ oz
Laudanum Lond. – 2 oz
Laudanum Liquid – 4 oz

Dried Leaves
Sennae – 1 oz

Electuaries [Confectons]
Diascord. – 4 oz
Lenctive – 2 ½ oz

Powders
Rad. Jalapp – 1 oz

Roots
Rhubarb – 1 oz

Salts   *Equipment*
Prunel – 1 oz   Sheets – 6
Cathart. Amar. – 1½ oz
Mercurii dulc. – 6 oz

Note

[1]   BL Add. Mss, 61335, fol. 184.

Appendix F

The Hospital Establishment and Staff in Flanders, 2 April 1693.[1]

One Governor, or Director: Ibid. Samuel Venner

Three Director's Assistants: Capt. Joseph Shedd
　　　　　　　　　　　　　　　Thomas Gardiner
　　　　　　　　　　　　　　　John Hudson

Four Physicians: Dr Thomas Lawrence (Physician General)
　　　　　　　　　Dr Jacob Herwaenden
　　　　　　　　　Dr Jonothan LeCaan
　　　　　　　　　Dr Bellone

Four Master Surgeons: George Pringle (Surgeon General)
　　　　　　　　　　　Hannibal Hall
　　　　　　　　　　　Jonathan Frederick Cichorius
　　　　　　　　　　　William Wallace

Three Chaplains: John Carpenter
　　　　　　　　　Henry Shute
　　　　　　　　　Edward Paget

Three Apothecaries: Isaac Teale (Apothecary General)
　　　　　　　　　　Michael Ibidlins
　　　　　　　　　　William Morris

Four Clerks   Samuel Keck
　　　　　　　Thomas Albritton
　　　　　　　Frederick Mathewson
　　　　　　　[Not named]

Eighteen Surgeons' Mates (including six 'foreigners')
Five Apothecaries' Mates

Note

[1]　TNA, WO 25/3138, fols 339–40.

Appendix G

Examples of Battle Injuries Received by Applicants for Admission to the Royal Hospital Chelsea, 1715–1732[1]

A trooper of Mapper's Regiment of Horse, who applied for admission in July 1722, had been shot in the right arm at Blenheim (1704), shot in the back at Ramillies (1706) and cut over the head at Oudenarde (1708).

A soldier of Sabine's Regiment, who applied for admission in July 1722, had been wounded in the left hand at the Schellenburg (1704), in his left heel at Blenheim (1704) and his right hand at the siege of Ghent (1708).

A soldier of Howard's Regiment, who applied for admission in December 1722, had been shot in the right knee at Blenheim (1704), his left leg had been fractured by a bomb blast and he had been wounded in the left elbow by the thrust of a halberd.

A soldier of Harley's Regiment, who applied for admission in December 1722, injured his right hand during the attack on Vigo (1702), had received several cuts about his head and left eye at Almanza (1707) and had been stabbed in the lower abdomen and fractured his right clavicle at Tortosa (1707).

A soldier of the 3rd Foot Guards, who applied for admission in July 1723, had his right leg shattered. He was wounded in his left knee as Saragossa (1710).and later the same year he was wounded on the left side of his head at Brihuega (1710) while attempting to carry a wounded officer to safety.

A soldier of Sabine's Regiment, who applied for admission in October 1723, had been shot in the right arm at Malplaquet (1710). He had also been shot in the head at Maastricht with the bullet entering behind his right ear and exiting in his neck.

A soldier of Sabine's Regiment, who applied for admission in October 1723, had been shot in his in his left wrist during the siege of Lille (1708) and in his left side, under the ribs, at Douai (1708).

A soldier of Hawley's Regiment, who applied for admission in December 1723, had a left arm amputated after being wounded at Alamanza (1707). He was later wounded in the head at Brihuega (1710).

A soldier of the 2nd Foot Guards, who applied for admission in December 1723, had been blown up by a barrel of gunpowder at Tournai (1709) where he had also been wounded in his left shoulder and arm. He was later cut in the left thigh at Bouchain (1711).

A soldier of Wade's Regiment, who applied for admission in February 1724, was shot in his left thigh at the Schellenburg and in his right knee at Blenheim (both in 1704).

A drummer of Wood's Regiment, who applied for admission in November 1727, had lost his right eye during the siege of Lille (1708) and been shot in his right arm and neck at Malplaquet (1710).

A sergeant of Anstruther's Regiment, who applied for admission in November 1727, had been shot in the left foot at Steenkirk (1692) and in the head at Nether Hespen. He had later been wounded in the right arm at Blenheim (1704).

A soldier of the 3rd Foot Guards, who applied for admission in August 1728, had been wounded in the abdomen during the siege of Menin (1706) and in the left leg at Douai (1708). He had also received multiple wounds at the siege of Tournai (1709).

A sergeant of Harrison's Regiment, who applied for admission in August 1729, had been wounded in his right groin when he became impaled upon a palisade and, at operation later, had part of his 'caul' (peritoneum) excised.

Note

[1] TNA, WO 116 and 117.

Bibliography

Manuscript Sources

Berkshire County Record Office
    Trumbull Add. Mss 103

Bodleian Library
    Bod. L. Vet. A4
    Rawlinson Mss

British Library
    Add. Mss
    Egerton Mss
    Harleian Mss
    Lansdown Mss
    Lister Mss
    Loan Mss
    Rawlinson Mss
    Sloane Mss
    Stowe Mss

London Metropolitan Archives
    H1/ST/A6/4
    H1/ST/A91/1
    HO1/ST/B/001/001

National Archives
    Admiralty Papers
    Audit Office Papers
    Colonial Office Papers
    Exchequer Papers
    State Papers
    Treasury Papers
    War Office Papers

St Bartholomew's Hospital Archives
    Ha/20/36
    Hb/1/9–13
    Hb2/1–2

Shropshire County Record Office
    112/1: The Account Books of William Hill, Deputy Paymaster to the Forces, 1692–1699
    112/274–112/427: Hill's reports of events in hospitals 1694

112/274–112/424: Locations of nine military hospitals

Somerset County Record Office
DD/PH/211, ff. 40 and 248
T/PH/Wig 2, ff. 4 and 6

Staffordshire County Record Office
D 742/0/2/29

Wellcome Library for the History of Medicine
RAMC 205
RAMC 582-4
RAMC 1299

Printed Primary Sources

Barry, G., *Discourse of Military Discipline* (Brussels, 1763).
Bray, W. (ed.), *Diary and Correspondence of John Evelyn* (London, n.d).
Brooks, N., *A General & Complete List Military of Every Commission Officer of Horse & Foot now commanding His Majesty's Land Forces of England etc. ... as established at the time of the review upon Putney Heath the 1 October 1684* (1684).
Burston, G., *Abstract of the By-Laws, Rules and Orders of the Royal Hospital of King Charles II near Dublin* (Dublin, 1752).
Calendar of State Papers (Domestic).
Calendar of Treasury Books.
de Beer, E.S. (ed.), *The Diary of John Evelyn* (London: Oxford University Press, 1959).
Chappell, E. (ed.), *The Tangier Papers of Samuel Pepys* (London: Navy Records Society, 1935).
Cholmley, Sir H., *An Account of Tangier* (1787).
D'Auverne, E., *A Relation of the Most Remarkable Transactions of the Last Campaigne in the Confederate Army, 1692* (London, 1693).
——, *The History of the Last Campagne in the Spanish Netherlands* (London, 1693).
——, *A Relation of the Most Remarkable Transactions of the Last Campaigne in the Confederate Army under the Command of His Majesty of Great Britain: and After, of the Elector of Bavaria, in the Spanish Netherlands, Anno. Dom. 1692* (London, 1693).
——, *The History of the Campagne in the Spanish Netherlands, Anno Dom. 1694, With a Journal of the Siege of Huy* (London, 1694).
——, *The History of the Campaign in Flanders, for the Year 1695* (London, 1696).
——, *The History of the Campaign in Flanders, for the Year 1696* (London, 1696).
——, *The History of the Campaign in Flanders for the Year, 1697. Together with a Journal of the Siege of Ath and a Summary Account of the Negotiations at Ryswick* (London, 1698).

Bibliography 213

——, *The History of the Campaign in Flanders, for the Year 1691* (London, 1735).
Elton, R., *The Complete Body of the Art Military* (1668).
Grey, A. (comp.), *Debates in the House of Commons, from the year 1667 to the year 1694* (10 vols, 1763).
Gwyn, E., *Memoirs of Eleanor Gwyn* (1752).
Historic Manuscripts Commission
  Bath Mss
  Cholmondeley Mss
  Dartmouth Mss
  Duke of Ormonde's Mss
  Earl of Egmont's Mss
  Heathcote Mss
  Stopford Sackville Mss
Japikse, N. (ed.), *Correspondentie van Willem III en van Hans Willem Bentinck* (2 vols, The Hague, 1932–7).
Journal of the House of Commons.
Journal of the House of Lords.
Kane, R., *Campaigns of King William and Queen Anne from 1689–1712* (London, 1745).
——, *A System of Camp Discipline* (London, 1757).
Lacelles, R., *Liber Munerum Publicorum Hibernioe, or the Establishment of Ireland, 1152–1827* (1824).
London Gazette.
Mackenzie, J., *A Narrative of the Siege of Londonderry* (1690).
Millner, J., *A Compendious Journal of all the Marches, Famous Battles and Sieges* (London, 1712).
Murray, Sir G., *The Letters and Dispatches of John Churchill, Duke of Marlborough, 1702–1712* (4 vols, London: John Murray, 1845).
Palladio, A. *I Quattro Libri dell'Architettura* (New York: Dover Publications, 1570, republished 1965).
Parker, R., *Memoirs of the Most Remarkable Military Transactions from the year 1683 to 1718* (1745).
Proceedings of the House of Commons
Prothero, G.W., *Select Statutes and Other Constitutional Documents* (Oxford: University Press, 1913).
Orrery, Earl of, *A Treatise on the Art of War* (1677).
Story, G., *A True and Impartial History of the Most Material Occurences in the Kingdom of Ireland during the Two Last Years* (London, 1693).
——, *A Continuation of the True and Impartial History of the Wars of Ireland* (1693, London).
Slight, H. and J., *Chronicles of Portsmouth* (London, 1828).

Secondary Sources

André, L., *Michel le Tellier et l'Organisation de l'Armée Monarchique* (Paris, 1906).

Ashley, M., *Financial and Commercial Policy under the Cromwellian Protectorate* (London: Frank Cass, 1934, second edition, 1962).
Atkinson, C.T., 'The British Losses at Steenkirk, 1692', *JSAHR* (1938), XVII: 200–205.
Baillargeat, R. (ed.), *Les Invalides, Trois Siècles d'Histoire* (Paris, 1975).
Baxter, S.B., *The Development of the Treasury, 1660–1702* (Harvard: Harvard University Press, 1931).
———, *William III* (London, 1966).
Belhomme, V., *L'Armée Française* (Paris, 1895).
Cannon, R., *Regimental Records of the Sixth or Royal First Warwickshire Regiment of Foot* (London: Longman, Orme & Co, 1893).
Cantlie, Sir N., *History of the Army Medical Department* (2 vols, Edinburgh: Churchill Livingstone, 1974).
Chandler, D., *Sedgemoor, 1685* (Staplehurst: Spellmount, 1985, reprinted 1999).
Childs, J., 'Monmouth and the Army in Flanders', *JSAHR* (1974), LII: 4–5.
———, *The Army of Charles II* (1976, London: Routledge and Kegan Paul).
———, *The Army, James II and the Glorious Revolution* (Manchester: Manchester University Press, 1980).
———, 'The British Brigade in France, 1672–1678', *History* (1984), LXIX: 387–9.
———, *The British Army of William III* (Manchester: Manchester University Press, 1987).
———, *The Nine Years' War and the British Army, 1688–1697* (Manchester: Manchester University Press, 1991).
Clifton, R., *The Last Popular Rebellion: The Western Rising of 1685* (London, 1984).
Clode, C.M., *The Military Forces of the Crown; Their Administration and Government* (2 vols, London, 1869).
Contamine, P., *Histoire Militaire de la France* (Paris, 1992).
Corbett, J.S., *England in the Mediterranean, 1603–1713* (2 vols, London: Longmans, 1902).
Cotteslow, Lord, 'The Earliest Establishment, 1661, of the British Standing Army', *JSAHR* (1930), IX: 147–61 and 214–42.
Cowper, L.I., *The King's Own, The Story of a Royal Regiment* (Oxford: Clarendon Press, 1939).
Culver, H.B., *The Book of Old Ships* (New York: Doubleday, 1924, reprinted 1992).
Dalrymple, Sir J., *Memoirs of Great Britain and Ireland* (3 vols, London, 1773).
Dalton, C., *English Army Lists, 1661–1714* (6 vols, London: Francis Edwards, 1892–1904).
D'Alton, J., *The Memoirs of the Archbishops of Dublin* (Dublin, 1883).
Darby, H.C., *Historical Geography of England before 1800* (Cambridge: Cambridge University Press, 1936).
———, *King James's Irish Army List* (Limerick: The Celtic Bookshop, 1855, republished 1997).

Davis, Col. J., *The History of 2nd Queen's (Royal West Surrey) Regiment* (6 vols, London: Bentley, 1887–1906).
Davies, G., *The Early History of the Coldstream Guards* (Oxford: Clarendon Press, 1924).
——, 'The Reduction of the Army after the Treaty of Ryswick, 1697', *JSAHR* (1950), XXVIII: 15–27.
——, (ed.), 'Letters on the Administration of James II's Army', *JSAHR* (1951), XXIX: 69–78.
Dean, C.G.T., 'Charles II's Garrison Hospital, Portsmouth', *Papers and Proceedings of the Hamshire Field Club* (1947), 16, 280–83.
de Perini, Général H., *Batailles Françaises* (Paris: E. Flammarion, 1904).
Dunning, R., *The Monmouth Rebellion* (Wimborne: Dovecote Press, 1985).
Fortescue, J., *A History of the British Army* (20 vols, London: MacMillan).
Garrison, F.H., *Notes on the History of Military Medicine* (1922, republished 1970, Washington and Darmstadt, 1899–1932).
Goodwin, G., *A History of Ottoman Architecture* (London: Thames and Hudson, 1971).
Gore, A., *Our Services Under the Crown* (London, 1879).
Gretton, Lt Col. G. le M., *The Campaigns and History of the Royal Irish Regiment* (London: Blackwood, 1911).
Gruber von Arni, E.E., *Justice to the Maimed Soldier* (Aldershot: Ashgate, 2001).
Gutmann, M.P., *War and Rural Life in The Early Modern Low Countries* (Assen: Van Gorcum, 1980).
Guyot, G., *L'ancienne abbaye de La Ramée* (Brussels, 1978).
Haydn, J. and Ockerby, H., *The Book of Dignities* (London, 1890).
Hill, C., *God's Englishman* (London: Pelican, 1970).
Holmes, G. (ed.), *Britain After the Glorious Revolution, 1689–1714* (London: Macmillan, 1969).
Howells, H.A.L., 'The Care of the Sick and Wounded during Marlborough's Campaigns', *JRAMC* (1908), 11: 526–38.
——, The Story of the Army Surgeon and the Care of the Sick and Wounded in the British Army, from 1660–1688', *JRAMC* (1910), 14: 81–90.
——, The Story of the British Army Surgeon and the Care of the Sick and Wounded from 1689 to 1702', *JRAMC* (1911), 17: 643–58.
Keevil, J.J., Lloyd, C. and Coulter, J.L.S., *Medicine and the Navy, 1200–1900* (4 vols, Edinburgh: E&S Livingstone, 1958–1963).
Kempthorne, G.A., 'Some Notes on the Medical Service of the Restoration Army', *JRAMC* (1939), 72: 340–46.
Lediard, T., *The Life of John, Duke of Marlborough* (3 vols, London, 1736).
Little, B., *The Monmouth Episode* (London: Werner Laurie, 1956).
Luttrell, N., *A Brief Historical Relation of State Affairs from September 1678 to April 1714* (6 vols, Oxford, 1857).
Lynn, J.A., *Giant of the Grand Siècle,*(Cambridge: Cambridge University Press, 1997).

Macartney-Filgate, E., 'The War of William III in Ireland', *Transactions of the Military Society of Ireland* (Dublin, 1905).
Majno, G., *The Healing Hand, Man and Wound in the Ancient World* (London: Harvard University Press, 1975).
Min-Hsun Li, *The Great Recoinage of 1689–9* (London: Weidenfeld and Nicolson, 1963).
Moore, N., *The History of St Bartholomew's Hospital* (2 vols, London: Arthur Pearson Ltd, 1918).
Muller, P.L., *Wilhelm III von Oranien und Georg Friedrich von Waldeck* (2 vols, The Hague, 1873–80).
Ogg, D., *England in the Reign of Charles II* (2 vols, Oxford: University Press, 1934, republished 1956).
———, *England in the Reigns of James II and William III* (1955, Oxford: Clarendon Press, 1934 republished 1956).
Olms, G., Gabriel, R.A. and Metz, K.S., *A History of Military Medicine* (2 vols, New York: Greenwood Press, 1992).
Parnell, Hon. A., *The War of The Succession in Spain* (London: George Bell, 1905).
Parsons, F.G., *The History of St Thomas' Hospital* (2 vols, London, 1930).
Peterkin, A. and Johnston, W., *Commissioned Officers in the Medical Services of the British Army, 1660–1960* (2 vols, London: Wellcome, 1968).
Porter, R., *The Greatest Benefit to Mankind* (London: Harper Collins, 1997).
Powers, Sir D'Arcy, *A Short History of St Bartholomew's Hospital, 1123–1903* (London, 1923).
Preston, R.A., 'William Blathwayt and the Evolution of a Royal Personal Secretary', *History* (1949, new series), XXXIV: 28–43.
Ranger, T., and Slack, P. (ed.), *Epidemics and Ideas* (Cambridge: Cambridge University Press, 1992).
Robert, G., *The Life and Progress of James, Duke of Monmouth* (2 vols, London, 1844).
Robinson, J.R., *The Princely Chandos, A Memoir* (London: Sampson Lowe, 1893).
Routh, E.M.G., *Tangier, England's Lost Atlantic Outpost, 1661–1684* (London: John Murray, 1912).
Scouller, R.E., *The Armies of Queen Anne* (Oxford: Clarendon Press, 1966).
———, 'Clothing of Queen Anne's Armies', *JSAHR* (1969), XLVII: 211–14.
Slight, H. and J., *Chronicles of Portsmouth* (London, 1828).
Sopers, P.J.V.M., *Schepen die Verdwijnen* (Amsterdam, 1971).
Steele, R. (ed.), *A Bibliography of Royal Proclamations of the Tudor and Stuart Sovereigns, 1485–1714* (2 vols, Oxford, 1910).
Stevenson, C., *Medicine and Magnificence, British Hospital and Asylum Architecture, 1660–1815* (London: Yale University Press, 2000).
Stewart, Col. D., 'Military Surgeons in the 16th & 17th centuries', *JSAHR* (1948), XXVI: 151–8.
Taylor, F., *The Wars of Marlborough, 1702–1709* (Oxford: Blackwood, 1921).

Walton, Col. C., *A History of the British Standing Army* (London: Harrison and Sons, 1894).
Webb, S.S., 'William Blathwayt, Imperial Fixer, From Popish plot to Glorious Revolution', *William and Mary Quarterly* (1968, 3rd series) 25: 1–32.
——, 'William Blathwayt, Imperial Fixer, Muddling through to Empire, 1689–1717', *William and Mary Quarterly* (1969, 3rd series), 26: 373–415.
Wilson, C., *Anglo-Dutch Finance & Commerce in the Eighteenth Century* (Cambridge, 1941).
——, *England's Apprenticeship, 1603–1763* (London: Longman, 1965, republished 1986).
Wilson, T., *An Account of the Foundation of the Royal Hospital* (Dublin, 1713).

Unpublished Theses

Barker, N.P., 'The Architecture of the English Board of Ordnance, 1660–1750', unpublished PhD thesis (Reading University, 1985).
Burton, I.F., 'The Secretary at War and the Administration of the Army during the War of the Spanish Succession', unpublished PhD thesis (London University, 1960).
Gruber, E.E., 'Who Cared? Nursing Care and Welfare Provision for Soldiers and their Families during the English Civil Wars and Interregnum, 1642–1660', unpublished PhD thesis (University of Portsmouth, 1999).
Waddell, L.M., 'The Administration of the English Army in Flanders and Brabant from 1689–1697', unpublished PhD thesis (University of North Carolina, 1971).

Web Sites

http://www.newadvent.org.
http://www.ramee.be/uk/coomans.htm.

Index

Adams, Dr, commissioner, 159
Adams, Lt J., 165
Addison, T., commissioner, 102
Admiralty Commissioners, 99
Aire, hospital, 149
Alicante, 168
Alicante, hospital, 166
Almanza, battle of, 163–5, 172, 175, 187, 209–10
Amyand, C., surgeon, 113, 122, 133, 145, 148,
Amyott, Dr, physician, 167
André, L., 2
Angiban, Mons, apothecary, 65
Anglesey, Earl of, 54
Anguine, hospital, 80
Ankott, Joseph, surgeon, 172
Ankott, Jane, wife, 172
Anne, Queen, 1, 47, 111, 113, 150–1, 170–2
Antwerp, 37, 84, 112, 135, 141
Antwerp, French hospital, 116, 146
Antwerp, hospital, 141, 145
Archbold, Dr, Physician General, 58
Archbold, P., surgeon, 58
Argyle, Duke of, 173, 187
Arlington, Lord, 12
Arnott, J., 165–6
Asch, hospital, 93
Ath, 35, 142
Athlone, Earl of, *see* Ginkel
Aughrim, battle of, 71

Baden, Prince Louis of, 126
Ball, L., surgeon, 92
Barcelona, 159–60, 163
Barthelemy, Dr, physician, 137

Bath, 41–2
Bavaria, Elector of, 111, 124
Beja, misericordia, 177
Belfast, 59, 61, 64
Belfast, hospital, 60–1, 64
Belhomme, V., 2
Bellamy, G., surgeon, 41
Bellasis, Lord, 11, 13, 15, 43, 83, 85–7
Bellone, Dr, physician, 207
Bergen op Zoom, hospital, 78
Berkeley, M., surgeon, 45
Berwick, Duke of, 163, 165–6
Bijlander, 96, 124
Bijloke Hospital, 81–4, 86–8, 90–3, 129–30, 141–51, 184
Bladon, Colonel, 170
Blake, Lt, 126–8
Blathwayt, W, Secretary at War, 47, 70, 81, 85–8, 101, 122, 159
Blenheim, battle of, 1, 124, 128, 133, 166, 209–10
Blenheim, bounty, 130–2
Bouchain, hospital, 150, 210
Boufflers, Marshal, 111
Boyd, D., nurse, 61
Boyle, H., Secretary of State, 173
Boyle, N., clerk, 57, 171
Boyne battle of the, 65–6
Brabant, Lines of, 135
Breda, hospital, 78–9, 122–3, 136, 139
Bridgwater, 42, 45
Brihuega, battle of, 172–3, 175, 209, 210
Brown, E, widow, 132
Bruges, 37, 86, 144–5

Bruges, St John's Hospital, 36–7, 81, 84, 87, 91–2, 151
Brussels, 36, 78
Brussels, Grootleger Hospital, 78
Brussels, hospital, 37, 79–81, 84, 86–7, 90–2, 140, 143–9
Brydges, J, 160–1, 163, 175, 183
Buissiere, P., surgeon, 63–5, 71
Bulstrode, Sir R., 36–7
Burdett, R., purveyor, 19–20

Cadiz, 13, 157, 159
Cadogan, General W., 130, 184
Camlin, S., surgeon, 92
Cantlie, Sir N., 1, 88
Cardonnel, A., secretary, 114, 122–3, 125, 127, 137, 145, 148, 150
Carlingford, 60–3
Carr, G., quartermaster, 54
Carrickfergus, 59, 60, 65
Castille, 172
Catalonia, hospital, 160–2, 168
Cell Brothers, 81, 95–6
Chabane, V., hospital director, 177
Chambers, J., surgeon, 92
Chambron, P., apothecary, 87
Charleroi, 35, 85
Charles II, King, 1, 3–4, 9, 24, 28, 33–9, 43, 54, 57, 182
Charles, Archduke of Austria, 160, 162, 168
Chelsea, Royal Hospital, 6, 14, 25, 38–40, 43, 57, 94, 99, 102, 105, 120–1, 130–1, 133, 165, 181–2, 185–7, 209, 210
Chetwind, T., apothecary, 57
Childs, J., 1
Cholmley, Sir H., 10, 12, 13–17
Churchill, Col C., 83
Cichorius, J., surgeon, 207
Coatsworth, Dr, Apothecary General, 151
Coblenz, 125, 136
Cockburn, D., surgeon's mate, 122

Code, T., agent, 169
Cole, J., surgeon's mate, 177
Colyer, *see* Portmore, Earl of,
Commission for Sick and Wounded Seamen, 33, 48, 99, 102–3, 106–8, 121, 130, 146, 158–9, 175–6
Contamine, P, 2
Corning, Dr, physician, 57
Courtrai, 35, 142, 152
Courtrai, hospital, 143, 146, 149
Craig, J., surgeon, 92, 140
Crawford, D., hospital governor, 120
Crawford, J., surgeon, 93
Cromwell, O., 3, 53
Currer, Dr W., physician, 54

Danvers, T., surgeon, 135, 148
Darley, A., hospital overseer, 54
Dartmouth, Lord, 23–5, 28, 100–1
D'Auvergne, E., 84, 86
Davis, M., chaplain, 56
D'Ayrolle, J., hospital controller, 86, 92
De Brie, Mr, surgeon, 152
De Lantrelle, M., nurse, 141
De Luke, M., French hospital director, 116
De Mailly, J., apothecary, 152
De Mare, M., French commissary, 141
Deal, 107
Deal, hospital, 25, 28, 120
Deas, W, surgeon, 92
Dendermonde, 142
Denia, hospital, 166, 168
Dixmude, hospital, 83–4, 87, 90–1, 95
Donauworth, 126
Dordrecht, hospital, 78
Dort, 130, 140
Douai, 149, 209–10
Douai, hospital, 149
Douglas, General, 67 163
Dover, hospital, 169

Index 221

Drogheda, 62, 65
Dublin, 57
Dublin, Archbishop of, 53
Dublin, hospital, 53–4, 65, 69
Dublin, Royal Military Infirmary, 54, 73
Dummer, C., surgeon, 160
Dundalk, 59, 60–64
Dundas, G., surgeon, 92
Dunkirk, 6, 9, 151
Dunn, Dr P., physician, 57, 67
Dunoon, Dr, Physician General, 172–4

Earl, General, 169
Eccles, J., gunner, 28
Eeles, Mr, surgeon's mate, 135
Elphinstone, W, surgeon's mate, 177
Elton, T., surgeon, 107
Ely House Hospital, 3–4
Escrick, Lord H. of, 36–7
Estremos, misericordia, 177
Evelyn, J., 34, 43, 46–7

Fabricious, Mr, surgeon's mate, 135
Fairborne, Colonel, 23
Falconberg, J., hospital governor, 66
Falmouth, 121, 168–9
Farendale, R., surgeon, 22
Ferguson, Dr, physician, 65
Feversham, Lord, 41
Fountaine, J., Surgeon General, 54
Fitch, Sir T, contractor, 37
Flanders, 3, 33–4, 36–7, 43–4, 47, 67, 72–97, 102–4, 111–52, 157–8, 161, 163, 167–8, 172, 175–8, 183–4, 207–8
Forcade, T., Surgeon General, 35
Friend, Dr, Physician General, 160

Galway, Earl of, 152, 160–4, 166–72, 174–5, 187
Gardiner, T., surgeon, 135, 207
Garrison, F.H., 2

Garshore, A., surgeon, 92
Gash, S., surgeon's mate, 131
Gask, G., 1
Genest, W., surgeon's mate, 133
George, Prince of Denmark, 120
Ghent, 140–1, 144–5, 149, 209
Ghent, hospital, *see* Bijloke
Ghent, pest house, 150
Gibraltar, 159, 176
Gibraltar, hospital, 158, 168
Ginkel, General G. van, 67–8, 70–1
Goddard, J., Physician General, 53
Godolphin, S., Lord Treasurer, 121
Goldy, J., surgeon's mate, 122, 124
Gore, A., 1
Goringhem, hospital, 78
Gouda, hospital, 78
Gowdy, Mr, surgon's mate, 113
Granville, G., Secretary at War, 120, 165
Grey, Dr G., chaplain, 87
Grey, E., nurse, 93
Greyerson, A., surgeon, 124
Gutman, M., 82

Hague, The, 113, 140
Hague, The, hospital, 79
Hall, H., surgeon, 87, 207
Hampton, R., hospital controller, 86
Harbord, W., Paymaster General, 60, 63–5, 184
Harley, R., Secretary of State, 164
Harris, M., matron, 44, 47–9
Harris, Mr, surgeon, 151
Harvey, M., nurse, 93
Harwich, 93–4, 119, 121, 168
Hawkins, J., surgeon's mate, 177
Hazlefoot, R., transport official, 121
Hedges, Sir C., 161
Hedley, J., nurse, 92–3
Heidenheim, hospital, 125–9
Herbert, Admiral, 57–8
Herwaenden, Dr J., physician, 207

Hill, R., Deputy Paymaster General, 80–3, 87, 187
Hingstman, Surgeon Major, 17
Hobbes, T., surgeon, 41–2
Hopkins, M., matron, 44, 47–8
hospital ships, see
  Unity, 24–6, 8
  Virtue, 24
  Welcome, 23–7
hospitals, see
  Aire
  Alicante
  Anguine
  Antwerp
  Asch
  Belfast
  Bergen op Zoom
  Bijloke
  Bouchain
  Breda
  Bruges, St John's Hospital
  Brussels, hospital
  Brussels, Grootlegerhospital
  Bethune
  Catalonia
  Chelsea
  Deni
  Dixmude
  Dordrecht
  Douai
  Dover
  Dublin
  Dublin, Royal Military
  Dunkirk
  Ely House
  Gibraltar
  Gorngchem
  Gouda
  Hague, The
  Heidenheim
  Heilbronn
  Helvoetsluys
  Hôtel des Invalides
  Hounslow Heath
  Kassel
  Kilmainham
  La Ramée
  Liège
  Lille
  Lisbon
  Louvain
  Maastricht
  Mecklin (Malines)
  Namur
  Neuville
  Neuwied
  Nijmegen
  Nordlingen
  Oudenarde
  Portsmouth
  Roermond
  Rotterdam
  Savoy Hospital
  'sHertogenbosch
  St Bartholomew's
  St Ghislain
  St Katherine's
  St Thomas'
  St Venant
  Tangier
  Tirlemont
  Tournai
  Triers
  Venlo
  Workorn
Hôtel des Invalides, 6, 14, 181–2
Hounslow Heath, hospital, 43–9, 58, 100–2, 182
Howells, Colonel H.A.L., 1
Hudson, J., hospital contractor, 87, 112–151, 184, 187, 207
Hunt, Dr W, physician, 57
Hutton, J., Physician in Ordinary, 68–72, 79
Huy, 84, 136
Hyde, Captain T., 165–6

Inchiquin, Lord, 13

Inglish, A., surgeon, 113, 122, 148, 173
Innes, Dr A., chaplain, 177
Ireland, 53–75, 83, 167
Isle of Wight, 27, 94, 146, 169

James II, King, 1, 9, 39, 43–4, 46–7, 57–9, 101, 112, 182
Jeffrey, J., purveyor, 57
Jeffreys, Colonel J, 57, 66
Jenkins, Sir L., 23–6
Johnson, R., apothecary's mate, 65

Kane, R., 150
Kassel, hospital, 125, 128–9
Keck, S., clerk, 87, 207
Keevil, J.J., 3
Keggelaer, F., hospital contractor, 79, 80–1, 86, 184
Kempthorne, Lt Colonel G.A., 2
Kilmainham, Royal Hospital, 6, 14, 37, 39–40, 54–7, 66–9, 71–2, 83–4, 87, 182, 185, 193–7
Kinsale, 67
Kirke, Colonel P., 21, 24–5, 28, 58
Kirkwood, J., surgeon, 93
Knight, J., Surgeon General, 36

Lamb, P., hospital contractor, 86–7, 92, 94, 184
Landen, battle of, *see* Neerwinden,
Langley, T., Mayor of Harwich, 94
Lansdowne, Lord, 172
La Ramée, field hospital, 140
Laroche, Mr, surgeon, 141
Lawrence, Dr T., Physician General, 22, 27, 41–2, 44–5, 61, 64–7, 72, 80–1, 86, 92, 113, 123, 148, 163, 173, 182, 184, 207
Lawrence, R., apothecary, 173–5
lazarette, 13–14, 181
LeCaan, Dr J., physician, 57, 86–7, 136, 167–8, 171, 186, 207
Lediard, T., 127

Lee, E., surgeon's mate, 133
Lee, R., surgeon, 124
Legge, Colonel G, 35–7
Leigh, E., commissioner, 102
Lerida, 167
Liège, 112
Liège, hospital, 84, 87–92, 123, 136–40
Lille, 145, 209
Lille, hospital, 146–51
Lilly, W., apothecary, 173–4
Limerick, 67, 71
Lisbon, 160, 162, 168, 170–1, 174
Lisbon, hospital, 159, 176
L'Isle, Lord, 53
Livesy, Brigadier, 120
Llewellyn, M., Commissary-General, 157
L'Oke, Mr, surgeon's mate, 141
Londonderry, 57–8
Long, W., surgeon, 94
Louis XIV, King, 6, 33, 35, 54, 5, 77–8, 111–12, 182
Louvain, hospital, 79–80, 92–3, 142–3
Lundy, R., Governor of Londonderry, 57
Lynam, J., butler, 57
Lynn, J., surgeon's mate, 122
Lynn, J.A., 2
Lyttleton, Sir C., 37

Maastricht, 123, 136, 209
Maastricht, hospital, 78, 85, 114, 136, 138–9, 143
MacCartney, J., apothecary's mate, 122
Mackenzie, Mrs, nurse, 143
Madrid, 162, 164, 172
Maitland, R., surgeon's mate, 177
Malplaquet, battle of, 148, 152, 187, 209–10
Marlborough, Duke of, 1, 33, 67, 94, 111–52, 157, 161,

166, 182, 186–8
Mary, Queen, 58, 87, 102
matrons, 44–5, 47–8, 56, 92, 101–2, 115, 139, 151, 195
Matthewson, F., clerk, 57, 207
Maxwell, J., surgeon, 175
Mecklin (Malines), hospital, 36, 78–81, 84, 87, 92–3, 141, 146
Medlicot, C., commissary, 160
Menin, 142
Menin, hospital, 144–7
Miller, R., apothecary, 54
Minorca, 159, 167, 176
misericords,
  Beja, 176
  Estremos, 176
  Redondo, 176
  Vlla Vicosa, 176
Monmouth, Duke of, 33, 35–7, 41–3, 55, 100, 102
Moore, W., purveyor, 57
Morley, Dr, commissioner, 159
Morris, W., apothecary, 57, 87, 207
Morrison, J., commissary, 93
Musto, H., surgeon, 41
Mylne, J., surgeon's mate, 177

Namur, 79, 88–90, 104, 135,
Namur, French hospital, 85
Namur, hospital, 78, 88, 89
Napier, R., surgeon's mate, 177
Ne Plus Ultra, Lines of, 150
Neerwinden, battle of, 84–5, 103
Neilson, Dr W., 170–72, 174
Nelson, W., surgeon, 124, 133
Neuville, hospital, 150
Neuwied, hospital, 135–6, 138–9
New Model Army, 4, 181
Nieuport, 37, 85, 151
Nijmegen, 113, 125, 128, 135
Nordlingen, hospital, 126–9, 133–4
Norwood, Colonel H., 11–13, 15, 20, 28
Nottingham, Earl of, 58, 102, 158

nurses, 13, 27, 44, 54–6, 61, 63, 69–70, 87–8, 92–3, 115–16, 127, 129, 134, 139, 142–3, 149, 178, 183, 186, 193, 196–7

O'Farrell, Colonel, 80–81
Ogg, D, 183
Ogle, Dr N., physician, 122, 133, 145, 149
Oliphant, Dr, physician, 86, 113, 125
Ore, W., apothecary's mate, 122
Ormonde, Duke of, 53, 150–1, 157–8
Ostend, 37, 120, 122, 143, 146–7
Oudenarde, battle of, 144, 152, 209
Oudenarde, hospital, 144–5

Paget, Dr E., chaplain, 87, 207
Paige, G., clerk, 87
Palladio, A., 14
Parsons, T., clerk, 132–3
Paulet (or Pawlet), J., surgeon, 124
Peace, T., commissioner, 176
Pear, R., surgeon, 122, 124
Pearce, Major General J., 176–7
Pearce, J., Surgeon General, 41–2, 44, 103
Pearce, R., surgeon, 159
Penman, J., surgeon, 177
Pendennis Castle, 28
pensions, 38–41
Pepys, S., 9, 17, 20–1
Peterborough, Earl of, 10, 94, 152, 160, 162, 187
Pierce, J., surgeon, 24–5, 28
Portmore, Earl of, 170–1, 174–6, 187
Portsmouth, 34, 37, 107, 130, 147, 160, 164
Portsmouth, hospital, 34, 37–8, 50, 51, 165, 171, 187
Portugal, 33, 132, 152l, 157–8, 186–7
Pottinger, T., Mayor of Belfast, 64
Povey, T., Receiver of Tangier, 17, 158
Prelone, Dr, physician, 86

Price, H., clerk, 87
Pringle, G., surgeon, 87
Prior, M., diplomat, 85–6
Purvis, J., surgeon, 57
Puzey, R., apothecary's mate, 122
Pyne, L., nurse, 56

Quinn, R., surgeon's mate, 177

Ramillies, battle of, 138, 139–41, 152, 209
Ramsey, G, 92
Ranelagh, Earl of, 47–8, 86, 88, 95, 101, 183
Reed, J., surgeon, 45
Richards, Major General J, 166–7
Rochester, 107, 130
Rodham, R., surgeon's mate, 122, 124
Roermond, 114, 123
Roermond, hospital, 138
Romney, Earl of, *see* Sidney
Rooke, Admiral Sir G., 157–8, 168
Rotterdam, 117, 124, 135, 139
Rotterdam, hospital, 78, 84, 87, 92–3
Routh, E., 11
Rouviere, P., surgeon, 175
Ryley, P., Surveyor General, 48
Ryley, W., cook, 57
Ryswick, Treaty of, 94, 111–12

Sandford, S., Mayor of Harwich, 94
Sandilands, Dr A., physician, 148
Sandwich, Earl of, 9, 10
Saragossa, battle of, 172, 209
Savoy Hospital, 3–4, 34, 49, 56, 182
Scardevill, Dr H., chaplain, 61, 65
Schellenburg, battle of the, 126–7, 133, 209–10
Schomberg, Duke of, 59–64, 159
Scouller, R.E., 111, 152
Seaborn, J., surgeon, 45
Seaborn, T., hospital director, 59
Seaman, R., surgeon, 94

Sedgemoor, battle of, 41–3
Segard, J., chaplain, 65
Shadwell, C., hospital director, 171–3, 177
Shales, Captain J., commissary, 43–4, 46, 48, 58, 60, 63–4, 184
Shannon, Lord, 146
Shepard, A., commissioner, 102
Shere, H., engineer, 12, 15, 189–91
'sHertogenbosch, hospital, 78, 113–14, 123, 136, 138–9
Shirley, A., laundress, 54
Shoade, S., surgeon's mate, 122
Shrimpton, Major General, 165
Shute, Dr H., chaplain, 87, 207
Sidney, Col H., Earl Romney, 37
Size, R., apothecary, 177
Smallbones, Mr, surgeon, 143
Smith, W., Mayor of Tangier, 19, 27–8
Solmes, Count, 65, 68
Spain, 33, 111, 132, 152, 157–78, 186–7
St John, H., Secretary at War, 132, 158–9, 160–1, 164–6, 178
St Bartholomew's Hospital, 42, 45–7, 49, 56, 95, 99–109, 130, 182–3, 199–201
St Ghislain, hospital, 148
St Katherine's Hospital, 24, 100–2
St Thomas' Hospital, 25, 42, 44, 45, 49, 95, 99–109, 130, 182–3
St Venant, hospital, 149
Stair, Earl of, 188
Stanhope, Major General, 160, 168, 172–3, 187
Starenburg, Count G von, 168, 172
Steenkirk, battle of, 79–80, 103, 210
Story, G., chaplain, 68
Summers, E., Deputy Paymaster, 35
Sunderland, Earl of, 170
Sweet, B., clerk, 87
Sydney, Viscount, 70
Sylvester, Dr, physician, 61, 65

Talbot, *see* Tyrconnel, Duke of,
Tangier, 9–31, 34, 44, 58, 101, 181–2, 189–91
Tate, A., clerk, 171
Teale, I, Apothecary General, 87, 92, 117, 122–5, 148, 151, 159, 162, 173, 207
Tenders, *see* nurses,
Thomas, R., chaplain, 65
Thomas, R., surgeon's mate, 122
Thompson, C., Surgeon General, 62–3, 65–6
Thopp, P., purveyor, 57
Tiguell, Mr, surgeon, 135
Tiquet, H., surgeon, 148
Tirlemont, 137
Tirlemont, hospital, 93, 137–8, 146
Torlesse, Dr R., physician, 107
Tournai, 35, 149, 210
Tournai, hospital, 148, 150
Trant, W., surgeon's mate, 65
Triers, hospital, 135, 138–9
Trowman, nurse, 143
Tyrconnel, Duke of, 57, 64
Tyrer, T., Mayor of Liverpool, 59

Valencia, 162–3, 166
Valenciennes, 35, 165
Vandike, C., surgeon, 92
Van Loon, Mr, Surgeon General, 68, 71
Van Meurt, J., apothecary, 117–18, 142
Vaudemont, Prince de, 92
Vaudemont, Princesse de, 80

Vendome, Marshal, 144
Venlo, 114, 123, 142
Venner, Colonel S., 66, 69–70, 83–4, 86, 94, 184, 207
Vereeche, J., surgeon, 94
Vernon, J., Secretary at War, 36
Vigo, 157, 209
Villa Viciosa, battle of, 173
Villeroi, Marshal, 136, 140

Waldeck, Graf von, 78
Wallace, W., surgeon, 87, 207
Walpole, R., Secretary at War, 121, 133, 146–7, 171
Walton, Colonel C., 1
Waterford, 67
Wertheim, 125
Westwood, S., surgeon, 92
White, Captain H, 166
Whittle, R, Apothecary General, 34, 42, 45
William III, King, 1, 46–7, 53, 57–9, 65–9, 72, 77–97, 105–6, 111–13, 117, 123, 141, 157, 182–4, 187
Wills, Lt General C., 167
Wilson, Dr, physician, 145, 148
Wilson, T., surgeon, 92, 113, 124
Wren Sir C, architect and surveyor, 38, 44, 48
Wurtemburg, Duke of, 128
Wylley, J., surgeon, 23, 41–2

Zichorius, F., surgeon, 87